What the Experts are Saying

With a mixture of good sense, a sense of humor, stories from her personal struggle with weight control, and the insights from a bevy of health professionals (including myself), Susan offers up a winning recipe for successful weight control.

—Hope S. Warshaw, MMSc, RD, CDE,
Author of Diabetes Meal Planning Made Easy (American Diabetes Association) and
Eat Out, Eat Right (Surrey Books)

If you want to learn about nutrition and weight control, Susan is the perfect mentor—she shares her experience with honesty and humor and will help set you on a track for lifelong healthy living.

—Dr. Barbara Wilson, BSc Hons, DPhil,
Manager of Nutrition Services, www.tescodiets.com

This book is so different from most diet books, and, since my family and I maintain our weight by making smart choices, I found the testimonials from other seemingly naturally thin people inspiring and validating. We're never deprived, but we don't give in to over-eating either. I'm thrilled that many famous—and not so famous—experts, dietitians, and others all have ditched the diet mentality and advocate staying thin naturally.

—Merilee Kern, author of children's book Making Healthy Choices
- A Story to Inspire Fit, Weight-Wise Kids

Susan Burke March has set out to do something that is sorely needed here in over-weight America: To shatter the accepted myths about nutrition, weight, and dieting and to feed us the accurate information we need to make better choices with food and our health. We'd all like to be thinner, naturally. We now have a fighting chance, thanks to Susan's entertaining and informative new book.

—John McGran, Diet.com Chief Editor

Like Susan, I often speak with clients who tell me that they think that everyone else can eat what they want, and they feel like they're the only ones that need to be careful. It's not true. Almost all people need to work to stay thin—that's a necessary part of being healthy, too. It's similar to having financial awareness—if we just wrote checks and took money out of the ATM, never balancing our account—we'd probably end up broke. But, maintaining consistent consciousness and control, and never assuming that somehow everything will balance out in the end—that's how to maintain weight, too.

—Elizabeth DeRobertis, MS, RD, CDN, CDE,
Weight loss and diabetes expert, in practice in New York City

Susan's advice is inspiring because it is written from her own personal experience as well as her expertise.

—Joy Pape, RN BSN CDE WOCN CFCN
President of EnJOY Life!, Health Consultant, and
Nationally recognized Certified Diabetes Educator and motivational speaker

This is a balanced and comprehensive book on common sense nutrition presented in an accessible and engaging way. I recommend *Making Weight Control Second Nature* as a must read for everyone interested in basic components of good health for both the mind and the body.

—Colette F  *earch for*
ı Services

D1473476

An Important Message to Our Readers

This product provides general information and advice in regard to the subject matter covered. It is sold with the understanding that the product does not purport to render medical, legal, and financial or other professional services. If expert advice or assistance is required, the services of a competent professional person should be sought.

Making Weight Control Second Nature

Living Thin Naturally

Susan Burke March, MS, RD, LD/N, CDE

Mansion Grove House

Making Weight Control Second Nature: Living Thin Naturally
Copyright © 2009 Susan Burke March
More information: MakingWeightControlSecondNature.com; LivingThinNaturally.com
Published by Mansion Grove House LLC

ISBN-13: 9781932421194   ISBN-10: 193242119X

First Edition, 2009

Mansion Grove House. Box 201734, Austin, TX 78720 USA.
Website: mansiongrovehouse.com
For information on bulk purchases, custom editions and serial rights:
E-mail sales@mansiongrovehouse.com or write us, Attention: Special Sales
For permission license including reprints, excerpts and quotes:
E-mail permissions@mansiongrovehouse.com or write us, Attention: Permissions
Printed in the United States of America

Library of Congress Cataloging-in-Publication Data

March, Susan Burke.
  Making weight control second nature : living thin naturally / Susan Burke March. -- 1st ed.
      p. cm.
  ISBN 978-1-932421-19-4 (pbk. : alk. paper)
1. Weight loss. 2. Diet. 3. Health behavior. 4. March, Susan Burke--Health. I. Title.
  RM222.2.M3526 2009
  613.2'5--dc22

                          2008054293

Copy Editor: **Kelley Lorencin**
Cover Designer: **Ken Dawes**
Content Designer: **Ken Dawes**
Permissions & Reviews: **Maureen Malliaras**

Credits: See Appendix "References"

About Susan

Over the past 15 years Susan's professional initiatives reflect her passion for healthy living and smart weight management.

As a registered dietitian, Susan served as chief clinical nutrition manager at Mt. Sinai Hospital of Queens, New York.

She changed gears when in 1999 she accepted a position at eDiets.com, then a small start-up Internet weight loss company. As vice president of nutrition services, Susan worked to help create innovative features and services that are today commonplace in the online weight management industry. Susan led the nutritional development of a roster of online healthy weight programs, including the Heart Smart, Glycemic Impact, Vegetarian, and Living with Diabetes programs, as well as eDiets' digitized "partner diets", commercial weight loss programs including the popular Atkins Nutritional Approach and Zone Perfect program.

Susan holds two bachelors' degrees—one from Florida Atlantic University in Boca Raton, Florida in Communication, and from Queens College, New York, in Family, Nutrition & Exercise Sciences. She also earned her masters degree in Nutrition Education from Queens College. Susan is a certified diabetes educator, and holds advanced training certificates in Adult, Pediatric and Adolescent Weight Management.

Susan is the author of hundreds of articles offering advice about healthy weight management, online weight and fitness programs, research on health and nutrition, cooking and recipe modification and critiques new products and programs.

Susan shares her expertise as a volunteer media spokesperson for the Florida Dietetic Association and is frequently called upon by the health care industry and journalism community to comment on issues relating to nutrition and healthy eating, weight management, wellness and diabetes. Susan is currently serving as Secretary for the Weight Management Dietetic Practice Group, a professional practice group of the American Dietetic Association.

Susan and her husband Ken March live in Flagler Beach, Florida.

This book is dedicated to my husband, Ken

Thank you for your unwavering support, wise copyediting, and kindness. And thank you for being my biggest fan!

Contents

A MESSAGE TO READERS

Dear Reader,

Give up the old behaviors that made you overweight, and turn new behaviors into something you do "naturally", without thinking about it. "Naturally thin" people have learned this—and make healthy living second nature.

Weight loss—is just the beginning, and not the ultimate goal. No one goes on a diet thinking that they will return to their old overweight body—they want permanent, not temporary weight loss. They want to like their bodies, to feel attractive, and avoid the anxiety that "dieting" so often provokes.

Permanent weight loss happens only when you permanently change your usual lifestyle—when you deliberately take ownership of your usual habits, what experts call "behaviors", and take different steps toward fitness—maybe tentatively at first, but then more surely as you gain confidence.

This book was inspired by actual conversations with clients, and even friends and relatives who know me well, who have said to me that they thought that I never have to worry about what I eat, because unlike them, I'm "naturally thin". That speaks strongly to the assumption that as if by magic, I can eat with abandon without gaining weight—and speaks volumes about what that person thinks about their ability to change. These conversations inspired me to ask my dietitian friends as well as other friends and colleagues if they had ever encountered similar assumptions, and what they thought it meant about behavioral change.

I've included some of the many replies I received, to illustrate how "naturally thin" is a process. Learn how it's possible to stay that way, permanently.. My heartfelt thanks to the "naturally thin" contributors who so generously share their experiences for this book. They so clearly illustrate how most people who look thin practice similar habits that allow them to stay that way, naturally.

As with all advice books, this book is meant to be a guide to healthy living, not a substitute for medical advice. If you have a medical condition and especially if you are taking medications for any condition, please stay in consistent touch with your physician and speak with them about your plans before changing your diet or beginning an activity regimen, including the suggestions in this book. If you're pregnant, or trying to become pregnant, then good nutrition and weight maintenance (not weight loss) is your goal—stay healthy and stay in touch with your healthcare provider.

Your best guides to making healthy living second nature are registered dietitians (RDs), who are educated and experienced in personalizing meals and activity plans. Try and meet with a registered dietitian for personalized care—you deserve it. Log on to www.eatright.org (the American Dietetic Association) to find a registered dietitian in your area.

Susan Burke March

Susan Burke March
susan@susanburkemarch.com

Foreword

Since I didn't write *Making Weight Control Second Nature*, I can say with unfettered enthusiasm what Susan cannot: This is one helluva' great book! It's not a good book; it is a great book.

Making Weight Control Second Nature begins where the struggle with weight control must first be won—inside your head. To get you there, Susan generously lets us all inside her head to view the torment she once experienced with her own weight—up close and personal. The writing is clear and compelling—you will feel the pain and frustration Susan felt. It will doubtless convince you that she has felt your pain.

But this intimate view of demons past is simply the prelude to their exorcism, which is what the book is all about. To the extent that Susan's past struggles remind you of your own, her triumph indicates where you, too, can go.

And then, for someone writing with such crisp emotional intensity, Susan does a remarkable thing. She shifts into a new gear. She demonstrates that she is every bit as good at delivering the details as she is at inspiring you to go for it. I've read books and met people who are good at one or the other—but the perfect marriage of inspiration and application, of will and way, is very rare indeed. *Making Weight Control Second Nature* delivers the combination.

Susan spells out the challenges of behavior change and offers guidance based on both theory and her own experience to help you get there from where you are. She lays out as clear a case for distinguishing dietary sense from nonsense as I've ever seen.

And the practical guidance just keeps coming. From recipes to restaurants, cooking methods to cookbooks, nutrition facts panels to portion control, *Making Weight Control Second Nature* covers just about everything that matters. Somehow—and although I've read it, I'm not quite sure how—Susan has compressed an encyclopedia of information into a single book of ordinary size.

Other than its size, there is nothing ordinary about this book—it is remarkable. It is a veritable feast of useful information, with carefully prepared courses devoted to the why, what, and how of weight control.

Susan Burke March has every attribute you could possibly hope for in your mentor and confidante for lasting weight control. Want someone who knows what struggling with weight feels like? Susan spent years in those trenches. Want someone with the will and skill to overcome those challenges? You wouldn't know by looking at Susan today that her weight was ever an issue. Want knowledge, aptitude, attitude, kindness, firmness, empathy, discipline, and insight—all in the proper proportions? That's a rare recipe, indeed—this is its recipe book.

The secret ingredient in *Making Weight Control Second Nature* is the revelation that hardly anyone is! Being thin and healthy, eating what you like yet liking yourself, and controlling your weight without fixating on it for the rest of your life are not about natural gifts, but about the gift of knowing how. That's a gift you can give yourself—by reading this book. I hope everyone does.

David L. Katz, MD, MPH, FACPM, FACP
Director, Prevention Research Center
Yale University School of Medicine

Introduction

Thin doesn't come naturally to me, but thin did become *second nature.*

I know a lot about a lot of different diets. Personally, I've "gone on" dozens of diets—and professionally, knowing about diets is my business, because I've worked as a registered dietitian and in the weight loss field for more than 15 years. Each year, more than 50 percent of Americans start a diet and may lose a few pounds—some may lose more. But most dieters usually regain all the weight—and even more weight than they lost. Is that you? That was me, too. I lost and regained weight for years, and came to believe that I was destined to be overweight...I became resigned to sad fact that I was different from a chosen race of people who could eat as much as they wanted and not gain weight. I think this notion of "naturally thin" was keeping me fat. I would meet a slim person and immediately think, Gee—I can't be like them—I have to watch everything I eat, and I can never have any fun. Since I didn't have a "skinny gene," I'd never be thin—they were the lucky ones.

But "naturally thin" is a myth—I know, because this formerly fat person has lost more than 40 pounds, and I've kept it off for more than 25 years. I started losing by learning how to eat, and I lost my weight not by going on a fat burning diet or a belly busting diet, but by taking control and losing one pound at a time, staying consistent one day at a time, enjoying my diet—one bite at a time, and keeping active—one walk at a time. Today, I never diet, and I've kept my weight and waist size fairly constant—within a 3- to 5-pound range—some months up, some months down.

When strangers see me, they may think I'm naturally thin. But they couldn't be more wrong—I am most deliberately at a weight that makes me feel good. Whether or not it's more natural for me to be overweight, I made a deliberate choice not to be. It is much too easy to be overweight, but I'd rather stay thin, naturally.

I broke away from the myth of thinness and discovered how to enjoy my diet; I never feel deprived and have improved so many areas in my life that were suffering because I spent so much energy dieting.

Let's cut through the static and uncover your healthier lifestyle, so you too can stay "naturally thin" permanently.

I joined a group of women gathered poolside at my sister's house as they were discussing their *diets du jour*.

One said, "I have to eat fruit two hours before protein, and never with fat. I can't eat any avocado or mango, but cantaloupe and watermelon are good."

Another chimed in, "I'm doing low carb, but I cheated last night! It's so hard, because I go out to eat almost every night, and I just can't resist bread."

The next gal said the "nutritionist" at the local health food store convinced her to do a cleansing fast—she was starting tomorrow. This poor lady said she planned on drinking only lemon water with cayenne pepper and maple syrup—for five days. I glanced over at my sister, who was glaring at me with a look that said, "Be careful now...it's my party." I knew she was worried that I was about to set them straight about diets.

Suddenly one said in a loud whisper, "Shhhh---Susan's a dietitian!" They all turned and stared at me, and nodded in unison as one said, "Oh, Susan doesn't have to worry about her weight...she's naturally thin."

Well, there is nothing "natural" about my being thin. My weight is considered healthy for my height. But it wasn't always that way. And if I let nature take its course—if I allowed myself to be influenced by my environment—just living in America with the constant barrage of advertisements for fast food and availability of huge portions—and with the labor saving devices that people have come to take for granted and accept—well, I'd probably be overweight and dieting, too.

It's a rare person who is naturally thin. When close to 70 percent of adult Americans are overweight or obese, it's much more logical to say that it's natural for everyone to be *overweight*[1]. It's true—in our society, it's now more common to be overfat than thin, so when people look around, to their peers, family, and friends, they think that normal-weight people look thin—and they are, compared to everyone else.

This increase in obesity is stunning in its scope. Just a generation ago, more people were normal weight than overweight—today, two out of three Americans are overweight, and one in three are obese[2].

Our culture is keeping up with our expanding waistlines. Automobile manufacturers widen bucket seats because people can't fit comfortably, sports stadiums are ripping out rows of molded plastic seats to replace them with roomier ones, and undertakers are making bigger coffins. Cemetery owners think they'll run out of room because gravesites need to be larger.

It appears that our society is gradually accommodating obesity—reconfiguring to adapt as the majority of the people are overweight—but I don't accept that obesity is normal, or natural.

The Power of Words

I think that deconstructing commonly used terms describing food, diet, exercise, and lifestyle is valuable, because by doing this, I constantly remind myself to think about how I think. This helps me fight off the effects of where I live, and the pressures of staying thin are lessened—it's almost a game sometimes as I watch television or see advertisements for high calorie foods—and see how technology conspires to have me burn fewer calories.

You too can restructure your life. By believing in the power of words, you can change how you think about how you eat and how you live.

Natural and Natural

For instance, the word *natural* has a number of different meanings—and primarily describes what happens in nature, as in *present or produced by nature*, and conforming to the *usual course of nature*. We think about *natural* as being inevitable—plants grow *naturally*, and planets revolve in their *natural* path through the universe.

Another definition of *natural* is something not produced or changed artificially, not conditioned.

Television, print advertising, radio, and billboards all encourage us to overeat. So it's nearly impossible to not be influenced by our environment—it's almost unavoidable. And I don't accept that it's natural.

If I left it up to nature and ate what has become America's usual diet, then I would be overfat, too. Although you may not think so, healthful food is plentiful, and delicious, but we're bombarded with messages that show us how much fun it is to eat out and to drive–through, to eat more and spend less. Like most people, being thin certainly isn't *natural* to me.

Natural means effortless. And being thin takes effort. It may look inherent, it may look like I've always been this way, but that's because I've made a deliberate and conscious effort to make my usual behavior appear natural and spontaneous.

The definition of *natural* is also *self-generated, spontaneous—happening or arising without apparent external cause.*

Can you make something both deliberate and spontaneous? Perhaps. After more than 25 years of making deliberate choices—day after day, year after year—it may look as if I've always been slim. But I was once more than 40 pounds heavier. People who didn't know me as an overweight and out-of-control young woman may see me in a narrow focus and think I've always been this way. I haven't.

"Naturally Thin" takes work

We live in a time of huge portions, cheap food, and technology that contributes to our burning fewer calories—and that in itself is a cause for weight gain. We spend so much time sitting—at our desks, in front of computers, and in traffic. It's quite easy to overeat and under-exercise. Overweight isn't always from bad choices. Medical issues and sometimes medications can produce weight gain—or make it hard to lose weight.

There's a dearth of grocery stores in inner city neighborhoods, but no shortage of fast food restaurants serving up huge portions of high-calorie foods, noticeable especially in underserved, poor communities. You can't miss the ads for cheap burgers and oversized soft drinks, and when *two* double hamburgers costs less than one grilled chicken breast, it's all too easy to make bad choices.

Besides economical challenges, consumers don't have the time to shop for and prepare whole, fresh foods. People don't know how or are unable to carve out the time to do activities to burn off those excess calories.

However, there are long lines at fast food drive-through windows. Some franchises have two lanes—as much as 70 percent of all quick-food business is conducted through a car window—drive-through is powering the fast food business.

So how did I go from overweight to in-control?

Overcoming overeating didn't happen quickly—but once I finally decided to take control, I sought out help and found different avenues to continue. As hard as it was to change my behavior, it was the day by day commitment to new habits that helped me continue. I had to re-learn how to think about eating—to understand why overeating was so ingrained in my life.

Thinking differently happened in concert with *doing differently—I had to change my behaviors.* I took a clear look and saw just what I was doing to stay overweight. I was able to envision a better way, it was truly a light at the end of a long, black tunnel, but the light became brighter the longer I held out against my natural inclination to overeat. Each day, my deliberate activity became the means to an end—and gradually I felt stronger.

Many questions come to mind about the word *thin.* Is it possible to be truly naturally thin? And, does it matter if you are thin? What does *thin* mean? Are thin people always healthier than overweight people? Can you be healthy even if you are overweight? Underweight is decidedly not healthy, and can indicate risk for osteoporosis and malnutrition.

Yes, the rare person may naturally burn more calories just resting than the average person, but even people who may be naturally thin when young often gain weight as they age—naturally.

Most people report eating less than they actually eat—and are less active than they think—and if they accuse me of being naturally thin, I think they are talking more about **their** natural or **usual** behaviors. It feels as if they are afraid to confront the truth about their own behaviors—and they have already given up thinking about changing from the habits that are keeping them overweight.

People who make *mindful eating* second nature may appear *naturally* thin, but they are the people who are paying attention to what they're eating—and how much. They usually stop eating when they're full. They eat what they want—usually enough to support their current weight. Almost always, a thin person is someone who practices thin behaviors and will consistently monitor their weight—not necessarily by stepping on the scale—and take steps to reclaim their weight if they gain some. Throughout the book, you'll find stories of some others—my colleagues and friends—who stay thin, naturally, and never go on diets to lose weight.

Eating Without Hunger

My problem with food started in my late teens. I overate to deal with anxiety, boredom, stress, and even anger. I abused food as I eventually would abuse alcohol and other drugs, overeating to block the thoughts that were provoking anxiety.

For the longest time, I didn't enjoy food—even though I was eating large quantities of it—and couldn't even enjoy my favorite foods because I always felt guilty about overeating. Guilt provoked sadness, and I never felt able to even contemplate change—I just felt guilty for not trying. I used food to assuage my guilt, to bury my anxiety. It was hard for me to eat right when I had been eating wrong for such a long time.

But, I overcame this vicious cycle by learning new habits, new behaviors, reinforced by new thoughts and positive affirmations that help me every day. Today, my habits are second nature but these habits had to be identified, practiced, refined, and reinforced.

It is sometimes painful for me to remember being overweight and out of control. And yes, some things cannot be changed—you can't change your genes or your inherited risk for some diseases. You can't change your past and your family's influence on your habits growing up. But you can make changes to your behaviors—you can choose what you want to change, and you can work toward those changes. These choices are a gift to all of us—there are so many areas of our lives that are *not* possible for us to control. But we have some unique freedoms when it comes to what we eat and how active we are—amazing freedoms that are different from all other aspects of our daily lives. We are free to choose to be overweight, unhealthy, and inactive—we can choose fast food, processed and packaged refined junk, or we can choose fresh food. We can set the alarm early enough to get in some exercise before work, or we can roll over and snooze.

For me, just the act of working toward change improved how I thought about myself. That set me on a positive path, a path which I deliberately work hard to stay on, so that being in control has become second nature to me. I have also seen firsthand with my clients the excitement and joy that a new behavior brings. When you can identify a single behavior that can be changed, and then you change it—when you replace that old behavior with a new positive one——it is like the door is thrown open, and you can see into the next room.

I like to think about the person in that room—she's someone who is smart and savvy. She looks calm and determined and optimistic; she knows she made deliberate, smart choices that day. Adopt *your* naturally thin lifestyle, a way of living that puts you in control of your weight and health. *You* can be that person, who makes deliberate choices—one day at a time, one meal at a time, one food at a time, and one walk at a time.

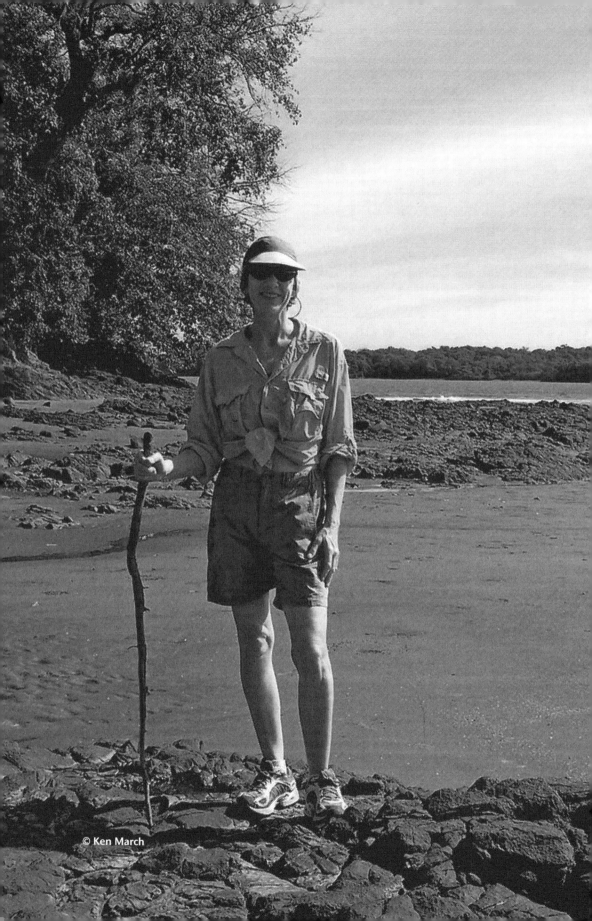

Chapter 1

My Transformation
From Naturally Thin to Compulsively
Overweight

If we did the things we are capable of, we would astound ourselves.
—Thomas Edison

My body dysmorphia started early, as I watched old movies on television entranced by voluptuous movie stars like Marilyn Monroe and Rita Hayworth. By age thirteen, I was still anxiously awaiting the first signs of maturity, envious of girls with developing curves who were attracting all the boys. My older sister mocked my flat chest, and I padded my bra and felt ugly.

Diet Lingo

I remember my parents talking a lot about "diets", but never talked about being fit. I didn't recognize the pictures of my father on my parents' bedroom dresser. In them, he looked like a slim, uniformed Clark Gable; I'd only known him as overweight. We'd always know when my father had visited his doctor because he'd tell my mother to "put him on a diet." Then he'd be 'good' for a day—maybe two—eating Spartan meals of Special K for breakfast, salad for lunch, and a small steak for dinner. No diet lasted long, and soon I'd hear, "Oh, I cheated on my diet today," and soon my father was back to eating cookies for breakfast, and I wouldn't hear anything else about the diet—until the next time.

My parents talked about overweight people as if they were somehow socially unacceptable—I got the impression that overweight people were deliberately that way, and because they made that choice they were somehow less than successful, and it was their fault. And here's the irony—although both my parents were overweight—and my father was obese, they'd criticize overweight strangers.

Wanting to Be Anywhere But Here

As an adolescent, I began to get into trouble—skipping school, not doing my homework. My mother was often angry with me for something, and many days, I dreaded my father coming home because I knew I'd be punished.

As I got older, I started staying out late, drinking and using drugs with my friends, and fighting constantly with my parents, going nowhere fast. Before my junior year, my parents offered the option of school in London, and I jumped at the chance to get away. The cool British school I thought I'd enjoy was instead a Swiss finishing school, and it felt like I was on the moon. I didn't speak French, I was lonely and angry, and food became my outlet for my anxiety. I began to binge, to stuff my feelings away, and gained about 20 pounds in just three months.

> People with eating disorders often use food and the control of food in an attempt to compensate for feelings and emotions that may otherwise seem overwhelming. For some, dieting, bingeing, and purging may begin as a way to cope with painful emotions and to feel in control of one's life, but ultimately, these behaviors will damage a person's physical and emotional health, self-esteem, and sense of competence and control
>
> *National Eating Disorders Association.*

Things may have turned out differently for me if I'd not gone away to school at sixteen—maybe things would have smoothed themselves out; perhaps I would have come to terms with my family; or maybe I'd have found a mentor or counselor who could have guided me. Of course, I'll never know. At 16, teenage girls often gain weight, and I may have gained weight just as easily living at home in New York. But, as a teenager alone for the first time, I floundered and began to use food to feel better—really, to avoid the frightening feelings. The more I used food to assuage my fears, the more weight I gained, the worse I felt about myself, and the more I ate. It didn't help that I had many advantages and opportunities. I was out of control.

In the 1970s, I had never heard the term *binge eating disorder*, and I didn't know about bulimia, a condition which classically appears during a period of intense stress and change. However, "stress" aptly describes my teen years and my relationships with my family. All the unresolved emotions that I felt—anger, loneliness, sadness, and frustration—I buried under mountains of food. Each time I began, it felt like falling into a black hole. I would start eating—and couldn't stop—and then felt worse than ever. I began to eat without tasting and then purged with laxatives. Within the year, I was smoking more than a pack a day and had gained more than 30 pounds by the time I returned home to finish my senior year.

Home to Bad Habits

By age 19, I was up to 170 pounds and couldn't remember when I had eaten normally. But when I suddenly came down with infectious hepatitis, I couldn't eat at all—couldn't drink or smoke either—and quickly lost about 20 pounds in just six weeks. I was weak and sickly—both from hepatitis and from such a dramatic weight loss, but when I got on the scale, I remember how seeing that new number strangely excited me. All that mattered to me was that I'd lost weight—the number on the scale seduced me into thinking I was "cured" of my obsessive overeating. Of course, I had not taken control. My weight loss wasn't because I'd identified why I was bingeing on food. I surely didn't develop healthy eating behaviors. As I began to feel better, I steadily regained weight, slowly but surely resuming my binge eating because the problems were still there—I still was unhappy, I still wasn't making any kind of healthy choices. I was the same old me with the same old problems. I never felt hungry, and no wonder—I was eating all the time. I deliberately avoided thinking about why I was eating—I ate because it was time to eat or because I hadn't eaten in a few hours or because I thought I *should* eat. Or I ate to distract myself, to soften my loneliness, anxiety, and boredom. I never tasted food once I started to binge; it was about feeling full, soothing my anxiety by stuffing it down, and my "drug" of choice was dry, refined carbohydrate foods—crackers, pretzels, and breads.

Well into my mid-20s, I would periodically attempt to lose weight by going on a diet, just like my parents used to do—and of course, each diet lasted a few days or, at most, a week. I tried eating only meat and chicken; I went on "juice fasts," drinking only fresh squeezed vegetable and fruit juices. Yes, I lost a few pounds, but of course I wasn't losing fat, and spent too much time in the bathroom. I tried the ill-fated liquid protein diet, which tasted so vile, I only gagged it down once and then threw it away. But I never addressed my reasons for overeating, so I was on the gain/lose/regain merry-go-round so familiar to chronic dieters.

The vicious cycle became even more intractable and harder to stop. Chronic overeating causes biological changes, and without help, it's hard to break that cycle[1]. I wasn't thinking about "normal" eating or eating naturally. I was preoccupied with food, overwhelmed by guilt, and I couldn't break the pattern. I wanted to stop bingeing, but I didn't know how to start. I had little experience with self-control. I couldn't identify any resources on learning how to deal with stress, and I further isolated myself from friends and family because I was ashamed of what I was doing.

Experts say that it is difficult to assess the number of people suffering with eating disorders. People don't like to talk about it—and I never did. I never told anyone, even when I began to reach out to get help with relationship issues. I worked with professional therapists and gradually developed coping skills to boost my low self esteem, but I didn't reveal to anyone that I binged and purged because it was too humiliating for me.

Eating Disorders
from a Family Systems Perspective

Research from a family systems perspective indicates that eating disorders stem from both the adolescent's difficulty in separating from over-controlling parents and disturbed patterns of communication. When parents are critical and unaffectionate, their children are more prone to become self-destructive and self-critical, and they have difficulty developing the skills to engage in self-care giving behaviors. Such developmental failures in early relationships with others, particularly maternal empathy, impairs the development of an internal sense of self and leads to over-dependence on the environment. When coping strategies have not been developed in the family system, food and drugs serve as a substitute.

Weiner 1998, 163-167

What is the Treatment for Binge Eating Disorder?

People with binge eating disorder should get help from a health care provider, such as a psychiatrist, psychologist, or clinical social worker. There are several different ways to treat binge eating disorder:

- Cognitive-behavioral therapy teaches people how to keep track of their eating and change their unhealthy eating habits. It teaches them how to cope with stressful situations. It also helps them feel better about their body shape and weight.

- Interpersonal psychotherapy helps people look at their relationships with friends and family and make changes in problem areas.

- Drug therapy, such as antidepressants, may be helpful for some people.

National Institute of Diabetes and
Digestive and Kidney Diseases.

Getting Better

But, I never gave up, and never resigned myself to being out of control. I thought hard about change; I *contemplated* change. I wanted to be better and kept trying to get better—reading books and attending lectures, trying to learn more about why I couldn't maintain a relationship, why I couldn't stop using food so self-destructively. I had a lot of success by signing up for face-to-face weight loss program that, most importantly for me, invited me to come as often as I wanted—even daily—which helped me enormously, especially during the first few weeks of trying to change my usual behaviors.

And although I lost weight and became more physically fit, I still hadn't dealt with my emotional eating.

Like so many who "go on" diets, the weight loss didn't signify an understanding of healthy living, and I began to regain weight a few years later. While living in New York City I tried the route of self-discovery—first by signing up for a weekend seminar where I (and hundreds of other strangers) heard that the path to controlling my destiny lay in signing up for a series of similar seminars (an investment of hundreds of dollars). But, luckily, I heard about a workshop by Carol H. Munter and Jane R. Hirschmann called "Overcoming Overeating," and from there, joined a women's support group to talk about the difficulties we all had accepting that "dieting" doesn't work and the angst that hating your body produces. But, taking care of your body, and accepting that "thin" wasn't the goal could lead to permanent healthy living. I stayed with this group, meeting weekly for months, and this experience helped me turn around. Getting to know other women who were facing the same problems—successful women from all areas of the city and from all professions—and focusing on identifying positive behaviors, accepting ourselves, our frailties and complicated personal relationships, made it possible to reach out for support rather than isolating ourselves and obsessing about food and dieting. This group (**www.overcomingovereating.com**) led me to identify *how* to begin to change. I admitted *why* I was overeating and began learning to lower my stress. It wasn't the food that was the problem; it was how I was using food to avoid dealing with my problems that created a different, distracting problem.

My eventual weight loss resulted from developing a "like" for my body, wanting to feel stronger and more athletic, and deciding to take control. I set goals for eating better and for activity, and I asked for support from professionals and from my peers, again and again. I learned that *doing* the planning and preparation for healthy eating helped me focus positively on eating well and staying active. The process helped me avoid indecision and mitigate the frustration and anxiety that had frequently triggered binges. I began to develop the self-esteem that resulted from the smallest victories—the day-to-day living instead of day-to-day dieting. Over the years, I went longer and longer without giving in—first without purging after a binge, and then without bingeing at all. Days without self-destructive behavior became weeks and months and years, and I count them a huge victory—a hard-won battle to make healthy living second nature.

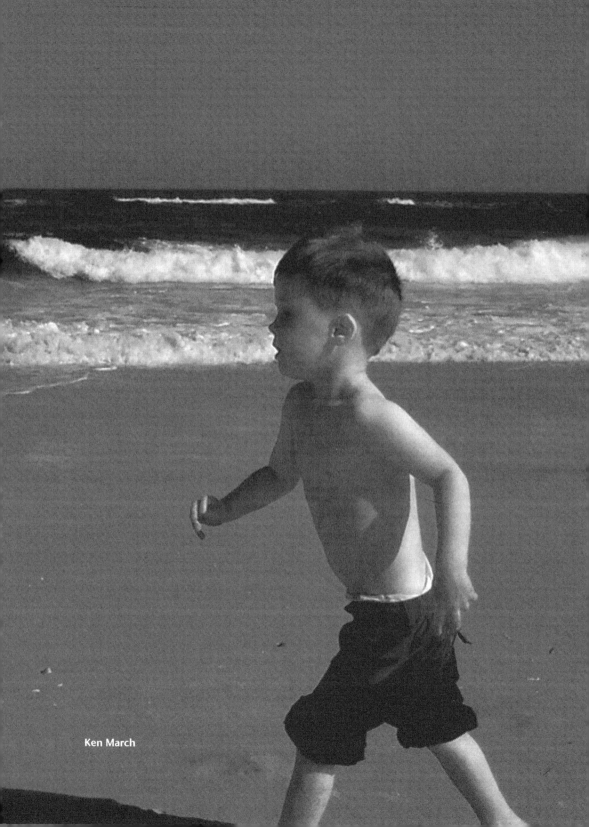

Ken March

Chapter 2

The 'New Normal':
Growing Up in an Overweight World

Events are called inevitable only after they have occurred
—Mason Cooley

Y ou may have been overweight as a child, or maybe the weight crept up gradually, pound by pound, candy bar on top of hamburger. Do you chalk it up to your genes? Do you say, "It runs in my family"?

While there are genetic markers that can predict some diseases, researchers still haven't found the "obesity gene," if one exists. You are statistically more likely to inherit a greater risk of being overweight if one (or both) of your parents is overweight, and it may have nothing to do with your DNA. I think behavior can overcome an inherited risk, I know I overcame mine. Maybe you have inherited your tendency to overeat because it was "normal" to eat that way at home, maybe your school encouraged overeating, or maybe you didn't grow up with a foundation in fitness, and never developed an exercise habit. Our environment compounds any genetic component of risk for overweight and obesity, but even if both your folks are overweight, even if your entire family is overweight—including grandparents on both sides—don't give up. Overweight does not have to be your fate.

DEFINITION

Destiny

—noun

1. An event (or a course of events) that will inevitably happen in the future

Epidemic

—noun

1. A widespread outbreak of an infectious disease; many people are infected at the same time

Good Girl! You Finished Everything!

Overeating is learned behavior.

When children learn that they'll get a positive response from Mom for continuing to eat, they keep eating. I know I did. I learned that I'd get a lot of positive reinforcement from finishing everything, even finishing my sister's leftovers. Many moms overfeed their children during bottle feeding, encouraging them to eat on an arbitrary schedule instead of when they're hungry. Toddlers learn to expect Mom's smile when they "eat all gone," and they learn that the reward for finishing their vegetables is dessert. When children gain parental favor from finishing everything on their plates, they learn that it's normal to keep eating despite being full. Pretty soon feeling full is the norm.

So why do people overfeed their kids? Perhaps parents worry their child won't be properly nourished or they don't want to have to stop to feed them later—both reasons are bad reasons for overfeeding, but they do it anyway.

Childhood obesity is a global phenomenon—and in the United States, at least 33 percent of kids are obese or at risk of becoming obese. According to the National Health and Nutrition Examination Survey (NHANES), the prevalence of childhood obesity is more than triple the targeted five percent set for their *Healthy People 2010* initiative (Centers for Disease Control and Prevention), and shows no sign of slowing.

- The rate of American childhood obesity is soaring; in 2005, the CDC reported that childhood obesity has tripled in the past 20 years, topping 17 percent, and is on track to double by 2015[1].

- American experts predict that by 2010, more than 50 percent of all adult Americans will be in the "obese" category. Economic costs of treating medical conditions associated with obesity were already in excess of $117 billion in 2000[2]...what will it be by 2010?[3]

- Australian health experts predict that if nothing happens to interfere with their continent's weight trajectory, by 2026, at least 50 percent of Australian children will be obese[4].

As recently as the middle of the 20th century, "chubby babies" were considered cute, and it was assumed that they'd outgrow their "baby fat" in time to emerge—like a swan—beautiful. Today, I see a chubby babies and worry about their future health; instead of growing leaner, they are likely to grow even heavier. Studies show that children who are overweight before age 5 are five times more likely to be overweight at age 12 than those who were not overweight before age 5. Overweight children don't "grow into" their weight[5]—they grow into overweight adolescents and obese adults[6]

Adolescence and Teen Years: Self Esteem and Self Control

Overweight takes a psychological toll on kids. Overweight kids may be more likely to be depressed, to do poorly in school, and to be "picked on" than normal weight kids. Puberty means a constellation of changes, physiological and psychological. For some girls, the combination of hormones and new feelings about femininity can mean

What's a Healthy Weight?

Body Mass Index (BMI) for **adults uses height and weight to calculate** risk for disease associated with being over-fat. BMI is only one measure of risk, and where you carry your weight (around the middle is riskier) and whether you smoke or drink excessively is also predictive.

BMI doesn't reflect how fit or muscular you are—some professional athletes would be called "overweight" because their BMI is high, and they couldn't be healthier. That said, BMI is a general diagnostic tool to predict increased risk of type 2 diabetes, hypertension, and heart disease, as long as it is not used independently of the other measures.

Adult BMI

- Underweight   below 18.5
- Normal   18.5 – 24.9
- Overweight   25 – 29.9
- Obesity   30.0 and Above

Further Assessment: If BMI is 25 or above, measure waist size. For Women: 35 inches or above indicates increased risk for obesity-related diseases; Men: 40 inches or above.

If you know your weight in **pounds** and your height in **inches**, you can calculate your BMI using the equation below:

BMI = 703 X [weight/height (squared)]

So BMI = 703 X [(weight in pounds) ÷ (height in inches X height in inches)]

If you know your weight in **kilograms** and your height in **meters**, calculate your BMI by using the following equation:

BMI = [weight/height (squared)]

So in the metric system, BMI = [(weight in kilograms) ÷ (height in meters X height in meters)]

Go to **http://www.nhlbisupport.com/bmi/** for a **BMI calculator**.

Children:

Health experts use a different method to assess risk for **overweight in kids ages 2 to 20**, called BMI-for-age. Growth patterns and body compositions are different for boys and girls, especially as kids grow into adolescence and puberty, so the child's calculated BMI is plotted on sex-specific growth charts, rather than a specific number (as for adults). The Centers for Disease Prevention and Control (CDC) and the American Academy of Pediatrics (AAP) recommend this yearly from age two.

The child's **percent BMI** reflects his weight and height compared to normal children his age.

- Underweight - BMI less than the 5th percentile
- Healthy Weight - BMI 5th percentile up to the 85th percentile
- At Risk of Overweight - BMI 85th to less than the 95th percentile
- Overweight - BMI greater than or equal to the 95th percentile

disaster for their waistlines; girls who grow up inactive may be less likely to learn to compete the ways boys do. They also have less opportunity than boys to build lean muscle: studies show that by the age of 15, almost 25 percent more boys than girls are involved in activities aerobic enough to work up a sweat, and that means that more girls miss out on some of the positives of being part of a sports team, including learning assertiveness, teamwork, and competitiveness, which builds confidence.

Does poor self-esteem lead to overeating and obesity? Or does overweight and obesity predict low self-esteem?

For me, it was the former. Even as a small child, my view of myself was fragile. I felt uncomfortable in my family, often alienated from my parents. I didn't fit in—I can remember my father dismissing my ideas as bad. He preached that girls should be feminine, which I thought meant they should not be too pushy and should defer to boys. On the other hand, boys should be "men," which meant they should be strong, decisive, and never cry. My impression was that there was no greater insult than to call a boy feminine. Boys were on the football team, the basketball team, and other letter sports teams; girls got to cheer from the sidelines.

When I was 12 and in junior high school, I thought that it was unfair that boys were able to build usable household items—like bookshelves—in woodshop class, but girls baked cream puffs in "home economics lab." I felt uncomfortable and humiliated, especially because we had to wear aprons and ugly hairnets. I'd pass the wood shop and

Lose the Labels—Health at Every Size

Even if people fall into the "obese" category, I think it is counterproductive to label people, especially children. In my practice, I see mothers "turn off" and become defensive to messages that label their kids as overweight, even if it is the truth. As a result, I have seen frustration and shame from clients and more barriers to achieving healthy behavior change.

I advocate the paradigm of Health at Every Size—where the counselor assesses the client's whole picture of health to make appropriate nutritional and lifestyle recommendations...not just weight. I believe that it encourages acceptance of one's self at that moment in time. It does not mean the individual stops working on being healthy through lifestyle change, but encourages realistic perceptions and goals for individuals.

I believe these are the messages we also need to be sending to children and adolescents.

Let's not paste a label on children and risk damaging their self-esteem and self-image, potentially contributing to future eating disorders. Instead, our goal is to improve quality of life through improvement in health behaviors.

Amy D. Ozier, PhD, RD, LDN, CHES
Northern Illinois University
Dekalb Illinois

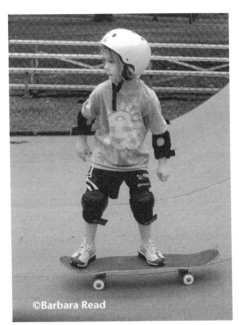

©Barbara Read

peek in—the boys were working so intensely, and I'd never seen them so focused on anything. Boys were usually such pests in the classroom—always joking and playing pranks. But something changed for them in shop class. It looked like hard work—they were dirty and sweaty—but they were having fun. Boys got to fix things, and girls sewed useless, un-wearable dirndl skirts and made complicated, inedible confections that were dumped into the garbage can on the way out of the classroom. Boys went home and worked on home repairs, but we (girls) never attempted to duplicate the archaic stuff we learned at school. For us, it was a torturous waste of time. But that's the way it was, and no one fought the status quo.

Kids from the suburbs may be less active than city kids, although it might seem like having backyards should hold an advantage. I recently moved from a suburban South Florida neighborhood of mostly single family homes and town homes, and each morning and afternoon I'd walk the dog, and see the same contingent of idling cars parked at the bus stop. These families lived less than a quarter-mile from the bus stop, but parents dropped their kids off every morning and picked them up every afternoon. Why weren't the kids walking? This was a safe neighborhood, with a bus stop at the top of a cul-de-sac and no traffic. This was gorgeous South Florida, where people go for the winter because the temperature is so wonderful. And this was a perfect opportunity to make sure the kids got at least a little activity. After all, most kids sit all day: they sit in school (most schools don't offer daily mandated physical activity); they sit on the bus; they sit in their parents' car; and then at home, they sit some more in front of the television or computer. Sometimes parents even "dial for dinner" and have it delivered, or they drive-thru and eat in their cars. Some families never get any regular activity.

Nielsen Media Research shows that the average American watches 4.35 hours of television daily[7]. The American Academy of Pediatrics recommends NO TV for kids less than age two but sadly, the organization reports that most parents set their infants in front of the television daily. It's no surprise that parents use the television as a baby sitter—parents have their hands full, and parents appease their concerns by believing the advertisements promoting programs as making kids smarter.

Television, though, isn't a benign form of entertainment, and viewing habits influence buying and eating habits. The Kaiser Family Foundation reports that programs targeting "tweens"—kids ages eight to 12—advertises sweet stuff in about 50 percent of the commercials. Unfortunately, there's almost no advertising for fruits, vegetables, or whole grain cereal[8]. Kids won't see favorite cartoon characters aligned with fresh salads and broiled fish, unlike high fructose corn syrup-laded junk foods. And since these kids are spending so much time watching television, they're not spending time playing outdoors or playing together. These days, kids—especially inner-city kids who are more likely to be obese—don't have the opportunity to spend time outdoors developing lean muscle and a healthy metabolism. American kids grow less fit each year, and today's kids are 15 to 20 percent less fit than their parents were at their age[9].

Is Overweight Contagious?

Type 2 diabetes affects the circulatory and nervous systems, increasing the risk for heart attack, stroke, amputation, blindness, kidney failure, and death. Diabetes experts predict that one in three Americans born today will develop type 2 diabetes, due primarily to the unremitting increase in overweight and obesity in children. The International Diabetes Federation estimates that 200 million people worldwide currently have type 2 diabetes, which will explode to more than 330 million by 2025[10].

Furthermore, today's generation is predicted to be the first to have a lifespan shorter than their parents.

Health officials have described the drastic increase in the diagnoses of type 2 diabetes in adults—and now in children—as an "epidemic." That's interesting, considering that most of the time, the term *epidemic* is applied to the flu or smallpox or any other disease transmitted by personal contact.

Is type 2 diabetes a contagious disease? Somewhat similar to a virus or bacteria, diabetes is *socially* transmittable—that is, constant exposure to people who are overweight or obese seems to increase your risk of contracting it. People are more likely to "catch" obesity if their family members—and especially if their friends—are overweight or obese. However, the reverse is true as well, and if your best friends and family take steps to gain control—getting healthier and losing weight—that's contagious, too[11].

The idea that obesity may be catching makes some people uncomfortable. I read an editorial where the writer complained that the "food police" in New York City were making his life miserable, and that the ban on trans fats in restaurant foods was unnecessary and wrong. He complained that, unlike second-hand smoke, obesity is not "communicable." He beefed that the government shouldn't put its nose in anyone's burgers and fries and that it's "un-American" to try to legislate how foods are made. After all, he argued, people know what's good for them. They are free to make healthy choices, right?

Perhaps—or maybe not. Advertising is ubiquitous—and the billions spent on influencing buying and eating habits takes its toll, and we don't even realize it. Advertising works—it helps change opinion, and it's hard to ignore. Persistent messaging is designed to promote purchasing, and insidiously guides behavior. Commercials that target kids show normal-weight, lively and engaged children eating snack foods—but who's watching? Perhaps overweight, unhappy children stuck inside their homes. Studies show that kids who have televisions in their bedrooms are significantly more likely to be overweight—regardless of their activity—and are likely eating more high calorie foods, and fewer fruits and vegetables[12].

Fight for the Future

Starting with video games in the '70s, kids have spent increasing hours glued to electronic screens, and today are less active than any generation in history. The American Academy of Pediatrics (AAP) reports that young people view an estimated 40,000 ads a year, linking oversaturation to obesity, poor nutrition, and cigarette and alcohol use.

I think television viewing is a privilege—for kids and for me. I used to let the tube blare at me whenever I was home, but no more. Lowering exposure to television made a difference in how I think and is one of the first changes I made to my new *naturally thin* lifestyle. If you have kids, or even if you don't, don't let television rule—take control of the tube. Take out the TV schedule and, as you would with any activity, schedule any shows you want to see. At the same time, schedule some time to workout; pencil in your Pilates or Yoga class or video. I like to "multi-task" and keep a resistance band and balance ball nearby. Make it a habit to do something besides sit while you watch, and get more bang for your viewing buck. When television viewing is purely sedentary, then it's no surprise that it correlates with childhood obesity, and reducing time in front of all electronic screens—televisions, video games, and computers—helps kids and adults avoid overweight[13].

Alternatively, let the technology support a *naturally thin* lifestyle. Some new music video games like *Dance Dance Revolution* are cool—if it means getting off the couch, it's a good thing and better than just exercising thumbs. Playing and interacting with other kids is what it's all about, and these indoor games can be a lot of fun. Nintendo's Wii Fit sports video games are good examples of how to use technology to work for your fitness, instead of against it. I've watched little and "big" kids having a blast, really burning calories as they interact with the screen. No doubt, getting outside to breathe fresh air is ideal, but some communities are not safe, and bad weather can limit outdoor activities. Let's take advantage of the digital age, and if it's fun, if kids will use it, if adults can benefit from it, then add it to the arsenal of strategies to prevent overweight.

Safe Routes to School

Today, only about 15 percent of schoolchildren in the U.S. walk or bike to school.

Community leaders, parents, and schools across the U.S. are using Safe Routes to School programs to encourage and enable more children to safely walk and bike to school. The National Center for Safe Routes to School aims to assist these communities in developing successful Safe Routes programs and strategies. The Center offers a centralized resource of information on how to start and sustain a Safe Routes to School program, case studies of successful programs, and many other resources for training and technical assistance.

Go to http://www.saferoutesinfo.org   to learn how to start a Safe Routes to School (SRTS) program in your community.

The "New Normal"

When everyone around you is overweight, you may think overweight is *normal*. Manufacturers are changing their product templates to accommodate fatter adults, and how sad it is that many American children are too heavy to fit into car seats appropriate for their age. When training as a dietitian, I spent the food-service rotation of my dietetic internship working in a large suburban school system, where the director had led the profitable initiative to make school lunch more like fast food. After all, that's what kids like, right? The objective was to sell more food, so just like the fast food franchises, they started offering "value meals" featuring larger portions of fries and sodas—the initiative significantly increased sales. They invited soda companies to place vending machines outside the cafeteria. Even elementary school kids were allowed to "opt out" of the hot lunch line and buy a bag of chips, a soda, and ice cream instead.

Although some schools have outlawed fatty fast food, and have switched out sweetened sodas for water and milk, many American schools continue the practice of merchandising fast food, even leasing space to major restaurant chains within their cafeterias. Adolescents can order a cheeseburger, large fries, and a 16-ounce soda—and eat two-thirds or more of the fat and calories an average kid needs for the entire day. Soda consumption, linked to obesity, has tripled for teen boys and doubled for girls over the last 20 years. American children now consume twice as much soda as milk, and as girls age, the increase in soda and decrease in other healthy beverages such as calcium and vitamin D-rich low fat milk may predict higher risk for obesity and osteoporosis[14].

Although fast food can have a place in a healthy diet, making a habit of fast food makes it hard to maintain a normal weight. And providing schoolchildren with healthier food and vending options takes commitment from the community and administration. When I was a kid, if I had a choice between a sandwich and an ice cream sandwich, I would have picked the ice cream, too. But it makes better sense to instill some good habits at an early age, and parents can get involved by contacting their schools to advocate for good eating.

It Doesn't Happen by Accident!

I can recall a moment in my early life when three realizations hit me: (1) I was six-weeks post-partum after giving birth to twin daughters, and, having never really exercised in my life, I was anxious to get back to pre-pregnancy weight; (2) A YMCA had just opened up in our community and offered child care for moms who wanted to join class; (3) I was more aware of the health problems my family had experienced (high blood pressure, high cholesterol, excess weight, and emphysema) and of my desire for something different for my children.

I can recall quite clearly a CHOICE to do things differently because of my family's genes and for my children—to lower their risk. Over the next several years, we developed the following habits, and we continue!

- Regular aerobic exercise at least 3 times weekly
- Strength-training at least 2 times weekly
- Fewer desserts created and consumed
- Healthier food choices
- Family meals eaten together in the evening
- Soda was viewed as a "once in awhile" treat—never a regular beverage
- Weigh regularly—at least 2 x weekly
- Never keep snacks or food in my office or in sight on counters/tables at home
- Single portions—never double!
- Limited restaurant dining
- Pack lunch daily for work

We—nutrition professionals included—are humans with feelings, vulnerabilities, and we make difficult choices in a challenging environment on a daily basis. And it doesn't happen by accident!

Lisa Finley, RD, LD
Columbia, MO
Registered Dietitian
-Jefferson City Medical Group,
Jefferson City, MO

Bigger Isn't Better—But It's Cheaper!

Overeating is a habit, a learned behavior—some even eat competitively. I've noticed that, for some, it's not "all-you-can-eat," it's "eat all you can"! For some, approaching a buffet line anticipates eating huge amounts as if in response to a challenge. I think one reason we eat so much is because we are constantly reminded that the larger size is a "bargain"; that "upgrading" your order costs only pennies; and that for just a few cents, your order can be a "biggie." A study of fast food eaters showed that people consistently underestimate large or super-sized meals by 500 calories. Do that just once a week and you'll gain almost eight pounds a year. Most people who eat fast food dine out at least three times weekly[15]. It adds up.

What does it take to gain a pound...or lose one?

Theoretically, consume an extra 3,500 calories per week—it translates to an extra pound on your hips or thighs or belly. It's all too easy to do.

Consider:

Eating to Gain Weight	Add extra calories per week	Gain unwanted pounds within one year
Drink just two 20-ounce sodas in addition to your usual diet	Each bottle has between 250 to 500 calories	About 8 pounds worth of calories (and watch out for your teeth)
Drink just 2 specialty coffees or teas per week (you know, with whipped cream)	Can top 700 calories	Add 10 pounds, and very expensive! Spend at least $400 per year
Drive through for a double cheeseburger, fries and soda instead of a turkey on rye with mustard, lettuce and tomato	I'll be conservative at an extra 600 calories	About 9 pounds, plus a triple whammy of fat, sodium and cholesterol.

Kids At Risk

Although all overweight children don't have overweight parents, the majority of them do.

The U.S. Surgeon General's office says overweight adolescents have a 70 percent chance of becoming overweight or obese adults. When one parent is overweight, a child is 40 percent more likely to be overweight. When both parents are overweight, it doubles the risk to the child, up to 80 percent. Statistics don't doom you or your children to be overweight—and you can take steps to avoid becoming a statistic.

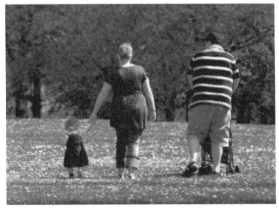

Overweight parents often set the stage for increased risk for kid's overweight

The University of Michigan conducts ground-breaking research in childhood obesity. Noting that Michigan has one of the highest rates of overweight and obesity, a recent study examined over 6,000 pediatric surgeries and found that more than 33 percent of the patients were overweight or obese—and, compared to normal weight kids, overweight kids have worse outcomes. The researchers noted that overweight adult patients are more likely to have conditions such as type 2 diabetes, hypertension, and asthma and other breathing problems, and they are more likely to develop infections in their wounds after surgery[16]. These conditions are also becoming common among overweight and obese children.

Another survey of parents of obese or extremely overweight kids showed that many parents are fooling themselves about their own kid's weight, especially parents of younger kids, from age six to 11. Parents of older kids will acknowledge the overweight much more often than parents of younger children, which leads researchers to conclude that these parents may perpetuate the problem by not addressing the factors that have led to their child's overweight[17].

- Childhood obesity doubles the risk for type 2 diabetes in children
- Behavioral problems in obese kids are three times more common compared to normal weight kids
- Kids who have behavioral problems are five times more likely to become overweight
- Weight loss surgery in kids has tripled
- What kids eat as infants and toddlers may predict overweight and obesity later on

When I was in junior high, President Kennedy's Council on Physical Fitness mandated that all children put on uniforms and run the track. We did pushups and sit-ups, and there were no excuses—we all had to participate. This was a new idea, because until this time, gym class for girls was like home economics—irrelevant and unchallenging. All the same, boys were supposed to be stronger than girls. Boys were expected to run longer and to climb the ropes in the gymnasium while the girls jumped rope. Boys had to do full-arm pushups; girls did bent-knee pushups that could be accomplished by the weakest of girls.

Currently, there is not a national program to prevent childhood obesity, and the amount of state-legislated activity varies from state to state. Most high schools don't offer regular gym classes, and elementary and middle school mandated gym classes aren't consistent. Even recess isn't guaranteed, and when it is, it can just involve standing and talking. Since so many kids don't have the chance to play or burn calories daily, it's not surprising that they're gaining weight. Many children don't have the opportunity to play organized sports; they return home from sitting all day at school and stay inside to play video games, watch television, or work on the computer. So many kids grow up without a foundation of fitness.

Take the Lead—Take Charge!

There *are* some things that we all can do, and family and community involvement are critically important for improving the health and nutrition of kids. You don't have to be a parent to speak with school administrators and local representatives. We can write to snack food and "kid's food" companies to stop advertising high-sugar foods on Saturday morning television. We *all* can turn OFF the television!   Join parents' committees and get the junk food out of school vending

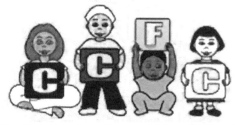

The Campaign for a Commercial-Free Childhood: Log on to www.commercialfreechildhood.org to get involved

machines—give the administrators a list of the low sugar snacks, nonfat milk and fruit you want your kids to eat—even in those vending machines. If you choose to become active, join the *Campaign For A Commercial-Free Childhood* (www.commercialfreechildhood.org).

This member-supported national coalition of health care experts and concerned parents, headquartered at the Judge Baker Children's Center in Boston, is working to change the way manufacturers unfairly target kids and unduly influence parents' purchasing habits[18].

We can all set healthy examples for our kids, our nieces and nephews, students, and our community by turning off the incessant television and scheduling time for favorite shows and computer use. Hang a family activities calendar right there in the kitchen, and schedule time for fun activities, and everyone can pick one fun thing to do each week.

Unnatural Eating	Eat Naturally Smart	Avoid Excess Calories and Pounds
Apple juice, 2 cups (232 calories)	A cup of low fat milk and a cup of water (88 calories)	Reduce daily calories by 144/ avoid 15 lbs/year (reduce likelihood of cavities by eliminating sugary juice and substituting teeth-loving milk)
Package of candy fruit chews (244 calories)	Apple slices (1 small apple) plus 6 oz. plain low fat yogurt (162 calories)	Reduce daily calories by 82 / avoid 9 lbs/year with higher protein snack—plus bone up on calcium, magnesium, and fiber.
Frozen peanut butter & honey sandwich – (210 calories) First three ingredients are different forms of sugar, including high fructose corn syrup, sucrose and "honey spread"	Natural peanut butter and apple butter on whole wheat pita (240 calories)	May be a few calories higher, but infinitely better nutritionally. Whole wheat bread without a laundry list of additives, colors, softeners, and other preservatives
Kid's lunch package containing ham and cheese and crackers: with fruit-flavored punch (high fructose corn syrup). The single serving has 660 calories, 22 grams of fat, and 1600 milligrams of sodium. That's 67% of the Daily Value for sodium—based on a 2000 calorie diet. Depending on your child's age, that could be much more than he needs for a healthy meal.	Roll-up lean ham (2 ounces) with sliced reduced-fat cheddar (2 ounces), fruit cup, and 6 ounces low fat milk (299 calories/9 grams fat)	Enjoy half the calories and twice the nutrition! These type of packaged lunch meals have more than two-thirds the maximum adult recommendation for daily sodium. Add some fresh fruit with more potassium to counteract high sodium choices. Roll-ups are great ideas for young and old: a fresh and fun lunch.

A Word About Kids

Kids need fuel for fitness and should never go "on diets" for the same reason adults should avoid a "diet mentality." Focus on fun fuel, stoking the engine with good quality food instead of junk, and never use food as a reward or punishment. Growing kids need calories from foods that will build their immunity and cell structure and ensure that their bones remain strong throughout adulthood.

When kids are small, they self-regulate what they eat and instinctually stop when they are full. This is the "secret" to avoiding overweight—adults, pay attention! Set an example and pay attention to your eating style; slow it down, because we all eat too fast—too fast to even recognize when we're full—so we keep eating and wind up overeating.

Never praise a child for overeating—stay away from the "more is better" mentality and avoid problems further down the road.

FAMILIES: Staying Naturally Thin

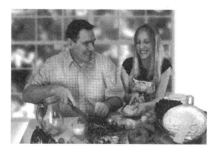

Some of the biggest obstacles to change may be right in your own backyard, so to speak. Unless you're living alone, your housemates—whether they are your family, spouse, kids, or friends—may not be willing to eat smart and stay healthy. But, *you* have control over what you eat, and you can set a naturally thin example.

NATURALLY THIN FAMILIES

All menus and snack ideas throughout this book are perfect for the whole family—adults and children. If you're a parent, your kids will appreciate being included in the meal planning, shopping, preparation, and serving: involving them as soon as they can hold a stirring spoon is the way to get them involved and help them learn about naturally healthy living. Pick up a copy of *Trim Kids*, by exercise physiologist Dr. Melinda S. Sothern, research psychologist T. Kristian von Almen, and registered dietitian Heidi Schumacher. This book is based on their clinically-proven program. It helps parents accurately assess their child's weight and understand the unique challenges of being an overweight kid. Together, parents and kids follow a 12-week program, exploring new ways of eating and interesting and fun fitness exercises. The book teaches parents to use kid-appropriate strategies to learn positive behavioral changes. Fun, fitness and fuel—in all, more of a "let's do it together" manual than a "do it like this" book, written for the parent with the kid in mind.

Although we're suffering from an epidemic of obesity, and our government recognizes the health care catastrophe waiting to happen, there are precious few dollars designated to fund healthy eating and activity programs in public schools and our communities. So, take charge! Of course it is difficult to compete with the billions spent on ad campaigns for processed and fast foods. And it is hard shielding kids from outside influences-- what I think are threats to your children's health and future. But, you can demonstrate YOUR commitment to healthy living. Choose your foods wisely, make physical activity second nature, and set an example of how to live naturally thin.

Change Right

I have many clients say to me "of course, you don't have to follow a diet, you're naturally thin." But no—I work at it and make choices everyday.

I don't follow a "diet," it is my lifestyle. It is a conscious decision I make daily to eat right and exercise. I tell my clients how we will slowly incorporate lifestyle changes into their life. I make sure they understand that I don't expect it overnight...they didn't get to the weight they are at now overnight and it will not come off overnight but, with the right changes it will come off and stay off.

Elizabeth O'Malley RD, LDN
Palos Heights, Illinois

Eat Together

Families who eat together stay healthier. Mealtime should be simple and enjoyable, a place for everyone to say "hello" without stress. Try your best to do as much preparation in advance to make meals less complicated and more enjoyable.

- Home-cooked doesn't have to mean complicated, and it is much healthier and—in the long run—cheaper than restaurant or take-out food. I love bagged salads; pre-cut vegetables; canned fish and chicken; frozen fish and vegetables; quick-cooking rice and grains; pre-baked pizza crusts; and bottled tomato sauce.

- Mix it Up: Who says you can't eat breakfast for dinner occasionally (hot oatmeal plus fruit and yogurt)? Some people do much better eating their main meal at noon.

- Sandwiches are Genius: If you're too busy to cook but still want a family meal, organize a submarine party. When made right, subs make super suppers. Buy whole grain rolls (buy 100% whole grain instead of "enriched wheat"), lean meats, some lower fat cheese such as provolone (a thin slice has about 80-100 calories), lettuce, tomato, and maybe some jalapeño peppers. Top with some fresh ground pepper and a sprinkle of very good olive oil and wine vinegar. Slice into 2-inch servings and serve with fruit salad. That's a meal!

- Make it Interesting: Eating the same foods day after day is not only boring, it's not as nutritious as eating a variety of different vegetables, fruits, fish, and even poultry (think turkey—it's not just for Thanksgiving!). Try a Mexican night—set the table with a colorful tablecloth and candles and serve fajitas and corn tortillas—or an Italian night with wine and fettuccini. Explore different cuisines: visit the library or bookstore or cruise the Internet for interesting and healthy new recipes from different cultures…your family will love it.

- Be Persistent, Not Pushy: Kids need to be offered the same food more than eight to 10 times to accept it, so don't be put off if your kids (big or little) reject a new food or if they only want the same foods all the time. As long as they're not pushed too hard, most kids will eventually begin to explore new foods. Plan a "new night" twice a week and offer two types of vegetables—the "favorite," plus a new variety, and eventually, they'll get it. How about you? Are you stuck in a rut of iceberg lettuce and tomatoes? Break through and explore deep colors and different flavors.

- You Can Say No: I think it's smart to just not buy some foods—just don't keep them in the house. Say "No" to regular soda or sugar-sweetened juice drinks or teas; say "yes" to water, club soda, your own slightly-sweetened iced (and hot) teas. Say "No" to trans fat-laden margarine or cookies, cakes, and crackers that contain partially or fully hydrogenated fat; say "yes" to fruit smoothies, frozen fruit bars, and trans fat-free cookies. Forget breakfast cereals with more than 8g of sugar per serving; most foods labeled "fruit flavored" only pretend to have real fruit.

- Sometimes is Fine: Even Sesame Street's Cookie Monster says, "Cookie is a sometimes food." Some foods are "sometimes" foods, others are only "very occasionally," and some are "always." Even big kids (adults!) can use this to think positively about all food. Some foods are too fatty and full of sugar and preservatives to fit into the "sometimes" category…just put them in the "very occasionally" category and leave them there, permanently.

- Don't Be Fooled: You know what they say, "Fool me once, shame on you; fool me twice, shame on me." Read ingredient labels first and don't be fooled by the pretty pictures on the front of the box. There is no fruit in Froot Loops. Most "fruit roll-ups" are just sugar; dried fruit is a much better option.

- Set an Example: Everyone around you—everyone you touch—will learn from your own good example. By demonstrating your willingness to spend the time preparing a healthy, home-cooked meal; to try new foods; and to be adventurous in the kitchen, your loved ones are likely to participate, too.

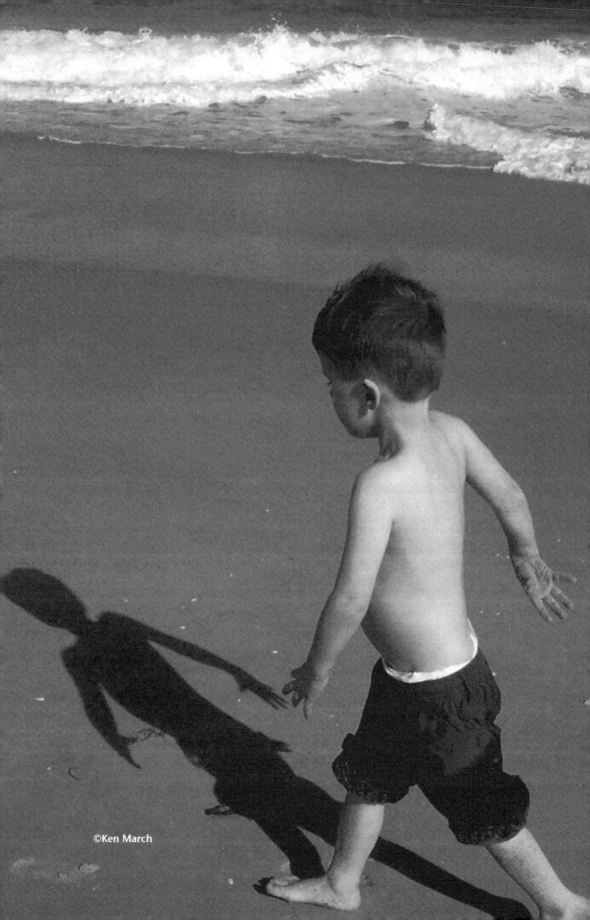

©Ken March

Chapter 3

Food Is Not the Enemy
Changing the Focus from Food to Behaviors

Your vision will become clear only when you look into your heart.
Who looks outside, dreams. Who looks inside, awakens.
—Carl Jung

I f you told me 25 years ago that I could keep weight off without dieting, I would not have believed you because I couldn't imagine not using food to feel better. When I felt stressed or anxious or bored or distracted, I turned to food. But on a cool night toward the end of March, 1982, I began to break away from my bad habit of using mental excuses for overeating. I had just signed the lease for an apartment on the upper level of a small, wooden-frame house on Long Island. The landlord gave me a break on the first month's rent in return for my giving the rooms a fresh coat of paint. There I was, alone on a Tuesday evening, feeling fairly positive—the way a fresh coat of paint makes you feel. After I had painted for hours, I decided to get some Chinese takeout from the place down the street. Back at home, I sat on the floor of the living room—I had no furniture yet—eating greasy lo mein noodles. After the first few bites, when the fat started to coat my tongue, I started to berate myself, the way I did every time I overate. Why was I eating this stuff? There was a grocery store just down the

DEFINITION

Instruction
—noun

1. The act or practice of instructing or teaching; education.

2. Command, mandate.

—Synonyms

1. Tutoring, coaching; training, schooling

Habit
—noun

1. An established custom; "it was their habit to walk together every evening"

2. (Psychology) an automatic pattern of behavior in reaction to a specific situation, and incorporated through daily repetition—something that has become ingrained resulting from conscious thought

street. I could have gotten some salad—I could have eaten better. Oh, why couldn't I eat healthy, why couldn't I get a life! I felt awful. I felt dejected, depressed, and angry.

In the old days, this script would have provoked me to just keep on eating, finish everything, and then go get some ice cream. But this time, I didn't.

I had been thinking about joining the new Diet Center® franchise that had opened in a storefront down the street from my office. Every day I'd pass by and think, "I really should join—maybe I could lose weight," and keep on driving. That evening, I deliberately stopped eating and threw out the rest of the food, put on my sneakers, my windbreaker, and a scarf. I went down the stairs into the cold air and walked in the dark for over an hour, all the way to the end of the road and back. I drank two glasses of cold water and felt great.

I've held on to that decision for the past 25 years and often think of that moment when I returned from the walk in the dark—I was cold and scared and happy and exhilarated all at the same time. For the first time, I made a deliberate and positive choice about my lifestyle. After that March evening, I cleaned out my cabinets and, the next day I decided that my discretionary income was destined to support my weight control. I had some money saved for a vacation, and instead, I joined the gym closest to my home, and signed up for a structured weight management program that provided me with a framework that I used to lose weight. This wasn't the first time I had tried a calorie-controlled plan, but this was the first time that I thought about what happens *after* the diet. And this is the first time that I committed to "checking in"—to monitoring my weight, and writing it down. For the first weeks, I visited the center just about every day, and saw the same weight loss counselor. The process was so different than anything I'd attempted before. At my first visit, before she handed me any information about what I was going to eat, we spent time talking about realistic weight goals, and importantly, identified behaviors to change. She asked me to keep a lifestyle log, and to write down everything I ate every day, and what type of activity I did—any deliberate exercise. Every visit she weighed me, and every other week she took my measurements. This is what I needed—I needed support, daily contact, and someone to cheer me. I opted for a real-foods diet, instead of buying frozen products, and I chose a very simple menu and stuck with it—I didn't count calories, but instead counted portions. I ate about 12 ounces of lean protein (egg whites, fish and turkey), *all* the vegetables I wanted (crunchy, that is—not starchy), at least three fruits a day (at least one of them a big, whole grapefruit), approximately two servings of high-fiber bread, and NO alcohol. Lots of water—unlimited herbal tea. Yes, very simple meals, but that's what I needed at the beginning—simplicity meant taking the anxiety out of eating.

Most people can lose weight by following a calorie-restricted diet—or by exercising long and intensively to burn enough calories to create a calorie-deficit. The best way is to incorporate both—restrict calories and rev up your metabolic engine. But, it's what you do after the "diet" that will create the scenario for permanent weight loss and control.

Face to face counseling can be fairly expensive and won't fit everyone's busy schedule and budget. Another option is logging on to the Internet for a free or subscription online weight management program. Online, it is possible to interact at a reasonable level of personalization and consistency—for a very reasonable cost. As long as you have Internet access you can maintain contact, get comprehensive information and support.

It wasn't a straight line to being in permanent control, however. Yes, I lost weight, and for a long time I made good choices and most importantly, stayed loyal to my activities. I loved being fit—I loved how my body felt, and that wasn't a problem. But the food still was.

Not a Straight Path to Naturally Thin

A few years later, I was living in Manhattan, running every morning and going to the gym to workout. I was much improved in my eating and activity habits, but I still hadn't taken control—and because I was unhappy in my relationship and my career, I fell back into using food to distract me. I was holding on to a favorite food, one I knew was too high in calories and fat, one that provoked me to feel bad about myself after eating it. Every morning, I went down to the corner coffee shop and bought a huge bran muffin. I'd cut it in half, wrap one half in tin foil, and put the other in the refrigerator, vowing not to eat it. And then I would, and I'd feel awful about myself, and I'd promise tomorrow I'd "be good" and have cereal and milk. And the next morning, I was back at the coffee shop. They were happy to see me: "Good morning, Susan—one bran muffin?"

I decided to see a nutritionist. I knew that I needed help, and I fantasized that I would get a diet, follow it, and then I'd be thin. I'd conveniently forgotten about the work with my diet counselor just a few years earlier, how much effort it took to change behaviors—I wanted a quick fix. I looked in the yellow pages and called to make an appointment. When I arrived, she handed me a clipboard and asked me to fill out a form titled "Diet History."

She said, "Be as detailed as you can," and sat there while I completed it. Then, she weighed me and made some notations on the paper I'd handed back to her.

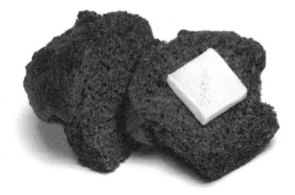

"Here," she said, handing me a double-sided piece of paper. "Here is your diet. Follow this, and I'll see you in two weeks. Oh, and stop eating the bran muffins. They have way more calories than you think."

The next morning, I had cereal and milk. But, the following morning, it was back to the Big Bran Muffin, and back to my usual self-talk, castigating me for *bad* behavior. I realized I needed help, again. I was lonely and using food to feel better.

Portion size counts! A 500-calorie-plus mega-sized muffin became my nemesis

Joining an eating support group made an enormous difference in how I felt about myself. When I felt frustrated or lonely or stressed or anxious, I connected with friends and supporters to talk about the emotion instead of stuffing it down with food. I kept on working on what I could do daily to reduce my stress, and I stayed active and continued to workout in the gym by using hand weights, exercise bands, and balance balls. The benefits of the structure of a pre-planned menu and activities schedule; of support and consistent activity, (especially the muscle-toning exercises), got me back on track—and over the past 25 years I've cemented my healthy behaviors into my *naturally thin* lifestyle.

Deliberate Good Health

Growing up, my family didn't have a TV, so I spent my childhood either reading books or playing--I was active. We ate our meals sitting down as a family, and it was mostly home-made—no frozen pizza or 'mac 'n cheese', and dining out was very infrequent. I was very thin as a child, but as I grew older I became much less active, and I actually started to gain weight. But then I was diagnosed with type 1 diabetes and eating healthy became a necessity. I learned how to count carbs and I paid attention to what I ate, and I think that's what kept me on the right path when I was old enough to make my own food choices.

I don't routinely keep cookies and chips at home, and I learned early on how to make healthy meals. I try not to set myself up for failure--I know my limits. I can stop eating after two Hershey Kisses, but I can't stop at two Oreo cookies. So, I keep "Kisses" at home for a small treat, but I avoid Oreos like the plague!

I believe—strongly—in the concept of moderation, but I also know that it's important to stay attuned to how my body and blood sugars react to how much and what types of foods I eat, and how much activity I do—and I pay close attention. When I don't feel like working out, or when I'd rather have French fries instead of a salad, I tell myself "My body deserves this" (meaning the healthy choice). Sometimes that's the ONLY thing that helps me make the right choice when it comes to diet and exercise.

Suzanne Fleming, RD, LD
McPherson, KS.

I Can't Talk You Thin

Today's dietitians often have better counseling training than when I was in school, and certainly better than the nutritionist who handed me a piece of paper without even having a conversation about my behaviors. Instead of an authoritative approach, dietitians have embraced *motivational interviewing*, a client-centered approach that evolved from behavioral treatment of other addictive behaviors including alcohol and cigarettes, and now more recently, overeating[1]. Being overweight didn't happen automatically—and weight loss is a complicated process, but can be best accomplished by understanding and first addressing the stages of change. For example, has the client even accepted that they need to lose weight, or are they not yet contemplating it? Counselors need to work from the client's stage—on the client's schedule—and not impose their weight biases, their own expectations, disappointments, or frustrations on the client. Although that person may be sitting down in my office asking for a "diet," she may first need me to listen to and accept her.

Motivational interviewing helps clients identify their own expectations and define their priorities and fears. Clients define their own goals—it may first be a weight goal, but ideally, the goals will be accomplished by adopting new behaviors and then weight loss and maintaining a healthy weight becomes a natural and permanent result[2].

The Stages of Change Model[3,4]

Experts say that it takes many efforts to make new behavior permanent. For example, you may not even be thinking about changing behavior at all—but then you start thinking, "Gee, I'd feel better if I lost some weight." You may buy a diet book—you may even "go on" a diet—but it may take you a few times before you finally accept that you have to make those diet changes a permanent part of your living to keep the weight off permanently.

Stages of Change Model
Stage in transtheoretical model of change
Patient stage

Precontemplation

- Not thinking about change
- May be resigned
- Feeling of no control
- Denial: does not believe it applies to self
- Believes consequences are not serious

Contemplation

- Weighing benefits and costs of behavior, proposed change

Preparation

- Experimenting with small changes

Action

- Taking a definitive action to change

Maintenance

- Maintaining new behavior over time

Relapse

- Experiencing normal part of process of change
- Usually feels demoralized

Benefits and Conflicts of Weight Management

Overweight and obesity increase risk for arthritis and joint degeneration, type 2 diabetes, heart disease, hypertension, stroke, some cancers, and even depression. The American Society for Reproductive Medicine notes that being overweight or obese reduces chances of getting pregnant and increases risks associated with pregnancy, including increased risk for gestational diabetes and miscarriage. However, just a five to 10 percent weight loss dramatically improves the chances of a successful pregnancy[5]. A conscientious physician who determines their patient needs to lose weight may refer his patient to a registered dietitian, but not always. Maybe the doctor will hand the patient a printed diet—or maybe not. Maybe the doc will just say to the patient, "Lose weight."

As a hospital dietitian, usually the only chance I had to speak with patients was at their hospital bedside, often while they were recovering from an angioplasty or open heart surgery. If I was lucky, when I arrived, they'd be there in their room—hopefully awake and able to converse. But often the patient wasn't in her bed—she could be away for a test or asleep or even discharged before I even had the chance to visit. It was never the best time to practice *motivational interviewing* techniques, which is the best way to prepare patients for behavioral change.

Instead of the old confrontational approach, where the counselor points out all the "wrong" things the client does, and then tells her what to do, motivational interviewing recognizes that most people need to express their frustrations and fears of change before they can focus on goals and strategies for behavior change.

There are very legitimate reasons that make it difficult to lose weight. If you're not able to exercise, weight loss will be more challenging—but almost everyone can do some type of exercises, even sitting down in a chair. Some medical conditions and medications make weight loss difficult—some meds even cause weight gain. Family obligations, work and school responsibilities, everyday life can make it difficult to schedule regular activity.

"Stacy," a 48-year-old mom of three, told me that she'd recently seen her doctor for her annual physical and he said she had "impaired fasting glucose" (fasting glucose equal to or greater than 100mg/dL—a precursor to type 2 diabetes). I noticed that she carried extra weight around her middle. She was also taking medication for high blood pressure. She said her doctor warned her that she was at risk for heart disease and type 2 diabetes.

Stacy said she was ready to lose weight, and that she "wanted to go on a diet," but she didn't ask me for help. I asked if I could help her pinpoint some places to make changes in her diet, but she just shrugged and said she knew what she needed to do. A month later, I saw her at the mall, and before I barely said, "Hello," she told me she hadn't lost any weight.

She said she had too much "bad food" in her house that she didn't want to throw away, but when she finished it all, she'd go out and buy "good food." Stacy was contemplating change, but she was not yet ready to make changes.

A Balancing Act

Often a client will tell me that they think that everyone else can eat what they want, and they feel like they're the only ones that need to be careful. It's not true. Just about all people need to work to stay thin, and that's a necessary part of being healthy.

I like to illustrate this balancing act by comparing calories to finances. If we turned off our financial awareness, just wrote checks and took money out of the ATM, maybe making a deposit here and there, but never balancing our account, we'd probably end up broke. We need to maintain consistent consciousness and control and never assume that somehow everything will balance out in the end, and that applies for maintaining weight too.

Elizabeth DeRobertis, MS, RD, CDN, CDE
Scarsdale, New York

"Stanley" has high blood cholesterol and one day he told me that his father had died of a heart attack before he was 60. Without my saying anything, Stanley pronounced that he didn't want to give up his favorite foods, and began listing them: bacon, cheeseburgers, French fries, steak and potatoes, and lobster and biscuits...he said he loved them all.

He said, "Susan, I just have to lose 20 pounds, and I'm going to do it!"

"Great!" I said, and told him to contact me if he needed help. I knew he was conflicted about losing weight—he was concerned enough to tell me about his health risks, but he feared that "dieting" would mean deprivation—and he hadn't yet reached the stage where he could even begin making changes to his lifestyle.

A few weeks later, I saw him at the grocery store, and he did it again.

"I need to lose weight," he said, so this time I asked him if Friday was good for him to meet. "No," he said, "let me call you. My doctor gave me pills, and I will call you soon." I haven't heard from him yet—maybe some day I will. Sometimes medications are necessary to control blood pressure and cholesterol, but most of the time doctors will recommend a lifestyle change to improve his health and lower risk.

Stanley has not committed to positive lifestyle changes and will choose medications rather than change his diet or lifestyle. He's unwilling to throw away the habits that made him overweight; he isn't ready to identify new habits that will allow him to enjoy a naturally thin lifestyle.

When a client says, "I want to lose weight, but I've tried before, and nothing works," they may be expressing their fear of failure. Simply giving them a "pep talk" doesn't address their very valid concerns (especially if they have repeatedly dieted and regained) or solve their problems. In fact, I can't talk them thin.

I too was conflicted about food and overeating. I wanted to lose weight, but I had been using food for a long time to help me cope, and it was hard imagine what life would be like without that emotional aid.

Behaviorists try to help their clients identify their own fears and behaviors that they want to change; then, they are more likely to come up with solutions that work best for them. For example:

- It's not about what I want the client to do. The client is there in my office, so I respect their participation.
- I want to hear what my client thinks. They need to be heard—and they don't need to hear about what I think. They need to know that I hear them.
- I am not there to judge them; I'm there to listen. I had a lot of ambivalence about my own weight, and if they can identify that ambivalence, that is a first step.
- I will help them define the pros and cons of being overweight; I'll help them define a healthy weight based on their personal medical history.
- I will help them define an agenda for change. By summarizing that agenda, they can agree to it, and I can help them negotiate their agenda.
- I am there to provide knowledge, information, and support.

Metabolic Syndrome

If you have any **three** or more of the following symptoms, then according to the National Institutes of Health, you have Metabolic Syndrome. The more of these risk factors you have, the greater your chance of developing heart disease, diabetes, or a stroke. The NIH says that, in general, a person with metabolic syndrome is twice as likely to develop heart disease and five times as likely to develop diabetes as someone without metabolic syndrome[6]. Although risk for some of these symptoms may be inherited, you can change your behaviors and lower your risk for heart disease and diabetes by changing any or all of these symptoms. If you are overweight, losing five to 10 percent of your current weight by modifying your diet and increasing activity can greatly lower your risk, and make you feel better too.

Risk Factors:

- Waist size: You carry excess weight around the middle (men greater than 40 inches; women greater than 35 inches)

- Plaque: Your lab tests indicate a risk for plaque buildup in arteries:

    - High triglycerides (at or above 150 mg/dL)

    - Low 'healthy' HDL cholesterol: women below 50 mg/dL; men below 40 mg/dL)

- Blood Pressure: You have high blood pressure (at or above 130/85 mm HG)

- Blood glucose: You have high fasting blood glucose (at or above 100 mg/dL)

- Pre-diabetes: You have insulin resistance or glucose intolerance (the body can't properly use insulin or blood sugar)

Your total cholesterol should be below 200 mg/dL, and your HDL (good) cholesterol should be 40 mg/dL or higher. LDL (bad) cholesterol will depend on other risk factors: the AHA notes 100 mg/dL as "optimal".

Old Confrontational Approach The Counselor says—	New Motivational Approach The Counselor listens first and then reflects—
You have a problem, and you need to change	Tell me what you think is your problem: I'm here to listen
Tells client what they need to do; doesn't ask the client what changes they are willing to make	Actively listens; expresses interest and respect
Counselor lectures client as the "expert"; client is passive recipient of instruction	Counselor encourages client to express his own concerns and desires, to pinpoint his fears and accept the need for change
The Counselor is the teacher—all the information comes out from him, and the client listens.	Counselor always stays in the 'now' with the client, and responds to his direction, working with the pace of the client and not on a pre-imposed schedule
The Counselor imposes labels or critiques based on his own judgments	Counselor continues to respect the client's work and remains open and supportive.

Habits are at first cobwebs, then cables.

–Spanish Proverb

I Broke the Mold!

I remember it clearly: I was in third grade when I ran up to say hello to my first grade teacher after not seeing her for two years. She looked at me and gasped "You have gotten so fat!" I was devastated.

At the time, my home life was quite stressful, with both my mother and younger brother hospitalized. The nanny who was supposed to be taking care of us wasn't nice. Friends and neighbors kept stopping by with homemade cakes, fried chicken, lots of fatty foods. I was getting a lot of positive feedback for eating—and found comfort in feeling full.

But, I didn't want to be fat. Between fifth and sixth grades I figured out that if I didn't eat I would loose weight, and I got noticed. The more weight I lost, the more positive comments, such as "You look great!!" and "Joey thinks you're cute." Very powerful messages for a 12-year-old girl.

Eventually, I started eating again but changed from eating "normally" (the way the rest of the family ate) to "better." I turned to low fat milk and whole wheat bread. I pulled the skin off the fried chicken; I ate vegetables with a vengeance! But, my family never got the message about healthy eating. They never gave up the 'southern cooking' that kept them overweight.

Over the years, I've had to work hard to maintain my weight. The pattern of unhealthy and compulsive eating that ran in my family was hard to break, and making a career in nutrition was a natural extension of my lifestyle and interests. .

I loyally walk or run almost every day or I play tennis and try to fit physical activity into just about everything I do. I take week-long biking vacations; I protect my feet by using good athletic shoes; since I live in Florida, I stay conscious of the heat and avoid activity during the hottest hours of the day. I go through gallons of sunscreen! I try and balance my meals, never skip meals, and enjoy a glass of wine with dinner. If I have a big lunch, I make dinner much lighter. Although I have sweets occasionally, I hate to waste calories on any that aren't really, really, good. I don't routinely keep them in the house and don't order dessert in restaurants for myself, but I'll share if the opportunity arises.

I weigh myself once a month. I find my motivation to keep my weight under control in being able to fit comfortably into the pretty clothes that I love to wear. This makes me happy and motivates me to keep active and fit.

Stephanie Norris MS, RD, LD/N
Orlando, Florida

Invest in Yourself

The desire to be thin seems universal. Just look at who's featured on the cover of many of the best-selling women's magazines *and* note how *men's* magazine covers feature unnaturally thin models. More than 35 billion dollars are spent yearly in America on weight loss products, programs, and supplements, and none of it has made a dent in the increasing rate of overweight and obesity.

When people were asked if they'd give up a year of their life rather than be overweight, more than 46 percent said they would, and almost 15 percent said they'd give up 10 years[7].

Permanent change takes work, and weight *gain* is easier than weight loss for most people. Taking control takes longer for some. This is especially true if you're not eating *to live*—if, like I was, you are eating without hunger, to soothe, to distract, or to block any bad feelings.

Of course, I didn't wake up one morning instantly "changed." Prior to that cold, March evening, I constantly thought about changing and constantly talked about it— how I wanted to change, how I needed to change.

Examining your attitude about "thin" is a good idea. Do you think people are *naturally thin*? Or maybe they're doing something special that keeps them that way. Well…there's truth to both of these statements.

Yes…some people are "naturally" thin. Some are genetically programmed to be able to eat more calories than the average Joe or Jane without storing the excess as fat. But history tells us that we are more like our hunter and gatherer ancestors, who feasted when they had food because they never knew when the next antelope would jump into their nets. Genetically, we're not able to overcome the fact that we eat like warriors—way more than we need—and spend most of our time sitting instead of chasing after game.

If someone says to me, "You don't have to worry about what you eat—you're naturally thin," it more reflects what they think about themselves—their fears and attitude about their body—than the reality of my weight. My *old* response might have been, "Oh, you're wrong—there's no such thing as naturally thin. I work hard to stay that way!" But I try to avoid talking about me—that isn't why the client is seeking out my services, and it doesn't address her fears and issues about being overweight.

A better and more effective approach to address this misconception might be to say, "What I hear you saying is that you think that no matter what I eat, I never gain weight?" And if she agrees, then it gives me the opportunity to say, "It's interesting, but for all the rarest cases, people who maintain their weight monitor their portions— whether consciously or unconsciously—and they stay active. Let's talk about what *you* can do to identify some of the challenges you have for adopting new healthy living behaviors."

Someone telling me that I'm naturally thin expresses a lot about what that individual really thinks about her own weight—and her ability to be "naturally thin," too. It can be an opportunity to understand the frustrations and fears that she has expressed, probably unknowingly, by stating something that she believes, but that may be holding her back from moving forward toward change.

The "naturally thin" statement could be clients' fear that they won't succeed, no matter how hard they try. I emphasize that *trying* to lose weight is not a specific behavioral change, but *doing* something different may be the ticket to weight loss. For me, giving up the bran muffin in favor of low sugar cereal and nonfat milk demonstrated behavior change and showed that I was moving forward.

So, when someone asks me directly for advice about how to change, I'll ask her to talk about what lifestyle behaviors she thinks are keeping her overweight and what changes she wants to begin with.

Trust & Perceptions

I was speaking with a dietitian colleague and asked her if she found her clients perceived her as "naturally thin."

She said, "Sharing some (minor) personal information has opened an avenue of communication with some of my clients and really deepened the trust – but I don't automatically share with all my clients that I'm not 'naturally thin'. The "it's easy for you" comment comes up often, however, and many patients are having trust issues with talking to someone about their weight. If they understand that I have genuine empathy for their situation because I have managed to lose weight as well, then maybe I can bridge the gap in the session and actually accomplish something with them.

It's not 'easy' but it is daily—I really do practice what I preach. What helps me control my weight are the very same things I recommend to my patients: I exercise almost daily; I fill "half my plate" with vegetables (I think this has made one of the biggest differences for me - it helps me feel full on fewer calories because of the high water and fiber content.) I also plan in advance for what I will eat: I make sure that I know what healthy options are available at restaurants before I go, and I make sure to shop for healthy ingredients to have at home to prepare meals. I definitely keep treats out of the house: out of sight for me is, truly, out of mind.

My colleague continued, "I'd like to share an interesting example of people's perceptions. We were sitting with a bunch of colleagues in the hospital cafeteria, and I said something about taking the stairs instead of the elevator.

One obviously overweight doctor said "Well, taking the stairs is easy for you, because you're skinny."

I said "That's WHY I'm skinny," and it was like a light bulb went off in his head. I have no idea if it made an impact on his own habits or his advice to his patients, but it got him out of his mindset that "I can't do that" or "only people who are skinny to start out with can exercise."

Thin is just a four-letter word.
A better three-letter word is 'fit'.

By definition, a habit is *a behavior or practice so ingrained that it is often done without conscious thought.* Thin habits need to be **permanent** to be **positive**. Habits practiced by thin people are not something they do just for a little while and then stop. Nope... thin people's habits are forever. That's what keeps them thin! Think fit, think smart choices, and thin will follow. A *naturally thin* person is most likely someone who makes a habit of eating well and staying active.

The Grammar of Diet

I used to think of a "diet" as something I had to "go on," as a verb. For example, "I'll go on a diet tomorrow (or Monday, or next week)." And for the longest time, I did this every Sunday. Of course, **all** diets can work, if by "dieting" you mean reducing the calories you take in so that you create a *calorie deficit*. But **no** diet works **permanently** unless you permanently adopt the healthy habits you used to lose weight! If you go on a diet to lose weight but abandon the healthy eating and activity once you see the "magic number" you've dreamed about on a scale, then all too soon that weight will start creeping back—one mega bran muffin, one burger, and one French fry at a time.

There are no bad foods, just bad habits. When I was growing up, my mother, grandmother, and other adults who were "dieting" talked about "being bad." I often heard them say, "I was bad today: I ate a potato."

Isn't that ridiculous? I mean, how can eating a potato make you a bad person? Wait a minute...what if that potato is slathered with butter and drowned in sour cream? Does that make the potato "bad"? Oh, the poor potato—never did any harm, just sitting there waiting to be eaten for its delicious flavor, in its own lovely, bare skin, without all that added fat.

Say you add lots of "good fat" to your potato. Olive oil is healthy, right? So, you drizzle oil instead of saturated fat-laden butter and sour cream. Does that make it a "good food"? Well, we know that diets high in saturated fat increase risk for heart disease, but since all fat is similar in terms of calories, and if you're trying to maintain your weight, adding either "good" fats or "bad" fats—brings extra calories to your food, even if it is "healthy" unsaturated fat from olive oil, or avocado or nuts. Stay calorie-conscious, not calorie-obsessed, and enjoy that potato like I do—scrub it, prick it, bake it (or microwave); then split it and brush lightly with olive oil, and pop it under the broiler until toasty brown. Instead of overloading with fat—even healthy fat— make it delicious, and naturally healthy.

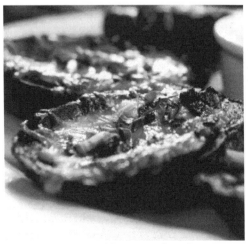

Poor healthy potato forced
to carry so much extra fat!

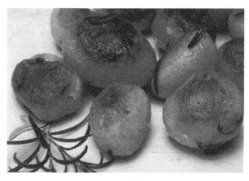

Oven Roasted Potatoes

There are bad people; people do bad things to other people, but food can't be "bad" or "good"—it's just food. You can make food fatter; by adding lots of calories, you can make a healthy food like a baked potato into a vehicle for fat, which can add a lot of unnecessary calories to your daily intake. But it's still not a "bad" food—it's a fatty food.

Make **your** natural diet a healthy one, and you can stay slim…naturally. Depending on my appetite, I eat more or less; sometimes I make a deliberate choice to eat something high in calories, but if I want it, I work it in—and eat a small portion.

And, I can do this is because my naturally thin lifestyle includes *daily* activity. Activity allows my body to naturally accept different amounts of calories daily, so I don't have to count calories as long as I maintain my activity. I eat and live like a "naturally thin" person.

You Can't Change Your Weight Until You Change Your Mind

I was overweight in college and I remember the day that I decided to do something about it. I was looking in the mirror on one Friday evening getting ready for a date when I suddenly felt uncomfortable with what I saw in that mirror. It was one of those moments of truth when the light went on and it was at that very moment that I decided to take charge. The next day I began an eating and exercise routine that I still adhere to today. With that said, when someone says to me, "Oh, you don't have to worry about what you eat, you're naturally thin," I always say something like the following.

I don't have to worry because I do everything necessary to control my weight. I've taken luck and worry out of this formula because I eat mindfully and I always make time to exercise. My being in shape is not a matter of being "naturally thin." It's a matter of being nutritionally alert and physically active. At the end of the day, the shape of your body and the condition of your health is intimately tied to the choices that you make and the actions that you take. I can sum up the answer to becoming thin in one word… Change! You have to change because you will never become who you want to be by remaining who you are. And this change all begins in your mind because, as the motto to my Inner Diet program so aptly states: You can't change your weight until you change your mind!

Dr. John H. Sklare
Atlanta, Georgia

Dr. Sklare is the President/CEO of Inner Resource Corporation and the creator of The Inner Diet (www.innerdiet.com), a program that addresses emotional eating.

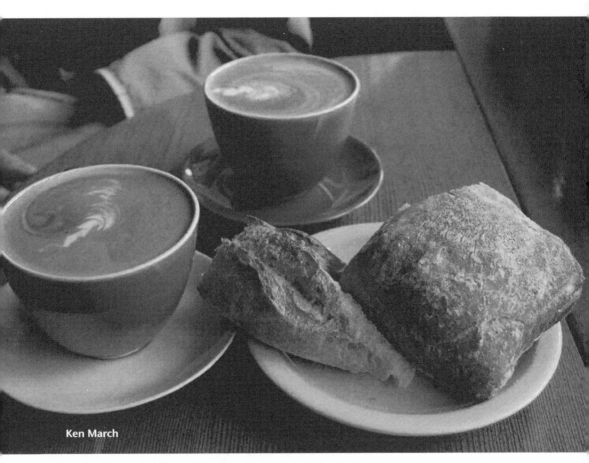

Ken March

A favorite treat--'skinny' latte made with nonfat milk, and a fresh sour dough roll. Walking in Freemont, Washington

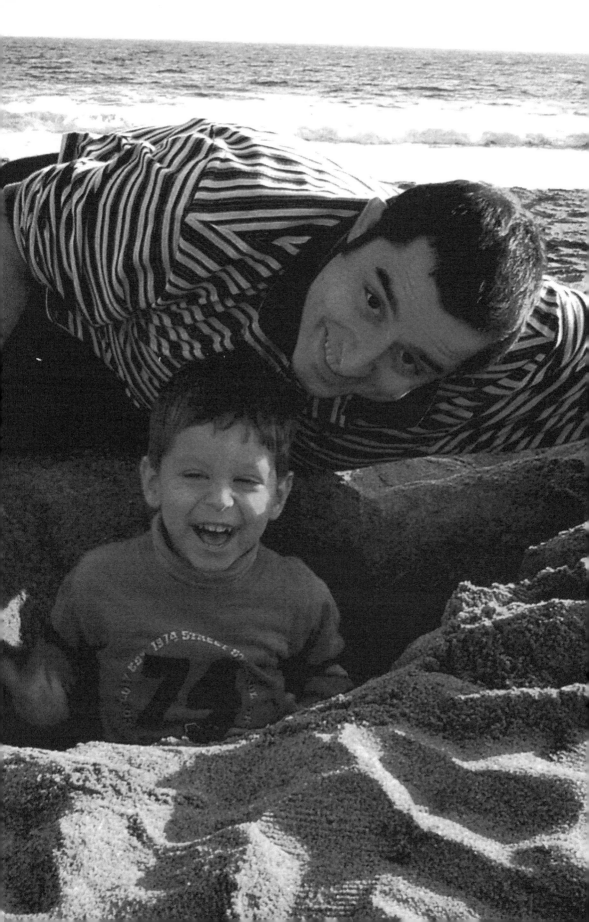

Chapter 4

Motivation Doesn't Just Happen
How I Turned Excuses into Opportunities

Motivation is a fire from within.
If someone else tries to light that fire under you,
chances are it will burn very briefly.
—Stephen R. Covey

"I don't have the motivation." How many times have I heard that complaint from clients as well as friends and family? The sentence continues…"I want to lose weight—but I'm just not motivated." Ah, if only I could go out to the store and buy them some motivation.

It wasn't as if I was unmotivated to change one day and motivated the next. For me, finding motivation to change was like learning a new language—it was that foreign to me. I started from scratch because I'd never before set out to accomplish a personal change; I'd never identified a goal before; I'd just been going along, letting life happen to me. Change took psychological preparation; it took multiple attempts before the change "fixed" into a new lifestyle. There may be backslides and detours; these are normal and natural. But perseverance leads to cementing new behaviors.

Motivation takes preparation. Alfred Hitchcock was an awesome example of a how preparation makes the project run smoothly and efficiently; before the camera ever rolled everyone on the set knew exactly what was expected of them. Hitchcock exquisitely planned and storyboarded every scenario, so that once he yelled, "Action!" he was able to execute—quickly, often in "Oscar-winning" form.

As I developed preparation habits, I found weight loss became so much easier, and I credit this new behavior for my ability to sustain the loss. Preparing for each day took the stress out of making the right choice. Later on, as I felt more in control of daily living, I began to relax, knowing that I could make better choices wherever I would go.

DEFINITION:

Motivation
—noun

1. The reason or reasons for engaging in a particular behavior, and may be internal, based on needs and desires, or external, based on potential for rewards and praise.

All Day, Every Day

At 4'10" my response to someone who assumes that I'm 'naturally thin' is, I'm careful about my weight—only all of the time and every day. I believe I've been able to maintain my 100 pounds for all of my adult years, other than one pregnancy, because I do practice what I preach.

But, I'm by no means perfect. I enjoy sweets, a few times a week – albeit in small portions. I may have a half-cup of my favorite, super-premium ice cream or a piece of chocolate or share a great dessert. I don't waste calories on sweets, or any foods for that matter, that aren't worth it. I don't have enough calories to spare on less-than-excellent foods.

I eat three to four restaurant meals each week, but I rarely cast caution to the wind. I practice portion control to the max – splitting and sharing entrees, ordering appetizers as main courses, splitting desserts and even asking for a half glass of wine on occasion. My husband and I enjoy going to great restaurants on occasion. We split menu items from appetizer to dessert – right down the middle. Lots of great tastes and just about the right amount of food. Otherwise I cook dinner most nights of the week – pretty much from scratch. It's a value to me to provide my husband and 11-year-old daughter with healthy meals. I want my daughter to grow up learning how to cook and how to eat healthy.

The other half of the equation is being physically active. I believe at my size and getting older by the day, being physically active is my only fighting chance to keep my weight where I want it and be able to eat more than a small amount of food. My husband and I are out four to five mornings a week, including chilly winter and hot summer mornings, at 6:00 a.m., walking about two miles. This year I also joined a gym. I'm managing to make it there about twice weekly for additional aerobic workouts and weight machine training.

I well recognize that as I age, to keep my weight where I want it I need to continue to keep up my routine, and perhaps escalate it. What keeps me going? Knowing that I feel better everyday and the hope of staying healthy for years to come.

Hope Warshaw, MMSc, RD, CDE
Author of Diabetes Meal Planning Made Easy, 3rd ed. (2006)
and Eat Out, Eat Right, 3rd ed (2008)

Changing Gears: My "Light Bulb Moment"

At age 34, I was running a small insurance office, but I felt like I was spinning my wheels—not looking forward to work at all, just tooling along the highway, barely keeping up with the traffic. I was paying my bills, but I was just going through the motions, and felt stuck, unproductive and restless.

Every kid has seen a cartoon character suddenly have a "light bulb moment," when the character sees something—or perhaps reads a posted sign. The head jerks up, the eyes open wide, and *Eureka!* They *do* something different. Something they saw or something they read made them react pretty dramatically.

Well...I had a light bulb moment when I read a book called *What Color Is Your Parachute*[1]. Of course, light bulbs don't go off all by themselves. In fact, there needed to be a lot of infrastructure in place so that reading the book could generate electricity to power that light bulb. But, my success in changing my lifestyle was responsible for my changing my career.

Looking back, I think that because I had taken the risk to change my lifestyle and was happy with my diet and my activity, I felt encouraged to change my life. I give credit to the daily lifestyle habits that by then had become *second nature* for giving me the strength to make a decision that changed my life.

As before, when I changed my habits to lose weight, I was trying to proceed from contemplation to preparation—the stage I needed to accomplish before I could progress to the action stage. I was constantly thinking about how little enthusiasm I had for my job (contemplation) but I hadn't taken any steps (preparation) toward a new career. *What Color is Your Parachute* suggested that I take a look at what I enjoyed doing in my free time—what were my favorite books, my hobbies, my interests? I had to overcome my beliefs, especially the one my father had instilled in me—he always said that only fools make careers out of hobbies. But, I decided to try anyway.

My interests—that was easy. I subscribed to healthy eating and women's fitness magazines, I went to the gym, and I rode my bike. I enjoyed modifying recipes—lowering calories by cutting fat and sugar, making them tastier by increasing spices and flavors. So, I went back to school to become a registered dietitian. I identified a new career, and set out to learn what I needed to do to accomplish my goals. Lucky for me, Queens College was just up the road from my office, and I could work while attending classes, eventually earning my degree.

I wanted to be more involved in promoting smart living, better eating, and supporting people's attempts to overcome overeating. *The Nutrition Action Healthletter,* published by the Center for Science in the Public Interest advocates for truth in advertising, for food safety and portion sensibility, and their research and writing is inspirational. Many food manufacturers shamelessly promote processed foods as if they are healthful—remember the oat bran craze of the early '80s when manufacturers put oat bran in potato chips and beer? As if those foods were suddenly "healthy" because they had fiber. Beer is beer—enjoy the brew, but oat bran doesn't change the alcohol content. Potato chips may have a gram of fiber, but as long as they are deep-fried and loaded with salt—they're still chips! Billions of dollars are spent promoting unhealthy foods, but few are spent promoting and teaching about healthy lifestyles and making good nutrition choices. CSPI's edgy articles influenced my career goals.

CSPI is now working to[2]:

- Get junk foods out of schools nationwide;

- Rid the food supply of partially hydrogenated oil, the source of artificial trans fat that promotes heart disease;

- Reduce sodium in processed and restaurant foods;

- Improve food safety laws and reduce the incidence of foodborne illness;

- Advocate for more healthy, plant-based, environmentally-friendly diets;

- Ensure accurate and honest labeling on food packages;

- Require basic nutrition labeling on chain-restaurants' menus and menu boards;

- Provide responsible information about the benefits and risks of agricultural biotechnology;

- Obtain greater federal funding for alcohol-abuse prevention policies; and

- Expose industry influence over the scientific process and in government policy-making (Center for Science in the Public Interest).

Dreams and Goals

What other changes have you made in your life? You may be motivated internally, but motivation can also be external. Maybe your husband or wife or your partner is urging you to get healthy; maybe they are worried about you. Their concern may motivate you to change because you want them to be proud of you. If you have kids, maybe they are your motivation; you want to be a good role model so they stay healthy, too.

My dream—my goal—became more specific than the vague "I want to lose weight." I wanted to take control, to admire my control, and to love myself for taking control. My goals to accomplish my dream were specific and writing them down makes them real. For example:

- I want to control my desire to overeat—it's interfering with my self esteem!

- I want to eat good food when I'm hungry and stop when I'm full.

- By eating better, I will lose weight and be more attractive.

- I want to exercise every day; I want to be more muscular, have better arm definition, and lose the bloat.

- I want to stop bingeing when I feel tired or anxious.

All these goals supported my dream of being healthy—I wanted to develop the self-esteem that would come with caring about me. I wanted to deserve my own admiration. I wanted to be true to the best part of me...the part that cared about me.

Why do you want to lose weight? Just to lose it? Or do you want to change your eating habits because you're tired of being out of control?

No one can "give" you the motivation you need to make changes. But when you understand your motivators, you can bring them forward into the spotlight and call on what motivates you to keep you going throughout this process. Every time you pinpoint a motivating thought, such as "Walking makes me feel better," or "Eating more salad and less starch makes my jeans fit better," you'll be able to save it and add it to your arsenal of motivating mantras.

Motivation needs to be practiced daily or it disappears.

Overcoming Family History

Today, I'm within a 'normal' weight for my height, but when I was in college I weighed 20 pounds more. Both my parents have type 2 diabetes, and this and my extended family history of overweight and obesity means I am more at risk for getting diabetes—so I am mindful of my weight. I think my family history may be part of the reason I became a Registered Dietitian.

I am motivated by the fact that exercise reduces risk for diabetes significantly. For each one hour of brisk physical activity per day, you reduce your risk for diabetes by approximately 35 percent! So when I don't feel motivated to exercise, I remind myself of this positive statistic. Like so many people, I have a weakness for sweet foods. But I also know that excess weight increases risk for diabetes. So I have learned I am better off not buying or throwing away foods rather than eat what is going to harm me in the end. It is cheaper to throw it out than end up taking insulin or medication for diabetes.

Our environment works against us. I recently left a job that I felt was too stressful: the environment was unhealthy—the wrong foods everywhere. Wish I would have left it sooner. I've already lost six pounds since I left that job for the job I have now.

Everyone, no matter if they are thin or overweight, has to work on eating right every minute of everyday. No one is able to stay healthy without effort. Everyone has challenges—from lack of time to having to face down the wrong foods.

If your job is keeping you from being healthy then it is time to find a new job. If your attitude is keeping you from being healthy—then you need to find a new attitude.

Susan H RD,
Minneapolis, MN

From Motivation to Action:
Your Contract with Yourself

Weight loss can feel overwhelming, especially when you have a number in mind—a number that you haven't seen in a long time. You know that activity is the best predictor of weight loss and maintenance, but we all have incredible time challenges, and skipping it is mighty tempting sometimes. If you're working outside the home, you normally come home to your second "job"…taking care of your family. Worse, you may feel expected to work 50-hour-plus weeks or take home work from the office on weekends.

I'm motivated to stay healthy because I like the way I feel now, and I don't let myself forget that every day counts. Don't be scared that it won't happen. If you don't start, then you'll never succeed, and simply taking the first step indicates your willingness to give yourself a chance. Each day you continue is definitely a victory over your past, and a step toward a better future.

You may find that connecting to a spiritual side of yourself can provide inner strength and motivation to change bad habits. For example, Janie decided to join a church group that met each Saturday, and she'd use that time to remind herself that she was a part of a much larger community. As the weeks went by, she found that she didn't think so much about herself and started thinking that maybe she was overeating just to avoid feeling lonely.

Carolyn was another client of mine who found a way to add motivators to her arsenal. She realized that connecting a financial motivator to behavioral change really excited her. For each pound she lost, she donated 10 dollars to her local food bank budget. Sometimes finding motivation in giving back to the community can help you get to your goals and help others, too.

Motivation can come from something in your life that you want—a new job, a new bathing suit, or even a new partner. But ultimately, the motivation to change will come from within. Gather your motivators, write them down, but make room on your chart for more. Turn those negative motivators into positive ones and keep them with you. New motivators come up all the time.

Rose Tremain said, *Life is not a dress rehearsal.*

I like this quote because, to me, it emphasizes the need to make every day work for you. Although you may feel like little decisions don't matter, they do matter—both to you and to your family. Just like you really can't take a vacation from your family (they're always going to be with you), your goal is not to "go on" a diet, or to leave your life behind when you make the changes necessary for permanent weight loss. You bring your diet and the fun things you do to keep fit along with you. You can take an occasional detour; you can eat a rich dessert or sleep late once in a while. But this is *your* one and only life. Live it—fully and healthfully—right now.

Facing the Facts

It wasn't until I was in my 40's that I faced the fact that I needed to lose weight. I got on a scale only at my annual physical—I was always a little anxious beforehand. Although I exercised consistently three times as week, and ate mostly healthy foods, I also enjoyed my sweets—and was eating them daily.

I gradually picked up 15 pounds between ages 30 and 45. At my highest weight I decided to lose weight for the first time in my life. I did it the way I tell my patients to do it—I increased my exercise to five or six days a week, and added variety— different activities to my usual three-times weekly. I limited my "extra" calories (sweets, chips, etc) to a maximum 100 a day—this worked to cut my calories without eliminating my favorite foods. I paid closer attention to my hunger level at meals and stopped eating at the point of satisfaction. I drank more water. My husband had similar goals at the same time so we motivated each other to keep going. I weighed myself frequently and while I realized it was normal to bounce around a few pounds it motivated me to keep going as I saw a downward trend. It took about eight months to lose the weight and I feel very good. I still weigh myself almost daily to make sure I maintain my loss. I look and feel much better about myself being a little lighter.

Marcia Pell, RD, LD/N
Panama City, FL

Getting Un-Stuck

Use your excuses to identify paths to change. Maybe you feel "stuck," unable to even get started. I know…I was there. I used excuses every day, in the scripts that played over and over in my head. Every day, I woke up thinking, "This is the day that everything will suddenly change, and I'll be strong, happy and thin." I was waiting for a magic wand to pass over me, and I'd suddenly have a clear path toward thinness.

I imagined I would go out to my favorite restaurant, and my eyes would amazingly skip right over the burgers and fries—I would magically choose grilled chicken and steamed vegetables. Then, I'd skip over to the gym and workout for two hours. Hah! It didn't happen. Without a plan, wishes were just that—wishes. I didn't identify resources, so I couldn't execute plans, which made me more frustrated, angry, and unhappy—so I'd eat. I was uncomfortable, so I ate more. Of course, I didn't lose any weight; I gradually and consistently packed on more pounds.

If, at this moment, you feel resigned to always being out of shape, take a deep breath, and begin challenging yourself.

Make Your Excuses Your Challenges: Do you recognize any of these common excuses for avoiding change?

Peer Pressure

Have you ever heard anyone say, "He (or she) made me eat it"? Think of the time your friends all got together for pizza and it worked out to three pieces per person. You felt uncomfortable not eating that third piece—everyone else had three. Or the time you were with Alice and Dave, and they insisted on stopping at the barbeque joint. It wasn't what you wanted, but you wound up eating what everyone else was eating—big meat sandwiches and fries—way more than you'd planned. Peer pressure is kind of safe, in a way—after all, it takes the pressure off of you to make healthy choices, and you can relax—someone else made the decision. Well, no one can put that fork in your hand and make you chew and swallow. It's your choice—you can say, "No," to food you don't want to eat and, "Yes," to what you choose to eat. Make the choice that's best for you. Make it nicely, make it firmly, and make it consistently.

Eating For Two Means More of You

Eating for "two" or for you? Some women use pregnancy as an excuse to eat all they want but never get back to their pre-pregnancy weight. Experts warn that women are gaining too much weight during their pregnancy and not losing that weight, putting moms at risk for a lifetime of illness[3].

Obese moms are more at risk for gestational diabetes, preeclampsia, Caesarean section, and post-partum infection; they're more likely to give birth to a child more at risk for metabolic syndrome with an increased risk for type 2 diabetes and heart disease[4].

Breastfeeding provides both short- and long-term benefits for both women and babies, and although babies do grow up healthy if they are exclusively bottle-fed, there are health and psychological benefits from breastfeeding. For babies, the benefits of breast milk include increased immunity and lowered risk for infection. And babies who are breastfed have a lower rate of childhood and even adult obesity. For moms, health benefits include reduced risk for breast and other types of cancers and osteoporosis, and an earlier return to pre-pregnancy weight.

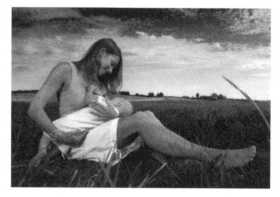

Permission to Eat

What if your doctor doesn't talk to you about your weight, even though you know you should make changes? As a new dietitian working in a cardiac hospital, I counseled patients at their bedside, often (too soon) after open heart surgery. One patient, "Myra," was pretty regretful that she hadn't taken care of herself—most people are totally unprepared for the shock and pain that follows cardiac procedures.

She said, tearfully, "I wish I'd listened to my doctor 20 years ago when he told me to lose weight...I can't believe I'm here!" Suddenly, from across the room, her surgeon called out, "Don't worry! You can eat anything you want now!" Poor Myra—when the "man in charge" gives you permission to eat, it's up to you to make the change; you won't get any support from him. Although it's never too late to make changes, making them now—when you're young enough to avoid complications—is a much better idea than waiting until you end up in the hospital. Maintaining activity helps you stay young and vital.

Food as Love: What Happens In Relationships

In your romantic relationships, do you try to impress your partner or spouse with your domestic skills? In the attempt to duplicate complicated (and fattening) recipes, the weight comes on—for both partners. Lovebirds indulge in decadent desserts, finding pleasure in seeking out and providing favorite foods for each other. Dining out becomes more frequent, and every birthday and anniversary is an excuse for celebratory foods. Family pressures can be intense—maybe you're dealing with the in-laws who won't take "no thanks" for an answer. You feel guilty if you decline Aunt Bea's apple pie that she made "just for you." You can't refuse Uncle Henry's banana daiquiri for fear of offending. On the other hand, once married, maybe you feel that the pressure is "off," that you've captured your mate, and now you can relax and enjoy your life, instead of worrying about how you look all the time. I've seen many women—and men—who diet like mad to get into a size six wedding dress or sleek tuxedo, but when you see them a few months later, they've obviously reverted to old habits and regained more weight than they lost. The day they walked down the aisle was the last day they paid attention to what they were eating.

My Family Refuses to Cooperate

If you and your family are used to eating lots of junk, you're right on track with the rest of the country, consuming huge quantities of manufactured foods daily. Food manufacturers and media conglomerates seem to have precious little conscience when it comes to pushing junk food, and billions are spent yearly just to get people to overindulge. But if you and your family regularly walk, jog, bike, or skate, you'll be up to the challenge. Change yourself first—and lead the way. When the ship is sinking, the captain has to take charge. Strategize your life first, then your family's. Yes, it's easier when you're all on the same page, but someone has to start. You're it! This is where the going can get very tough. Here's where tough love pays off.

My Family Sabotages Me

Why does it seem that sometimes the people who love you the most can be your biggest obstacles to change? "Jill's" husband seemed to love her too much. She said, "I don't get it. "Bill" was all gung-ho when I told him that I was going on a diet. He even said he was going to work on his diet too, and no doubt, his love handles were getting a little too generous to hold. He promised that we'd both go shopping for new bathing suits as soon as we lost 20 pounds. But can you believe it?! The very next day he came home two gallons of ice cream—my favorite, and a gallon of his favorite, too! When I got angry with him, he got really defensive. What gives?"

Oh, he certainly tested Jill's resolve. Poor Jill was left feeling lonely and insecure— doesn't he love her enough to help her? Why would he deliberately try and trip her up? This is all too common between couples. Either one partner or the other may demonstrate that *they* are not ready to change—they may be unwilling or even unable at the moment to take action, and they'll quietly demonstrate their reluctance by bringing home treats and suddenly wanting to eat out more often than usual.

Say you decide to join a gym and start getting up early to get there before work. Is your partner, husband or wife supportive? Do they ever say, "Hey honey, I'll come with you"? If you say, "Let's take a walk after dinner tonight," do they say, "Sure dear, I'll put my boots on—don't forget your scarf because it's cold tonight"? Or do you just hear silence—no feedback. So you ask directly, "Want to go for a walk?" They say no—it's too cold outside. What do you do? Do you sit down on the couch and feel depressed about not getting the support you need?

Maybe your partner is insecure and afraid that you'll be too attractive to others, or it could be that they're just lazy. Or maybe they just don't feel like going and don't have the motivation—and they could be envious that you have the motivation and will power to make the hard changes. It's much easier to stay on the couch; it's so easy to indulge in ice cream nightly. Let's give them the benefit of the doubt. It just may be they don't want to see you struggle with feeling deprived. But ultimately, it is your choice.

It is **very important** to identify what you can change and what you cannot change. You can only change you, and you can demonstrate your commitment to your change by telling your partner your intentions, or you can just demonstrate them if you think your partner is uncomfortable with your activities and diet. I adopted this mental "script" to think about food and activity. No one can make you eat it; it's your choice to eat it—or you can skip it. No one can put your shoes on and walk you out the door and down the street. It's up to you. One footstep at a time, one bite at a time, one day at a time.

Whether your partner or your family is enthusiastic or not, listen politely, and gently but firmly take control. When you have a goal, it's a great idea to communicate it. Tell your family what you're doing and why you're doing it. You can list the reasons why—you want to be stronger; you want to be trimmer and have more muscle and get rid of excess fat; you want more energy; you want to sleep better; you want to live longer; and you don't want to have to take medications for diseases that are related to being overweight. Your changes are for positive reasons, and the changes you make and the strategies you'll use to keep yourself on track can be incorporated by everyone in your family.

I Have No Time

I read in the paper about a senior mom who took up running at age 60. Until then, her idea of exercise was shopping in the mall. She was overweight and had recently been diagnosed with high blood pressure. She half-expected this, because both her parents had high blood pressure and they were overweight until just before they died; her father age 63, her mother at age 71. When her doctor said, "Now *you* need to lose weight," she was scared and determined to get healthy. But unlike so many people who go from the doctor's office right to the pharmacy for pills, she went from the doctor's office to the sneaker store and started walking. For a while, her husband accompanied her, but she quickly got bored with walking and soon began to race-walk; then she started jogging. Her husband had to find another walking partner because this determined lady joined a running club, and today she gets up at 5:30 a.m. almost every morning for an hour of cardio and weight training. She says it's not a problem waking up early, because ever since she started exercising, her energy and mood are much improved. And this is how I did it too; I got up earlier. I find that if I wait until after work, I find excuses to put off exercise until tomorrow. So, you're not a morning person? That is fine, as long as you do it. Schedule your activity as you would your job: you need to find time during the working day or after dinner. Use your lunch time or a treadmill or stepper at home while you watch television.

I Can't Do It Alone

Aerobics and step classes are a lot of fun, and running and biking clubs are challenging and social. For me, I like to get out in the morning for my "quiet time" with myself. Sometimes it's easier to do it alone rather than rely on someone else to do it with you, in terms of strategizing your time. The problem with relying on someone else is that it's too easy to take up another person's excuses. If you're scheduled to walk with your neighbor and she cancels, does that mean you don't go? No! Always have "Plan B" in mind, and get your exercise regardless.

It Costs Too Much To Be Fit

If you're inclined to join a gym, that's great—it got me started on my road to naturally thin. Gyms have a variety of equipment, and I like them because they offer a structure for my routine. I go around a "circuit" of weight machines, free weights, and bench work in order to work different parts of my body. Gyms also offer a variety of classes, and if they are at times that are convenient for you, that is great. A locker room and shower—wow. I used to workout before going to the office, and I have friends who go after work. A gym is a great destination—it's social and structured. But I know many people who never set foot in a gym and are incredibly fit and active—it's not necessary to join a gym, but it's a great strategy for jump-starting a fitness routine.

On the other hand, I had a friend who decided that he was going to get fit and invested in a roomful of high-quality gym equipment—benches, barbells, weights, and a treadmill. He spent thousands of dollars, and for a few months, he worked out daily and got really fit. But he sold it all and joined a local gym. He decided that he was too lonely at home alone and was happier with the camaraderie and motivation he found at the gym.

There are lots of things you can do to be active; they don't need to be structured, just consistent. My friend "Deborah" has a routine that's simple, but effective. She gets up about 30 minutes before her kids, puts on her IPod, and jumps rope in her garage. Her kids get up, do jumping jacks and sit-ups to their favorite tunes in the living room for 15 minutes, and then eat a quick breakfast of cereal and milk and bananas before going to school.

You don't need the gym to get started. Tailor your activity to your lifestyle and budget. Fitness experts recommend walking as an ideal starting point since it only requires a well-fitted pair of walking shoes or sneakers, and measure your route by driving it first—gradually increasing the effort by shaving minutes off your time. (A pedometer is an inexpensive and effective tool you can use to measure your progress and create an incentive toward a goal. See Chapter 8, Simple Steps to Natural Fitness)

If you don't have the money to join a gym you may be able to workout at a local school, YMCA, or purchase day passes for the local hotel's fitness facility. You may be able to barter for a membership or passes. Many gyms have different membership levels. You may be able to buy a series of visits instead of a full membership—and if you determine that works better for you, that's ideal.

1. Take out a pad and pen to figure out how to afford your gym membership. Draw three columns on a sheet of paper. Title the left column "Pay to Play," the middle column "Payment Weekly," and the right column "Replay."

2. In the "Pay to Play" column, list all the "extras" you pay for weekly. Go out to dinner? Buy daily snacks in vending machines? Write down what you spend per item. How many times a week to you buy coffee? Once? Twice? Daily? Are you buying tea, or other take-away drinks daily? Total them up—you may be spending up to $50 more, every week! Total all your expenditures on incidental food and drinks for the week, and then multiply it by four. Compare that figure to the cost of a monthly gym membership. I bet you could take the difference and buy a new pair of high-test sneakers! Don't stop at food and drinks. Other extras may be weekly manicures, or maybe you pay someone to wash your car or your dog.

3. In the "Replay" column, write what you could do instead of paying for all those extras.

4. Total all your expenditures on the left column and compare to the total monthly amount you need to pay to belong to the fitness center closest to your house.

I gave up my "premium" cable television membership and used the dollars to pay for my gym membership. It works out about the same (around $40 per month). My neighbor really wanted to start taking Pilates (a method of exercise and physical movement designed to stretch, strengthen, and balance the body). She found that instead of buying a membership to the expensive gym, she could take out free Pilates DVDs from the local library, and now she does Pilates at home for 45 minutes, three times a week.

My Gym Membership: Approximately $40 per month		
PAY TO PLAY	PAYMENT WEEKLY	REPLAY
Starbucks large latte coffee: on the way to work: Monday through Friday	$4.00 DAILY = $20.00	Bring coffee from home in go cup
Mid-afternoon vending machine snack or soda: Monday through Friday	$5.00	Bring snacks: peanuts in shell; baby carrots; cup of yogurt; diet soda
Lunch at Subway on Tuesday	$6.50	Bring your own sub: scoop out whole wheat sub and stuff with turkey breast and spouts; mustard and club soda
Lunch: take out Chinese on Thursday	$4.75	Bring plastic tub of tuna, chopped celery, and carrots: Save $$$: take a walk
Popcorn at movies on Saturday	$4.50	Movie popcorn is made with trans fat—skip it
Buy a bottled water from the vending machine: Monday through Friday	$5.00	Most bottled water is just filtered tap water: use home refrigerator filter and bring your own
Drinks after work with the girls on Thursday (1 Cosmo plus tax and tip)	$12.00	Instead of top shelf cocktail, order glass of wine or light beer
TOTAL	$57.75 per week or **$231 per month!**	Save $$$$!

I Don't Know How to Exercise

Perhaps you are intimidated by the word "exercise" and think it means "no pain, no gain" or some other such myth. But as long as you can put one foot in front of the other, you are moving toward your second nature. Exercise just means moving, getting your heart rate up (exerting yourself) and keeping it there for at least 20 minutes. It doesn't matter how you do it—you can jog, climb stairs, or you can dance around the house! You can skate, bike, or just walk fast. You just have to do it, and do it every day—just like you would check the mail, take out the garbage, or even kiss your sweetie goodnight. It's a good habit to get into. Don't be intimidated by the word "exercise"...just think of it as "activity."

Good Food/Bad Food

When people think about diets, they think they'll have to eat only "good" foods and give up their favorite "bad" foods. I hate when people attach human attributes to food—it sets them up for feeling so confused! After all, if you only like "bad" foods, does that make you a bad person? And if you're a bad person, then you don't deserve to be thin, right? So you may as well just keep eating!

Turn it around and say farewell to that type of thinking.

Instead of thinking that you have to eat that cake or finish everything on your plate, you can choose what to eat—and what to leave. You have the power to choose, and choice is a powerful thing. Food can't jump off the plate and into your mouth. You can't blame food for making you fat. You must pick food up off the plate (with a fork or with your fingers) and put it into your mouth, then chew and swallow it. We're made to enjoy food. We have taste buds that are sensitive to different tastes and flavors, and just as people living in Alaska get used to the cold and people living in Florida become accustomed to high temperatures and humidity, taste buds become accustomed to different tastes and textures. If you only eat salty, fatty and sweet foods, then you'll always expect those flavors. My breakfast habit was pretty strong—that bran muffin was sweet and fatty, and I grew to expect those tastes. It took a while, but I gradually re-trained my taste buds to enjoy the taste of fresh foods—unsweetened cereals and naturally sweet fruit. Now if I eat something that's coated with fat or loaded with sugar or overly salted, that's what I taste first. You can do the same—re-train to taste.

Food Is My Only Friend

I used food as a "friend" to deal with loneliness, anxiety, and even anger. I buried my emotions with food, and then the guilt set in. "Why did I eat that?" was a constant reminder that I was out of control. It's a hard habit to break, and it's cyclical. I felt bad, so I ate foods that made me feel better (my comfort foods), but overeating made me feel worse. Overeating can be both physiologically and psychologically addicting. Food may have a chemical effect on your psyche—stimulating the release of calming hormones—but the act of overeating also distracts you from the problems at hand. Food can be fun, and even fattening foods, high calorie treats, or special occasion foods are fine in the right portions at the right time. But food can't be a substitute for dealing with a problem that's keeping you anxious or stressed.

I'm Tired of Trying

"Jean" came into my office, sat down, and started to cry.

She said, "I can't do it—I've tried and tried, and it's too hard to follow a diet, and I'm sick of trying." I asked her to help me understand what she was feeling, and she talked to me for a long time about why she was so unhappy about being overweight and feeling out of control. I reassured her that she didn't have to lose all the weight in one week to be successful, and we identified some times of the day and evening that were most difficult for her. Evenings were the worst—she said that her habit was to sit down in front of the television after dinner, and after the second commercial, she'd have to get something to eat—usually a big bowl of ice cream. We also talked about when she felt good about herself. I asked her to identify two things that she felt were important to change—one food thing and one activity thing. For the first two weeks, she changed just those two behaviors. She stopped drinking a big glass of orange juice every morning; instead, she drank a big glass of water and a 4-ounce glass of orange juice—about half the size she was previously drank. She agreed to make the juice fresh every morning, and by doing this, she realized it took almost three oranges—much more than she realized. During her television viewing, she also changed from ice cream to sugar-free hot chocolate and an apple, sliced thin. And she added activity. She walked every day before she went to work for at least 14 minutes. Sometimes she walked at home, but most days she walked in the parking lot before she went into the building, and if the weather was good, she also walked at lunch. That's how it started. Every day that she prioritized her small changes, she felt better about herself. She began to ask me to help her make more small changes, and that's how it gets better and better. Change happens one day at a time. Every day is an opportunity to make stronger action verbs a part of your life. Instead of "trying," it becomes the process of doing.

Fat is in My Genes

If your parents were fat, are you doomed to be fat, too? If you have accepted that sentence, then have you also accepted that your children are destined for a lifetime of fatness and a shorter lifespan? Don't accept "genes" as an excuse for being overweight— you need to fight. Yes, a very small number of people have higher resting metabolic rates and may be able to eat more than the average person without gaining weight. But even if you have a medical diagnosis, a condition that makes it harder for you to maintain a healthy weight, don't give in. Even if you've inherited a tendency to be overweight, it doesn't mean that it's your destiny. It is your destiny to take control, be trimmer, and be healthier. By building lean muscle and changing your body type, you allow your body to work for you instead of against you. I do not look like my parents; I developed my muscles by exercising consistently and eating a diet that nourished my efforts. My second nature is my second chance.

Priorities

What's your priority? A big burger and fries, or avoiding disease? How many times have I heard a person say, "Yes, my blood pressure is under control...with medication." Or, "My cholesterol is within normal range...with medication." If you are over-*fat*, losing just five to 15 percent of your body weight can often bring your readings down to a level that's manageable without medication. Treating the symptoms doesn't eliminate the problem and may actually create secondary problems. For example, overweight is the most common cause of knee and hip pain, leading to chronic overuse of NSAIDs (non-steroidal anti-inflammatory drugs), such as ibuprofen and aspirin. This can cause stomach problems, such as bleeding ulcers.

Is your goal just a number on the scale? Are you dreaming of a number instead of a new lifestyle? Or is your goal to reduce your weight by permanently losing excess body fat? Is your goal to lose 20 pounds? Or is your goal to lose and maintain 25 pounds? Twenty five pounds sounds like a huge challenge, but most people won't settle for a smaller goal—they want it all gone, like magic. Set smaller, achievable goals and set up a personal rewards system. That way, you motivate yourself to keep going. I have achieved permanent fat loss and monitor my weight by using a scale and, more often, putting on a favorite pair of jeans. I've maintained my weight for more than 25 years by making permanent the habits I practiced while losing the excess fat.

What Can a Type 2 Do?

Although there is a genetic link to insulin resistance (about one in four people have a gene that increases risk), how you choose to live your life may increase—or lower your chances of getting type 2 diabetes.

- Be more sensitive. Make your body more sensitive to the insulin you do produce by changing your diet and lifestyle. Make your body work for you...treat your body with respect to get it to work more efficiently.

- Set a goal of five percent: Reducing your current weight by just five to 10 percent can improve your insulin sensitivity.

- Write down your personal goals for losing weight and increasing activity: Some include staying healthy to avoid complications; feeling more energetic; fitting into your clothes better...write them down and post them on your bathroom mirror, so you can see them every morning.

1. This week, choose one thing that you can change...permanently. Don't be overwhelmed by trying to do too much all at once: Each week, just choose ONE:

    a. I will change from whole milk to 2% milk (or from 2% to 1% or nonfat milk)

    b. I will change from a sugary cereal to one with no sugar added

    c. I will stop eating french fries with my burger

2. Set an activity goal for the week:

    a. This week I will walk for 10 minutes three mornings

    b. This week I will take 20 minutes to eat my lunch, and spend the rest of the time walking.

    c. This week I will take an extra 20 minute walk on Saturday and Sunday

3. Monitor: Frequent blood sugar monitoring helps you understand how your food and exercise are affecting your progress. Graph your readings so that you can easily determine where you may need extra help.

Your Motivational Arsenal

Let's get to work on your own motivation arsenal. Avoid negative motivators, such as "I better get into shape or else my husband will leave me," and employ positive ones, such as "I will get into shape, so that I **feel** more attractive and strong."

Write your positive motivators down on Post-It notes and put them up on your mirror in the bathroom, your car, and wherever they can do you the most good. Think frequently about your reasons to change, and stay positive. Put a checkmark next to all the motivations that apply to you.

Re-write your excuses and make them "uses."

Re-Write Your Excuses	Turn Them into Thin Behaviors
I didn't have time to shop this week.	I shop once a week and use a list—it makes shopping much easier and quicker, and I'm not tempted to buy stuff that isn't on my list!
I don't like to exercise—and don't have time.	I found activities that I like to do! I put my treadmill in front of the television so that I can watch my favorite program and exercise, too.
I'm expected to serve all those fattening favorites at my holiday dinner.	I've learned new recipes! They're delicious, and I feel great that I can eat healthier food and still enjoy the party.
I always eat terribly when I'm traveling.	I've gotten into the habit of packing a container of dry cereal and fruit so I never have to eat that junk at the airport!
I just can't give up my favorite fried food—it means too much to me!	Nothing tastes as good as fitting into my favorite jeans naturally, without having to go on a diet—I have lost my taste for foods that make me fat.

- **Appearance:** If you're like most people, you'll say, "I want to look better." Think specific—for example, "I want my arms to be firmer; I want to lose one inch from my waist in one month." Maybe you want to fit into your favorite jeans...the ones you put in the back of the closet, thinking that someday, maybe by magic, you'll be thin enough to fit into again. It's not all about the size of the jeans, any more than your weight should be an ultimate measure of your success. Each manufacturer makes their clothes differently, and what you're after is liking what you see in the mirror. By the way, don't even think about looking like one of those models in the magazines! They're usually 15 years old and air-brushed. Motivators that work best include becoming fit, firm, trim, and toned. These are much more positive than boney, frail, or waiflike!

- **Health:** Overweight is linked to some important health issues, and if you're overweight and have a family history of type 2 diabetes, high cholesterol, or high blood pressure, your risk for these diseases increases. Lose just five to 10 percent of your weight, and these conditions usually improve.

◆ Type 2 diabetes: Linked to being overweight or obese, you're 80 percent more likely to have type 2 diabetes if you're overweight and have a family history. You pass the risk on to your kids, which can be a motivator for you to get to your healthy weight now. For people with diabetes, keeping blood sugar within a normal range means balancing food, sometimes medications, and activity, and learning what's right for you means working closely with your physician and diabetes expert—such as a certified diabetes educator—to gain control. Does being overweight cause type 2 diabetes, or does type 2 diabetes contribute to being overweight? The answer may be a little of both. Overweight decreases cell insulin-sensitivity, and, since increased insulin sensitivity enhances the body's ability to store excess glucose as fat, some medications prescribed for type 2 diabetes promote weight gain. So, a lifestyle change incorporating a healthy diet and exercise is just what the doctor ordered for better blood glucose and weight control—it's especially important for people with type 2 diabetes.

◆ Heart Disease, high blood cholesterol: The Weight-control Information Network of the National Institute of Diabetes and Digestive and Kidney Diseases (http://win.niddk.nih.gov) notes that overweight increases risk for high blood pressure and high blood lipid levels—including high triglycerides and LDL cholesterol (the "bad cholesterol") and lower levels of HDL cholesterol (the "good cholesterol"). These are all risk factors for heart disease and stroke. People with more body fat are likely to have higher blood levels of substances that cause inflammation, which increases heart disease risk.

◆ Hypertension (HTN): According to the National Heart, Lung and Blood Institute (NHLBI), high blood pressure is "blood pressure equal to or greater than 140/90," but greater than 120/80 indicates pre-hypertension. Overweight and obesity considerably increase your risk for hypertension. Overweight with a family history of hypertension plus being a member of an ethnic minority (African, Hispanic, Native, or Asian American) vastly increases the risk. High blood pressure increases risk for stroke and diabetes, and because it's largely symptom-less, the first sign could be a stroke, even death.

◆ Arthritis: When you're overweight, it's more likely that you're damaging your joints and tendons. This can mean a "Catch-22," a vicious cycle in which it's harder for you to exercise, which makes it harder to control your weight, which makes it likely to worsen your arthritis. Your joints and tendons are made to carry a healthy, normal weight body, not a lot of excess weight. Overweight kids can suffer permanent bone and tendon damage.

◆ Overweight increases risk for breast, kidney, colon and esophageal cancer, gout, gastric reflux disease, and sleep apnea.

• **Mood:** Are you blue? If you think your weight and your low mood are related, you may be right. Studies show that overweight people may be discriminated against by employers, have less education, and make less money compared to normal weight people. Compared to normal weight kids, overweight kids are more depressed, have more trouble in school, get passed over for team selection, and may even be discriminated against by teachers.

- **Pride:** The act of changing is motivating. I found an amazing satisfaction and sense of accomplishment the first time I used the step machine for 30 minutes without stopping—and without leaning. Then, I felt so great when I was able to wear a pair of shorts without feeling like I wanted to hide. It grows—it gets better and stronger.

- **Financial:** If you eat out often, you're spending a lot of money! Cut back, put the money into your lifestyle—for example, invest in a gym membership or fitness equipment—and keep the weight off permanently.

What are your motivators? Maybe you want to look better, feel stronger, be more professional, run a marathon, or join a gym! Write them down.

YOUR MOTIVATORS	FIRST STEPS TO MAKE IT HAPPEN

I Like the Way I Look and I Feel!

Numerous times I have encountered people who seem to think I'm naturally thin, when in fact I work on my weight every day of my life. For instance, I recall mentioning to one of my obese patients that I had gone for a run the night before and she said something like, "But why? You don't need to do that." It never occurred to her that I looked the way I did because I exercise five days a week for more than an hour, and have done so for many years! When I was younger, it was more of a chore, but now it's just part of me.

Overweight is in my family, and I know I have to work hard to stay within my "comfort zone," about seven pounds is my limit. Because of my profession and my vanity, perhaps, I just never allowed those genes to express themselves. As soon as my weight goes out of that comfort zone, I do things like keep a food diary; step up my exercise; and pay more attention to portion sizes. Of course, this is exactly what people who lose weight and keep it off do. This is what I found to be true when I was writing about the "masters of weight control" in my Thin for Life book, and what the National Weight Control Registry has found—successful weight maintainers immediately reverse small weight gains.

How do I stay motivated? Honestly, a lot of it is vanity—I like the way I look and feel at this weight. When I'm tempted to overeat, I sometimes ask myself, "What do I want more—immediate gratification, or to feel good about my weight? I also really like the way exercise makes me feel. I don't always like doing it, but I feel great afterward, and exercise affords me daily treats, which I love.

Finally, I'm motivated by knowledge that as I get older, I have some health problems that will become much worse if I gain weight. I fully intend to live into my 90s or beyond!

Anne M. Fletcher, MS, RD, LD
Author, the Thin for Life books,
Weight Loss Confidential, and
Sober for Good (Houghton Mifflin Co.)

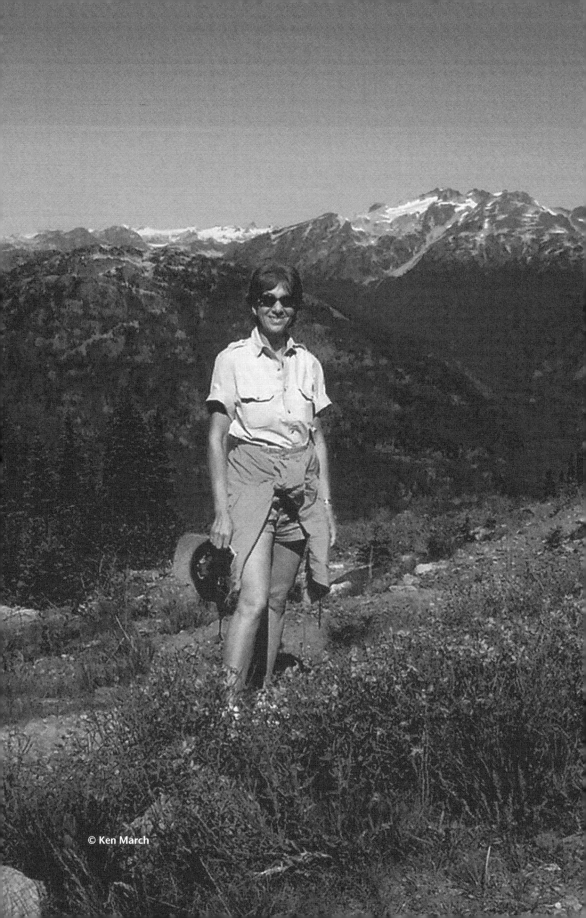

Chapter 5

Keep Moving the Goal Post
Why Change is a Naturally Good Thing

*What you get by achieving your goals is not as important
as what you become by achieving your goals.*
—Zig Ziglar

Wait a minute—you think, "I've gotten this far in the book, of course I'm ready to lose the weight." Well...not so fast.

Set Goals!

Have you ever set a goal? I hadn't. Oh, I'd wished and hoped for something to happen, and I'd lost a few pounds—the same few pounds, over and over—but I'd never *really* set a goal for change. But setting goals, writing them down, talking about them, and thinking about them were critical components of my taking control.

I remember when I signed up for the weight loss program, the program that finally got through to me, all those many years ago. Unlike the many, many times before, the times I had gone on a diet, this time I was asked to write down my usual diet and my usual habits. OK, I thought—although I really didn't want to do it. I wanted a diet, remember? I wanted to lose weight without changing my behaviors.

DEFINITION

Goal
—noun

1. The purpose toward which an endeavor is directed; an objective.

Intention
—noun

1. An act or instance of determining mentally upon some action or result.

2. The end or object intended; purpose.

The reason I kept coming back, week after week, was because this time was different. I was open to change; my counselor seemed really interested in me—not just my weight. She asked my permission to discuss the reason I was overweight to begin with. We didn't start at "a diet"—she asked me to identify what I was doing to keep the weight on. And she actually asked my permission to explore with her what I could reasonably expect from weight loss. Did I just want to lose pounds? Or did I want to look better? Did I expect my life to change just because I went on a diet, or did I expect that weight loss was a process? It was a revelation! And it prepared me for what I was about to undertake. A lifestyle change—not just a diet.

And although counseling professionals are urged to focus the session on the client, my counselor firmly but gently told me that what I was going through wasn't unique to me. She shared with me that she became a registered dietitian because she'd conquered overeating, and she was inspired to change careers and learn about nutrition, too. That was a "light bulb moment" for me. I was open to her suggestions and her support for my success.
That exercise—filling out a questionnaire and discussing my fears—began the process that moved me from preparation to action.

A Dietitian's Awareness-- 24/7

I can relate to your question about how other people perceive me, and have heard those "naturally thin" remarks. People assume you don't have to work at weight maintenance.

I operate in "awareness mode" 24/7. My techniques include exercise; jogging and or yoga most days of the week. I eat five to seven servings of fruits and veggies daily and I practice eating mindfully all day long. If I didn't do this, at 46 yrs, I most likely would not be able to maintain my weight of 135 lbs on my 5'6" frame.

This is not unique, most "thin" folks work at it. The good part is it has become a way of life, and so I'm not obsessed about what the scale says on any given day.

I also practice loving-kindness toward myself. I give myself lots of non-food rewards and I'm gentle with myself if my food choices are less than optimal. Yes, we all have those moments!

Sheila B. Clarke, RD, MBA, RYT
Healthier Way Nutrition Consulting Services
Riverside, CA

Preparation, I learned later, is the point at which I accepted that I had to change. And from there, I moved on to action. That's when I joined a program, got a plan and a shopping list, and got support. I joined that gym and scheduled time to go to the gym.

I stopped using the word "diet" as a verb. I stopped *being on a diet*. I began *to eat* to lose weight. This was a huge difference, a chasm of difference. From those first few sessions with my counselor, I learned—and accepted—that the weight loss program was only the first step toward weight maintenance.

I'd never thought of weight loss that way. Before, each time I "went on" a diet, I thought it would be the *last* time I had to diet. "Oh, no," she said, "you're not 'dieting,' remember? You're *eating!*"

I gradually accepted that the weight loss part of the program was only the preparation for maintenance. The eating plan for weight loss was to introduce me to the way I would be eating forevermore—never to return to my old way of eating. For the first time, I was asked to take responsibility for my own choices. Instead of following yet another diet with a list of foods to eat or not eat, this time it was up to me to identify my own areas for change. It was the first time I had taken such an active role in the process. Consequently, I wasn't following someone else's diet, I was making healthy changes within my own lifestyle.

It was the first time I had ever articulated a goal—but more importantly, I used a system that monitored my progress. I checked in regularly with my counselor for the first three months and then measured my progress. For the first time, I wasn't afraid of the scale because I knew that I was following a healthy eating program and working out. For the first six months at least, I weighed myself almost daily. I set activities goals for myself; as I lost weight, built muscle, and increased my endurance, I bought myself new clothes, and I eventually remade my career. I even returned to school to learn about nutrition. All these goals were interconnected, and I monitored my accomplishments.

Have you articulated your goal? Have you thought about what happens when you get there? I found that each time I reached a goal, I felt like setting another one. I first set a goal for five pounds of weight loss, and that took me about three weeks. Then I set a goal for another five pounds and started setting fitness and behavior goals, too. Each goal was small—it was attainable, and it fit into my lifestyle. For example, I set a goal to not automatically turn on the television when I got home from work; instead, I took a half-hour "de-compression" break. That small goal turned into a very important lifestyle changer. I found that I felt so much less anxious and stressed, and I felt healthier, too. If it was still light outside, or if the weather was fair, I'd go for a walk. If it was dark by the time I got home, I put in an exercise or yoga tape and, 30 minutes later, I felt energized and motivated to eat a healthy dinner.

Think:
Language:
Think of the language we use to describe weight loss diets. I used to say, *I'm going on a diet* or *I heard about a new diet that I want to try.* My old way of thinking meant that a diet would be a temporary change. Do you think this way? If going on a diet means you only follow it until you lose weight, and if you then return to the habits that made you overweight to begin with, you'll eventually regain the weight.

Think:
Future:
Evaluate how you think about the change. Can you accept that you're going to have to do things differently from now on?

Set a goal for the future

Don't set a goal to lose weight—if losing weight means you'll return to your old habits. You'll just return to your old weight.

I'd buy a new diet book—and might even follow the diet for a few days. But, soon, within a few days, I'd return to my 600-calorie bran muffin for breakfast, and that would knock me off my "diet" for good—until the next time. I wasn't prepared for permanent change.

This is a very important point that took me years to understand. For years, I just wished I could lose weight. I didn't translate my size 18 pants to my body storing all those excess calories as fat—it was strangely distant. I *wished* I could be thin, but stoked my fat cells by compulsively overeating.

Before beginning a new weight loss program, Stop—and think. *Am I "going on a diet" to lose weight, temporarily?*

Or are you prepared to say farewell to the past and to the habits that contributed to weight mismanagement. Habits are expressions of how you think about how you live.

Now, I wake up thinking how I need to live to love my life. Habits run my life—in a good way. I set a goal—*I set a goal—to lose excess fat and to not gain it back!*

Change is Good—Most of the Time!

The day you decide to do it is your lucky day.
Japanese Proverb

What we think determines what happens to us, so if we want to change our lives, we need to stretch our minds.
Wayne Dyer

If you are attempting to change and your family or friends aren't behind you, it can surely be discouraging. Maybe your husband says he likes you as you are, or your kids say, "Mommy, you get cranky when you diet." Maybe you and your best friend go on a diet at the same time, but you lose more than she does so she gives you the cold shoulder (it happened to me!). Maybe your husband goes out of his way to cook all the foods that you *shouldn't eat* because he resents that you're ready to change—and he isn't.

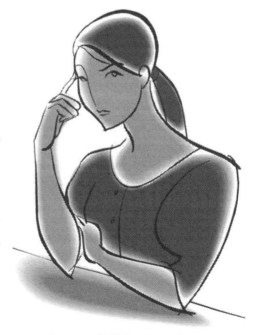

Stop-—and Think—About Change

What I Can Control

Ah…life can be complicated, and overweight is often a symptom of the difficulty you have dealing with issues in your life.

My overweight illustrated that I used food to try to lessen the anxiety I felt because I wasn't dealing well with many issues in my life.

Changing from out of control of your diet and your activity to in control of your diet and activity is excellent. And it can happen—one day at a time.

My mantra is the little saying, or script I have developed when I feel an urge to use food to relieve tension or anxiety. This is what I think—this helps me stay in control and reminds me to use other stress-reducers than food.

There is very little in my life over which I have control. Someone tells me what time I have to be at work—someone tells me when I can leave. Someone tells me what I have to wear. But no one can tell me what I have to eat—when I have to eat it—and how much I have to eat. I make the choice! And no one can tell me how much activity I can do daily—I can do as much or as little as I like. I can take control of my body—make it better and feel better—and do it daily. And I will!

Breaking the Cycle

When I was overweight and out of shape, unable to deal with anxiety, I was caught in the vicious cycle of feeling guilty about overeating, and then overeating because I was unhappy about being overweight.

My internal voice kept nagging at me, "You can do it, just do it, do it now!" But since I had no *plan* to change, just vague *wishes,* just about every Monday I went on a diet.

Each Sunday evening, I'd have the same internal conversation with myself: "I have no self-control; I'm bad; I need to lose twenty pounds. I'm going on a diet tomorrow." Maybe you have a similar dialogue with yourself.

Every Sunday I expected a miracle on Monday. So what happened? Nothing. While I beat myself up by thinking bad thoughts about myself, I neglected to do any planning or preparation for my Monday diet, other than to wake up expecting to instantly be twenty pounds lighter. I can tell you everything I was doing *wrong*—and it's no wonder there was no change.

- I didn't have a plan to change my bad habits.

- I didn't go through the pantry and refrigerator or freezer to get rid of tempting, fattening foods.

- I didn't call any friends to invite them to workout with me and didn't schedule walking or exercise for the next week.

- I didn't invest in any fun home exercise videos or equipment.

- I didn't see a dietitian. I didn't have a plan. Nope. I just had wishes—I wished for weight loss, and no surprise, it never happened.

And no surprise that by 3:00 p.m. on Monday afternoon, I usually found myself facing the office vending machine. Once I dropped the coins into the machine, all bets were off, and often the mental anguish that came from my internal conflict led to an eating binge that didn't stop until I went to bed that night.

This went on for years, and I remember feeling despondent, wondering why—even though I wanted to be thinner—I kept getting fatter.

- I wasn't facing the problems that were causing me anxiety.

- I didn't have a blueprint for what to do when I was tempted to use food to overcome anxiety.

- I didn't have a clear, visualized plan to create a lifestyle to reach a goal weight and maintain it.

- I had daydreamed about eating better and exercising, but didn't set specific goals.

- I had no way to measure my progress, and I never gave myself a realistic and usable plan of action.

- I didn't seek out professional help, didn't ask someone to help me devise a plan.

My Tipping Point

I had been in the **contemplation** *stage* for a long, long time. When I was 16 and beginning to use food to bury my feelings, even then I contemplated change. I wasn't clueless about my lack of control, and I didn't deny my responsibility for my actions, but thinking about what I needed to do to change—just "pre-contemplating" the change— actually made me feel worse for a long time. Although I was never resigned to being fat, it took years to get to *preparation.*

And looking back, I realize that even getting to *contemplation* was hard. Contemplating action and accepting that change would require sacrifices, well—I was afraid to even try. I was sure I would fail. Yes, I understood that I wanted to change—I'd even somewhat imagined doing things differently. I thought my life would be different—better—if I could stop bingeing, if I could BE different.

Contemplation meant imagining myself in different situations, how I would think when I went shopping for food or went out for dinner. This *other* Susan would buy fruits and vegetables and eat whole grains and lean meats—instead of boxes of crackers and fried foods. But I hadn't gotten to *preparation,* let alone *action.*

Nevertheless, I was building a foundation, because I was thinking about change. But because I didn't know about the stages of change when I was 40 pounds overweight, I didn't realize that I was on the right track. I had taken the first steps toward making changes, and accepted that I needed to change, but still, I can remember feeling nervous about it. And gradually I was getting closer, moving finally into contemplation and even tipping over into preparation—taking baby steps.

Once I got into the preparation stage, the planning and execution flowed much more easily than I had thought it would. Between preparation and *action* lay my commitment to investing time and energy into change.

For me, it was all about getting support. I learned that feeling that someone else was on my side helped me continue, and one day at a time, one step at a time, change happened. Success builds on itself, and each day that I ate a healthy breakfast—after I had walked or biked or jogged or MOVED for at least 30 minutes—was a day to build the rest of my life upon.

I invested in *me*. And I continue to bank my hours, and my habits, in my little personal investment account.

I believe that each person has an inner core of sensitivity, developing a point of view or creating a positive experience that they can draw on to help take control. For me, it was that first time I acted positively without thinking—I felt so amazed that I had taken that walk down the road that spring evening. It meant I had a future and could invest all my future experiences in myself in a positive way, leading to permanent change.

It's not always a straight line to the goal and once you are happy with your weight, it's important to never forget how you arrived there. Healthy weight maintenance means you may travel up and then down, right and then left. Life is like that, but remember, food is the fuel that keeps you going. While you're operating in an action phase, and being consistent about making healthy choices, look ahead toward your eventual progress toward the next stages—toward maintenance—and even an occasional lapse where you may regain. But you always make it back to your healthy weight, because it's *second nature* to be in control.

Notice—I didn't say "relapse". I think relapse is a harsh word—it almost sounds as if it means return! But, for me, there was no turning back. There was some regain, but not relapse into old habits—just a reminder that I needed to go back to what I'd learned *naturally* and redefine my goals again.

If you do it right, relapse will not be a return to where you started such a long time ago...it will just be a reminder to redefine your goals!

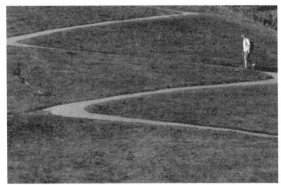

The path is not always a straight line to the goal. Stay with it—you'll get there

Daily Inspiration

It was a sunny Sunday morning, and I had finished my housework. I was riding my bike to the beach and up ahead spied my neighbor, "Linda," who was walking her dog.

Two things occurred to me: it was late in the morning for her to be walking, and unusual because Linda usually jogs with her dog, all the way from her home at the end of the street and back—nearly two miles. I stopped to say hello, and when she said she was feeling a little under the weather, I understood why she was walking and not jogging. I asked her, "Linda—have you ever been on a diet?"

Of course, this may seem like an intrusive question to ask of someone walking down the street on a Sunday morning! However, I was participating in the LITE Study[1], examining the habits of weight loss maintainers, and I'd already recruited four control participants—people who have always kept within ten pounds of their healthy weight. Linda said, "Well… actually, I need to lose about five pounds. Isn't it funny, but after I hit 40, my body changed. I used to be able to eat more, but I have to watch it closer now. If I gain five pounds, I take care of it immediately."

"What do you do to lose the weight?" I asked. She said, "I just give up my evening cocktail or wine with dinner—just cut out all alcohol for three weeks… it's amazing how quickly the calories add up. No alcohol, and I don't eat anything after dinner. After three weeks, I'm usually back in shape. Oh… and I keep jogging."

I said, "That's wonderful, Linda. And as a dietitian, I think you're doing it right, because you're not removing any important nutrients from your diet—instead, you're cutting out excess calories. By the way, you're just the perfect "control" candidate for a study of successful weight maintainers, and maybe you'd like to participate? All you need to do is talk with a registered dietitian and do a three-day diet recall, and wear an accelerometer to capture your activity for a few days. If you're interested, I'll email you the information."

Just before I rode away, I said, "I admire your consistency. Even though you're not feeling that well, you're still out here walking." She said, "I don't feel horrible and not bad enough to skip my activity. I don't feel energetic enough to run, but I feel OK to walk—and it makes me feel better just knowing I did it."

Linda has made her healthy habits second nature. She knows what works for her and if she gains a few pounds, she takes action before it gets out of hand. She has made these smart strategies second nature.

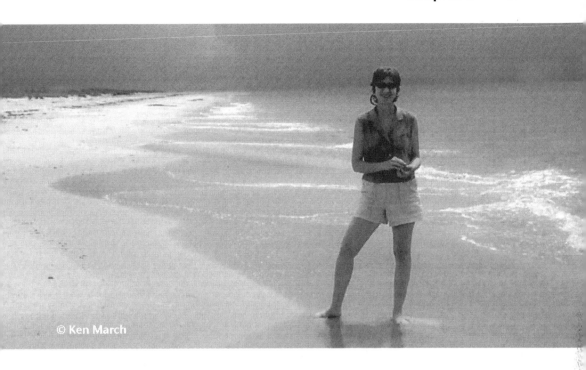

© Ken March

Next Steps: Remember the Motto "Prepare to Succeed"

> *"The path to our destination is not always a straight one.*
> *We go down the wrong road, we get lost, we turn back.*
> *Maybe it doesn't matter which road we embark on.*
> *Maybe what matters is that we embark."*

> — Barbara Hall
> Northern Exposure,
> Rosebud, 1993

I like to use this analogy, because many people can relate to the imagery.

Imagine you're going on a road trip from New York to California. You can see the map of the United States—it's a long way to go, and you're going to drive. You get out your map and a ruler and guesstimate how many hours you need to drive daily to get there. You can log on to the Internet and use a map/directions software program to get results in an instant.

Because you're smart, you will be prepared and have all the equipment you need before you get started. You make sure your tires are pumped up and have good tread; you have maps—maybe you even have a GPS in your car. You stock your cooler with water and healthy snacks. You may even have reservations at motels on the route so you will be well rested in the mornings.

You're not going to drive straight through, because you know you'll feel like hell when you get there.

Believe It

The more intensely we feel about an idea or a goal,
he more assuredly the idea, buried deep in our subconscious,
will direct us along the path to its fulfillment
—Earl Nightingale

I wanted to be different—I thought about it constantly. But, my *different* didn't mean "110 pounds" or a specific number that I expected to see on the scale. It was *never* only about the number on the scale. It was about control and about my having the strength and ability to make healthy choices.

It wasn't all about wanting to be thin. My desire, my need was to like myself more and to enjoy my life more because I could be in control of my choices—instead of letting the food and fear of not being able to choose differently paralyze me. The people I admired most were those who stayed thin *naturally*, and I realized that they never talked about how much they weighed. They were my friends who walked the healthy walk—literally— every day. They had regular exercise routines, and they didn't overeat—but, I noticed that at a party or special occasion, they'd have room for dessert. They might have said they were "addicted" to chocolate, but I noticed that they ate just one Hershey Kiss! Wow...that was amazing to me.

I admired people with self-control. That was what was missing in my life. I realized that if I never tried—really tried—to develop a personality that I could believe in—someone with self-discipline who didn't need to be perfect, but needed to make healthy choices— then I'd forever be unhappy. I believed that—I still believe it.

Your Personal Roadmap

When you're setting goals for weight change, make a roadmap for permanent changes that allow you to keep the weight off without having to "go on" a diet again. With good preparation, even if there's a detour you need to make, you'll overcome any obstacles and get to your goal. And the secret to staying thin *naturally* is that by the time you get to that goal, you will have learned so much from that journey—your journey will have affected you so completely—that going back will feel unnatural. You won't do it! Your healthy choices will become second nature.

Getting Started! What Worked for Me

Getting Started! What Worked for Me

Let me tell you how I got started. This is what worked for me.

- ▶ I understood that I was in a stage of change (preparation) that required that I **identify resources** including support.

- ▶ I set **multiple goals**.

- ▶ I **shared them** with my personal counselor (a very good idea to achieve behavioral change).

- ▶ I **kept track** of my progress.

My goals were: **Diet** Goals, **Activity** Goals, and **Personal** Goals

- ▶ Diet Goals:

  - ○ I spelled out what I was going to eat each day, how much I would eat, and when. **Make my usual diet a healthy one**

- ▶ Activity Goals:

  - ○ I charted what activity I was going to do, how long I was going to do it for, and when.
    Get some activity, at least 30 minutes, daily

- ▶ Personal goals:

  - ○ I wrote down positive self-talk replies to negative self-talk statements.
    Develop a sense of personal accomplishment by following my diet and activity schedule

The SMART Test

A common business strategy when planning a project is to make sure the goal or goals pass the "smart" test—they must be *specific, measurable, achievable,* and have a *realistic timetable.* What finally worked for me was that I made my body the kind of project I would undertake at work. I used business strategy and analyzed what I needed to accomplish, got my resources lined up, and got the job on track. This method of planning helped me to succeed at change.

Instead of simply thinking about weight loss, it is very valuable to think of your body as your project, as if you're beginning a new job. At first, there is some hesitation; you don't know for sure if you're doing everything right. You depend on feedback from your supervisors and peers....but after a while, the job becomes easier—almost second nature—and as long as you keep practicing what you trained for, you're going to be fine. And sometimes things change in the job...sometimes you need to learn new skills.

It's *natural* for things to change—that's part of life. What's *unnatural* is if you don't change to accommodate the changes!

Every year, my body changes naturally. With age, metabolic rate slows. Even if I don't change what I eat and how much I exercise, the weight will come on. I can accommodate a couple of pounds, but I want to keep my health as good as it is now and don't want my weight to interfere with it, so if I regain, I walk a little longer and eat less bread and a lot more crunchy veggies.

After a while, the job becomes easier. The idea is to think of your body as your job. Your job is to attain a lifestyle that allows you to stay at your desired weight *naturally*. Remember, it's natural to eat more if there's more to eat, it's natural to ride instead of walk, and it's natural that you'll gain weight if you eat more and move less.

What You Can Expect

My body responded once I started paying attention to what was going in and once I started making aerobic activity an everyday affair. Then, I found that the exercise bands and weights really made all the difference. I started getting stronger, building muscle, and I was enjoying food for the first time.

I saw the scale change pretty quickly at first—and after a few weeks, my weight loss stabilized. For the next few months, I lost one to two pounds every week, and in four months, I had lost over 20 pounds. Over the following four months, I worked at maintaining that weight loss—and realized that I could do it!

I weighed about 165 pounds at 5'7" when I started; my ultimate goal was 135 pounds. My first weight loss goal was 16.5 pounds (10% of 165). A realistic timetable for losing 16.5 pounds is approximately eight to nine weeks (approximately 2 pounds per week). I made that goal and weighed in at 148 about two months later. I set my next goal the same way as the first—10% of my current weight, which was 148, or about 15 pounds. Eventually, weight became less important than the way my clothes fit.

Sometimes it is helpful to give yourself a few weeks at each goal weight—just maintain that new weight and be comfortable in your new diet and exercise.

I've maintained my current weight for more than 20 years. But, it wasn't a straight, smooth path to 135 pounds—that happened over a period of years. Because I was building muscle and aging at the same time, the weight goal gradually became less important than the way I felt, my muscle tone, and my waist size. Once I felt great in my favorite jeans, I stopped weighing myself every week; instead, I put on those jeans once a week, whether I am wearing them or not.

Sandra's Story

At our first meeting, "Sandra" announced, "I want Sheryl Crow's arms, Catherine Zeta Jones' legs, and Demi Moore's abs, and I want them by Memorial Day, in time for the swim suit season." Wow, I thought, this is going to be tough.

People who have unrealistic expectations about their bodies are usually doomed to fail. For example, this conversation took place in my office on April 30th, which meant Sandra was dreaming of a totally reconstructed body in about one month. Her goals were specific enough, but her specifications had no basis in reality. She was at least 15 pounds overweight, but even if she could lose the weight—and she could—she had not exercised in years and she didn't even walk regularly.

Even the most gorgeous celebrity will admit that most magazine photos are retouched and colored. Don't be fooled by perfect skin, perfectly straight and white teeth, and absolutely no dimples on thighs—past a certain age, things change. Most magazines depict perfection, but this is fantasy. Even male models have plastic surgery to create more defined pecs, and their photos are just as re-touched as any female model's.

Perfection can never be a successful goal—we're changing all the time. Many fantasize about their bodies. What they need to become is a better version of themselves.

Better means trimmer, leaner, stronger—attainable by eating better, working out with light weights or resistance bands, and developing aerobic endurance. The most attractive women and men have firm arms and legs and look healthy, not skinny. They work at it—they dance, they go to the gym, they run. They work it! And it becomes part of their lives.

Sandra wanted a body that was someone else's, not hers, and celebrity bodies are different from yours and mine. Most celebs have personal trainers and nutritionists, and their entire daily focus is on being fit—it's their full-time job. Some people may never, ever attain the fantasy shape they want because their genes might get in the way. I knew a fit woman who wanted slimmer ankles and dieted constantly—but her body structure wouldn't respond to starvation. She had liposuction on her legs and was left with bruising for months, and she was never satisfied.

After all, even celebrities have to be content with Mother Nature's dictates. Could Sandra ever be content with "the best you can be"? Being fit and firm is a better goal, and she needs a realistic timetable to achieve it. Even if the goal is specific, measurable, and attainable, it also needs time—and I believe smaller goals make it more fun and exciting. Take it one day at a time, with fun rewards for meeting shorter milestones—that's the best route to permanent change.

Write it Down

Goals that are not written down are just wishes
Written goals have a way of transforming wishes into wants;
cant's into cans; dreams into plans; and plans into reality.
Don't just think it - ink it!

—*Authors Unknown*

SMART Goals	YOUR Goals
Specific:	1. What are your goals? List all the goals you wish to achieve. 2. Why are you working toward this goal? List the benefits you expect to gain from accomplishing this goal. 3. When will you begin? 4. Which equipment and materials do you need? In the Second Nature Fitness chapter, you'll find a list of tools and equipment. Use it to check off items to put into your personal toolbox. I have balance balls, hand weights, gym membership, and support group: what do you need? A personal trainer? Fitness videos? Dance lessons!
Measurable:	Set multiple goals. My first goal was weight loss, but really, I should have said "fat" loss. My goal was to burn stored fat. I used the scale to monitor my progress for the first few months, and so can you, as you reduce fat stores and build lean muscle. Remove the last digit from your current weight—the result is approximately 10 percent of your current weight. That's your first fat loss goal. For instance, if you weigh 150, your first fat loss goal is 15 pounds. You don't need to weigh yourself daily, or at all. You can measure progress by inches or by clothes size or by measuring your behavior—by logging each day's meals and fitness activities. You can do all of the above. In the beginning, I found that weighing myself helped me focus. Throw out that old dusty, rusty bathroom scale and get yourself a new digital model that's easy to read; consider the scale your friend, not your enemy. Your new scale will help you monitor your progress. Weight is just one measure of your progress, and if you are discouraged when you don't lose weight every day, don't worry about daily weighing. Measure your progress by measuring your behavior, too.

Attainable:	My goal? At first, all I thought about was losing weight to look better, but not just thinner—I wanted to look more fit and trim. Set a goal that's realistic for you—we can't all look like Ms. Zeta-Jones. But we can look firmer, leaner, and healthier— more in control. Setting exercise and eating goals helps you reach weight goals. It's not magic, but it seems like it. Just by modifying some usual habits and replacing them with healthy ones produces positive changes.
Realistic Timetable:	The faster the weight loss, the less permanent it is. Gradual weight loss—about one to three pounds a week—means you're doing it right. You're staying well-nourished and giving your body time to adjust to your new lifestyle. The rate of weight loss is dependent on a lot of factors, including your body type, your metabolism, and how much activity you get daily. Work in both aerobic activity (get your heart rate up) and anaerobic (light weight training). You may lose more than five pounds your first week, and as you start eating healthier food and taking in fewer calories, aim for a steady two pounds per week.

A Personal Challenge

As I teach people how to incorporate healthy choices and exercise into their busy lives, I find ways to include them in mine. There is no better way for me to learn than by doing it myself.

On a daily basis, I do the little things I advise my clients to do. For example on the day I go grocery shopping, I come home and immediately clean and portion my veggies and fruit into little snack plastic baggies, so they are ready for me to grab as I head off to work. I try to include something from each food group at lunch and dinner, and although I may eat part as a snack, I know I have made my diet balanced and nutritious. I have been a picky eater all my life so I try new foods all the time to include them into my meals because I know they are good for me. I think of food as fuel for my body—and before I eat something I think what nutritional value does this give me? I consciously evaluate if I am hungry or full when I am eating.

I make a point of testing and challenging myself. In September, completed my first triathlon and stay in training for more. I joined a soccer league even though I had never played before just to try something new. I do well having a goal, and something to work toward. Working out for the sake of exercise doesn't motivate me personally as well as taking on a challenge.

It's a never ending process, there is always something I can do to improve but I keep taking little steps to help me reach my goals.

I have seen first hand the struggles people have with managing their weight. I know this is not an easy thing but taking it one small step at a time can lead you to being healthy for the rest of your life!

Renee DeFrang, RD, CDE
Grand Rapids, MI

Taking Stock

My first priority for changing my habits was to gain self-control over my eating habits. My second priority was to become more physically fit. Before even starting a new diet or fitness program, it is time to stop and think about priorities. What are your priorities? Stop and prioritize your own personal reasons for wanting to lose weight and get in shape. Is it because you want to look better? Or improve your health? Maybe it's because you're afraid your kids will inherit your tendency to be overweight, or maybe it's because you're worried that your kids won't respect you if you don't take control. Is it because you're going on vacation and want to look good in a bathing suit? These are all legitimate reasons for you to change.

What is not legitimate is starting a sentence with, "I want to lose weight," and not completing it with the word "permanently." There's a big difference in setting a temporary goal and a permanent goal.

There's a big difference in saying, "I want to lose weight so I can fit into that sexy suit—but then I'll gain it back." I'm sure you mean, "I want to lose weight so I can fit into that sexy suit—permanently."

Would you say, "I'm going for health insurance, and I need to lower my blood pressure by losing weight, but then I'll take the risk for stroke and heart attack and gain it all back." Of course not! But people go "on" diets and think that they will magically maintain the weight loss. It's necessary to adopt those new healthy habits as your own.

Natural Goals

Specific: Avoid the deadly comparisons—they're self-defeating. Even the movie stars don't look like they do in the magazines. Instead of a goal like, "I want to look like (fill in your favorite celebrity)," set a goal that says, "I will tone my arms so that the loose skin underneath stops wobbling." Instead of "I want abs of steel," try a specific goal, such as, "I want to lose fat around my waist: My goal is to reduce my waist size by at least one inch within one month. When I reach that goal, I will set a new goal to lose one more inch."

Stay true to your goals in a positive way. Instead of saying *never*, say *always*. Instead of saying *oh, I can't do that*, say *I can*.

I changed how I think, and I think about what I *can do* instead of what I *can't do*. Incorporate positive living habits into your life permanently. Do it by being specific. For example:

- My first goal is to walk every day for 15 minutes for two consecutive weeks.

- My second goal is to add my Tae Bo fitness video every other day for two consecutive weeks.

- My third goal is to eat fresh fruit at breakfast and as an evening snack.

- My fourth goal is stop eating fried potatoes and eat baked, broiled, or grilled potatoes instead.

Measurable: Filling in a worksheet is a simple, positive act of commitment (Your Daily Diet Worksheet: Chapter 7). By writing daily I identified what I was going to do that day—that's preparation. I used one worksheet, that had my weekly meal plan printed on it, and then I added my activities, and a bunch of positive quotations to it every week.

The Internet is a valuable tool for information and support that I didn't have when I began my program 25 years ago. Today, you can sign up for a subscription weight management plan online, or you can use one of the many free websites that allow you to create your own personal program. Your registered dietitian may offer online support and e-tools. Log your weight, blood pressure, and blood glucose and produce reports and motivating progress graphs.

Remember that weight is only one measure of your progress. Just the action of writing or electronically logging your food, activities and thoughts is a positive behavior, and indicates your commitment to change.

Attainable: Of course you want to look like Ms. Catherine Zeta Jones—who wouldn't? But she's a unique individual with a whole lot of help and support, including full-time personal trainers and chefs. Her job is to look great—and you probably don't have her disposable income. But you can consider yourself an investment and dedicate resources to your body project that you may currently spend on stuff that isn't as important.

Your goals need to be realistic, but challenging. Looking and feeling good for us was easier when we were young, before we hit puberty and hormones seemed to get in the way of our best efforts to ignore them. If the goals you set are too easy, you'll get bored. If they're unrealistic, you'll also get discouraged.

Realistic Timetable: OK, you want to lose 20 pounds. So did I, and so do most people. When asked, "How much weight do you want to lose?" most people will answer, "Twenty pounds."

The question should be, **"How much fat loss do you want to maintain?"**

Do you want to lose 20 pounds? **Or do you really want to keep *off* 20 pounds of excess fat permanently?**

Regardless of the plan you choose, a diet that requires fewer calories than you need to maintain your current weight is the first step toward weight loss. Add daily exercise, and that deficit of calories will tip the scale in your favor. But not all diets are created equal—the only best diet is the one that you can stay on permanently. The best idea is to create your own diet—using the definition properly—and use it to maintain your weight loss permanently.

My usual diet has become second nature because I learned what I need to eat to maintain my weight. In the **Naturally Eating** chapter, I'll demonstrate what *I* eat and then show you how to create your own natural diet using a template that allows you to choose foods easily.

Sometimes life gets in the way, and I don't get to the gym as often as I'd like—or I don't get my one or two long bike rides in for the week. After a couple of weeks of doing less than usual, my jeans feel snug. Some may call it a relapse, but it's not—it's just a regain. So, back to deliberately adding fifteen daily minutes of really concerted effort—work that bike a little harder, cut out those nuts, and eat some fruit and vegetables.

I started out following a written plan. I learned about calories, fat, protein, and carbohydrates. I learned the best foods to eat and how to read labels. Today, I don't count calories or use a written plan, but I started with one and used it faithfully to lose weight; then, as I gained fitness, I learned that my body needed more calories to continue to lose weight because I was burning more.

My goals became second nature habits. You can be confident that your goals will be met if you make your new habits *second nature*. By accomplishing the small daily activities of healthy eating and activity, you are working toward accomplishing an ultimate goal of weight maintenance and increased fitness.

Your ultimate goal is achieved by accomplishing many small goals. Each goal is—in itself—a perfect pearl of self-worth and success. Over time, the weight goal becomes less important because the lifestyle goals will change you.

Examine that ultimate goal and the smaller goals you set to achieve that ultimate goal. Now, set a time frame to achieve each small goal.

Then give yourself the **rest of your life** to maintain your weight loss. The habits I've developed to lose the weight have become *second nature* to me and allow me to stay *naturally thin.*

What You Can—and Cannot—Change

Anatomy is destiny

—Sigmund Freud,
Collected Writings, 1924

Some things you just can't change, such as your bone structure; truly large-boned people may weigh more, and that doesn't mean they are over-fat. However, the extra inspiration for moving from the contemplation to preparation to action may come from your genetic predisposition for gaining extra pounds around your middle, which increases risk for diseases associated with obesity. Set goals for fitness and health, and you'll see your weight goals accomplished.

Why a Goal Weight?

Your weight is but one indicator of your progress toward behavior change. When I decided to make losing weight my first goal, the scale was helpful because it showed me that I was making progress. As long as I followed the program I had committed to, I could count on seeing the number gradually decrease. But my fitness goals gradually took over, and I stopped weighing myself as frequently. As I continued to workout, firming my muscles and losing inches, stepping on the scale meant much less to me than how my clothes fit. The amount of lean muscle you have compared to fat predicts your ability to maintain your weight. Your waist-to-height ratio is more predictive of health, especially for pear-shaped people who carry excess fat in their hips and butt.

Weight is only one goal and usually becomes increasingly irrelevant, as you achieve your fitness goals. Weight matters less as you become trimmer, and your clothes fit better, and as you have energy to exercise comfortably.

Don't settle for one goal, and don't draw a line in the sand.

Are You Overweight...or Overfat?

Body builders, men and women both, work hard to reduce their body fat, especially as they near the day of the event. The goal is to make their muscles "pop," so their diet is as rigid as their training, and they reduce their body fat drastically before competition. As they replace fat with muscle, their BMI goes up.

Now, that's strange, right? The higher the BMI, the more at risk for disease, isn't that what you've heard? But, when it comes to muscle mass, all bets are off.

If you have more muscle relative to fat stores, your weight for height, or Body Mass Index, is higher. To calculate BMI, you consider weight (in kilograms or pounds) compared to height (in millimeters or inches); however, the number isn't relevant for everyone, especially people with a lot of muscle (or pregnant or breastfeeding women).

Which weighs more: a pound of fat or a pound of muscle? Ah, a *trick question!* Yes, both weigh a pound, but they mean very different things to the way your body looks and the way your body operates. Once I began building muscle, I felt so much better, looked better, and had more energy.

Your weight is just a number on the scale, and it doesn't take into account your body type, how much muscle you have, or if you have a large or small bone structure. Just as a body builder can weigh more but be ultra-fit, a small-boned woman may have a normal BMI, but if she carries excess weight around her middle, she could be tipping the scale against her—abdominal weight increases risk for heart disease and diabetes.

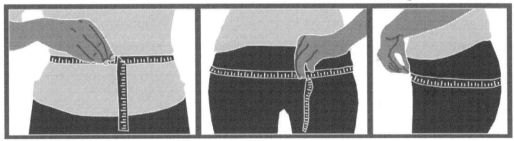

How to measure: Measure your waist with a non-stretchable measuring tape at the narrowest point between the bottom of your ribcage and your hipbones. Tension should be firm but not pulled so tightly as to compress the tissue underneath. Measure your hips at the widest point around your buttocks.

- Measure your waist at its narrowest point (over your belly button)

- Measure your hips at their widest (over your behind)

- Divide your waist size by your hip size. Women's waist-to-hip ratio should max out at 0.8, men's at 0.95.

- "Apple" body type: fat gained around the belly; "Pear" means fat gained on hips, thighs and butt. Women after menopause often gain weight around their belly, increasing risk for obesity-related health problems.

Waist is More Important Than Weight

Waist wins. If your BMI is over 25, but your waist size is less than 35 inches (women) or less than 40 inches (men), you're probably more muscular than fat. Can you be fit but fat? You can be fit and overweight—that is, if your body is muscular and trim. But, the greater the percent of weight from stored fat, the higher your risk for eventually getting diseases such as high blood pressure, diabetes, heart disease, depression, arthritis, and even cancer. Waist size is a better predictor of health than weight. Excess fat stored on the abdomen may lead to hormonal changes, inflammation and possibly arterial plaque buildup, and increases risk for type 2 diabetes and heart disease.

Weight is Just a Number on the Scale

In an unscientific survey, I asked a dozen different people if they made a resolution to lose weight last year. Ten of them said, "Yes," and eight of the ten said they wanted to lose 20 pounds; two said 10 pounds.

Everyone said that they lost *some of the weight*. And most had regained some of the weight back—some had regained all of the weight. Only one man reported keeping all the weight off

I asked, "When you resolved to lose weight, did you resolve to lose weight *permanently?* They all said they didn't think of that!

I used to think, "I want to lose 20 pounds." That didn't work. What did work was resolving to make *second nature* the healthy habits I used to lose weight.

When I changed my goals from "I want to lose weight" to "I want to lose fat and be fit, and I want to control my eating," that helped. Instead of focusing on 20 pounds, I said, "I want to permanently lose and never regain the first five pounds of excess fat that's sitting on my butt." You get the picture.

The Weight is Over

Your healthy weight? Here's how I define MY healthy weight:

- My healthy weigh is the weight at which I have no diseases associated with being overweight—high blood pressure, high cholesterol, type 2 diabetes, arthritis, gastric reflux, or sleep apnea, for example.

- Maintain a leaner body and replace excess body fat with lean muscle. My goal was to lower my body fat from over 30 percent to less than 30 percent. (Men, aim for less than 25 percent.)

- I'm able to do aerobic activity daily—I aim for at least 30 minutes and try for more on many days.

- I feel in control of what I eat and can go shopping for clothes without dreading the experience.

My Natural Life

Setting goals for change is just like planning a long trip. Goals need to be realistic and measurable. Think about the journey as your chosen destination, not a "round-trip". You're not going back...you're going forward, so get on board, and enjoy the ride.

I didn't become overweight overnight—it took years of ignoring my best interests. Set a realistic timetable for change—break it down into small, achievable goals.

Goal setting is smart strategy, because it helps build up your ego. Each time I reached a weight goal, I felt more excited about the process.

Have you ever used Google Maps? (http://maps.google.com) It's a very clever program—you can click on your destination, just about anywhere in the world, and see an amazing amount of detail—even the trees in the yard. But I think you're missing the bigger picture when you focus so intently on just one goal. Being prepared for the journey takes more than getting directions. Having resources to deal with contingencies is critical.

This Vehicle Only Goes Forward

I don't weigh myself as often as I used to. I get on a scale occasionally at the grocery store—they have this huge, old-fashioned step-on scale—and I get weighed at my doctor's office for my annual physical. I have a couple of pairs of pants that I use to monitor my weight. But when I was in fat-loss-mode, I did weigh myself, at first, every few days. I was excited to see the scale tipping in my favor. But, I became increasingly giddy at the daily success of writing down my daily accomplishments. I logged my good breakfast, my activity, and my workouts. I made those choices and went forward.

Of course, a lot of the time I struggled to stick with it, but kept my eye on what I could do that day, and tried never to think about giving up. I kept reaching out for support, especially when tempted to overeat to assuage anxiety.

Get Out Your Compass

Using a GPS to find your destination is great, but there's something to be said for using an old-fashioned compass, too. With a compass, you have to learn to navigate in all types of environments and find your way around the bumps in the road you're sure to encounter on the way to your destination. Think about preparing to meet your body goals as you would preparing for an automobile journey. You need good fuel, you need solid tires, and you need experience and navigational skills to make the journey successful. You can buy the car, but you need to equip it, fuel it, and drive it. You need to develop the traveling skills—just as I did—and make them second nature.

Ready, Steady—Go!

Before you get started on your journey, be prepared...mentally and physically. You're undertaking a big project, so gather your resources, including your **will.**

If you_____	Then you will_____
Want to lose weight, pick some smart reasons: for better health, energy, and to enhance your self-esteem.	Talk with your doctor about your intentions to begin a healthy weight program, especially if you haven't had a physical lately, or you're currently on any medications.
Are overweight because you use food for emotional support and to reduce anxiety.	Work with your support group or one-on-one with your counselor and take an unflinching look at your eating patterns. Identify the times that you overeat, and write down five new strategies to change that behavior.
Accept that "dieting" doesn't work.	You will start eating! Fresh, whole foods will brighten your taste buds—you'll see, food will become more enjoyable. Make eating healthy your hobby and it will become second nature.
Are ready to achieve permanent weight loss.	You will put structure in your life, and plan your meals and activities—structure helps define your needs, and makes possible permanent change.
Accept that support will make the process better and easier.	You will join a support group, and you'll find that being there for others helps motivate you even further.
Have a lot of weight to lose.	You will remember that weight is just a number on the scale—other goals including daily activity and stress reduction are just as important. Weight loss happens by changing the way you think about yourself—you can do it, one pound at a time.
Are ready to stop cheating.	Then you will win. Cheating is a word not found in a naturally thin dictionary!

A Mountain of Inspiration

I was listening to National Public Radio this morning. A young man was being interviewed. Born with a genetic defect, he was missing one leg, but he had just climbed Mt. Everest—on crutches! He and his father had trained for months. They were ready to go, but his father was the one who was unable to make the final ascent—he developed such severe altitude sickness that he couldn't go on. But he told his son, "You're ready. You go. You succeed."

The boy summited...he succeeded. He said in the interview, "I had trained for it—I developed the skills I needed. And I made it back down—which was almost as hard."

You can't say, "Beam me up, Scotty," and—poof!—be at your goal. It takes training and developing intellectual and emotional strength, but it happens—one day at a time. Once you're at your goal weight, it's just as important to stay strong so, as the young man says, you can come down from your mountain and participate in our world of temptation, continuing to remain healthy and *naturally thin* forever.

You're in Control Goal Sheets

You see...you can improve all these goals by working on Goal Number One!
Go From Overweight to In Control

Be creative and think of all the ways to modify your current behaviors and look forward to having the control to succeed.

Goal Number	MY GOALS	HOW TO? Details, Details!
	To Go from Overweight to In Control	
1	To Lose Fat	
2	To Get Stronger	
3	To Look Leaner and Have More Muscle Definition	
4	To Have More Energy	
5	To Feel More Physically Attractive (Sexier!)	
6	Have More Fun Going Shopping for Clothes	
7	To Lower My Risk for Illness	
8	To Set A Healthy Example	
9	Look Good for a Family Reunion (or other Social Event)	
10	To Look More Professional	

Now, How To?

To Go from Overweight to In Control	HOW TO? Details, Details! Journaling is a proven method for weight loss. Keep your food & fitness records current as a reminder to see how far you've come.
To Lose Fat	**Choose** a program that includes a healthy meal and activity plan and monitor your progress daily either using your own Goal Sheets or try an online program. Choose a program to suit your lifestyle, food preferences, and budget. Weight is just one measure of progress, and every 2 weeks log your waist and/or hip measurements. Keep your journal handy, and write in it daily (journaling works!). Don't forget to reward your new lifestyle.
To Get Stronger	**Invest** in a fitness plan. Use an online program, join a gym or local Y, or get some DVDs. Consider your lifestyle, your fitness level and your budget. If you can't get to a gym, invest in simple home equipment: a balance ball, hand weights, exercise bands, and a jump rope will get you fit and strong. Losing fat and toning up makes you not only look better, you'll feel better, too. Your body will LOVE it that you're creating more muscle—when you're stronger, you feel more powerful.
To Look Leaner and Have More Muscle Definition	**Choose** three days a week to do strengthening exercises, and enjoy the feeling of firm muscles—your clothes will fit better—an added bonus. Don't worry about bulking up—most women don't have the testosterone men do. The idea is to get toned and fit, not muscular and musclebound.
To Have More Energy	**Create** your personal calorie deficit—not by starving and eating too few calories, but by changing what you eat, eating for energy. Make deliberate activity your daily mission. You will sleep better, which means more energy during the day.
To Feel More Physically Attractive (Sexier!)	**Confidence** I think there is nothing sexier than a firm, toned body. Caring about how you look is attractive. When you take control, you feel confident, walk taller, and feel stronger!
Have More Fun Going Shopping for Clothes	**Fun!** As you become more confident with your control, you'll feel the power! It is a powerful and wonderful feeling to know that your clothes fit well because you are physically fit. I was motivated to continue as I began to be able to wear clothes that showed my arms rather flowing garments designed to hide.
To Lower My Risk for Illness	**Reduce** your risk: Just losing 5-10% of your current weight can dramatically decrease risk for hypertension and type 2 diabetes. You reduce the stress on your joints and tendons and lower risk for knee, hip and back problems. Just walking is easier when you carry less excess weight.

To Go from Overweight to In Control	HOW TO? Details, Details! Journaling is a proven method for weight loss. Keep your food & fitness records current as a reminder to see how far you've come.
To Set A Healthy Example	**Demonstrate** how you prioritize your foods and your activities, and your family, friends, and peers will look to you as an example of someone who cares enough to take control. Take a challenge: join an online group and start logging your new behaviors; join a running or walking club; take a fitness-oriented vacation, such as a bike tour. All levels of fitness are welcome, and you'll return home feeling fit, not fat.
Look Good for a Family Reunion (or other Social Event)	**Enjoy your life** It's not about "going on a diet," but instead being able to look forward to a social event rather than dreading it. Your confidence shows, because you are in control. No more do you make social events an excuse for overeating.
To Look More Professional	**Demonstrate** your commitment to working hard to stay fit and healthy. You reap benefits by setting a good example for your colleagues at work. If your office has a fitness and/or diet program, join up—and stay with it.

Your Personal Goal Sheet

Goal Number	MY GOALS	HOW TO? Details, Details!
	To Go from Overweight to In Control	
1	To Lose Fat	
2	To Get Stronger	
3	To Look Leaner and Have More Muscle Definition	
4	To Have More Energy	
5	To Feel More Physically Attractive (Sexier!)	
6	Have More Fun Going Shopping for Clothes	
7	To Lower My Risk for Illness	
8	To Set A Healthy Example	
9	Look Good for a Family Reunion (or other Social Event)	
10	To Look More Professional	

Risk of Associated Disease According to BMI and Waist Size from Partnership for Healthy Weight Management
http://www.consumer.gov/weightloss/bmi.htm

BMI		Waist less than or equal to 40 inches (men) or 35 inches (women)	Waist greater than 40 inches (men) or 35 inches (women)
18.5 or less	Underweight	--	N/A
18.5 - 24.9	Normal	--	N/A
25.0 - 29.9	Overweight	Increased	High
30.0 - 34.9	Obese	High	Very High
35.0 - 39.9	Obese	Very High	Very High
40 or greater	Extremely Obese	Extremely High	Extremely High

Note: BMI 30-39.9 is considered obese; but the risk changes from high to very high when waist increases to greater than 40 inches for men and greater than 35inches for women

Body Mass Index Table[3]

To use the table, find the appropriate height in the left-hand column labeled Height. Move across to a given weight. The number at the top of the column is the BMI at that height and weight. Pounds have been rounded off.

BMI	19	20	21	22	23	24	25	26	27	28	29	30	31	32	33	34	35	36	37	38	39	40
Height (Inches)												Body Weight (Pounds)										
58	91	96	100	105	110	115	119	124	129	134	138	143	148	153	158	162	167	172	177	181	186	191
59	94	99	104	109	114	119	124	128	133	138	143	148	153	158	163	168	173	178	183	188	193	198
60	97	102	107	112	118	123	128	133	138	143	148	153	158	163	168	174	179	184	189	194	199	204
61	100	106	111	116	122	127	132	137	143	148	153	158	164	169	174	180	185	190	195	201	206	211
62	104	109	115	120	126	131	136	142	147	153	158	164	169	175	180	186	191	196	202	207	213	218
63	107	113	118	124	130	135	141	146	152	158	163	169	175	180	186	191	197	203	208	214	220	225
64	110	116	122	128	134	140	145	151	157	163	169	174	180	186	192	197	204	209	215	221	227	232
65	114	120	126	132	138	144	150	156	162	168	174	180	186	192	198	204	210	216	222	228	234	240
66	118	124	130	136	142	148	155	161	167	173	179	186	192	198	204	210	216	223	229	235	241	247
67	121	127	134	140	146	153	159	166	172	178	185	191	198	204	211	217	223	230	236	242	249	255
68	125	131	138	144	151	158	164	171	177	184	190	197	203	210	216	223	230	236	243	249	256	262
69	128	135	142	149	155	162	169	176	182	189	196	203	209	216	223	230	236	243	250	257	263	270
70	132	139	146	153	160	167	174	181	188	195	202	209	216	222	229	236	243	250	257	264	271	278
71	136	143	150	157	165	172	179	186	193	200	208	215	222	229	236	243	250	257	265	272	279	286
72	140	147	154	162	169	177	184	191	199	206	213	221	228	235	242	250	258	265	272	279	287	294
73	144	151	159	166	174	182	189	197	204	212	219	227	235	242	250	257	265	272	280	288	295	302
74	148	155	163	171	179	186	194	202	210	218	225	233	241	249	256	264	272	280	287	295	303	311
75	152	160	168	176	184	192	200	208	216	224	232	240	248	256	264	272	279	287	295	303	311	319
76	156	164	172	180	189	197	205	213	221	230	238	246	254	263	271	279	287	295	304	312	320	320

Weight-control Information Network (WIN); www.win.niddk.nih.gov
http://win.niddk.nih.gov/statistics/index.htm#table

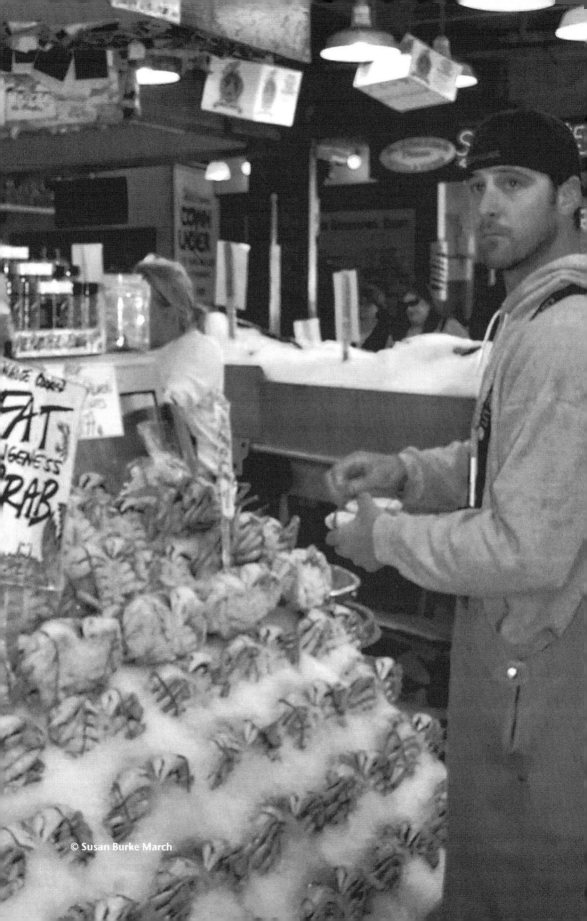

© Susan Burke March

Chapter 6

My Favorite Diet—is No Diet At All
How All Diets Work—and All Diets Fail

Motivation is what gets you started. Habit is what keeps you going.
—Jim Ryun

My feeling about diets is this: I'm not a fan of eating *less* food when dieting—because I don't like to be hungry. What worked for me was eating *more*—and especially eating *differently*. To lose weight, I ate a greater volume of lower calorie foods—I ate all the crunchy vegetables I wanted, and I changed my other food choices to get more bang for my buck—the "bang" being larger portions of lower calorie fruits and vegetables—and almost no fried foods, or foods made with added fat. I've maintained this strategy, and my usual diet keeps me where I want to be.

I may eat more frequently—but not unthinkingly. When I'm home, I stock frozen vegetables or buy pre-cut bags of crunchy veggies (if you're able, stock your office refrigerator). When I'm hungry, I microwave a bowl of green beans or broccoli and sprinkle on some fat-free dehydrated butter granules or nonfat salad dressing for a quick and very low calorie—but filling snack. I don't leave the house unprepared—I bring some fruit or carrots or a small baggie of peanuts in the shell.

DEFINITION

Instruction
  –noun

   1. The act or practice of instructing or teaching; education.

   2. Instructions, orders, directions, authoritative commands

Self-help
  –noun

   1. The act of providing for or helping or the ability to provide for or help oneself without assistance from others.

I stay healthy by monitoring "discretionary calories" from desserts, special foods, or even a glass of wine, and mentally account for them by maintaining my fun activities. If I don't get at least 30 minutes of aerobic activity daily, the scale is going to start to creep up. Even if I overindulge one day, the next day I stick to my guns, saying "no" to high calorie foods and "yes, please" to fun fuel.

I learned what portions are right for me and make portion control a habit even when dining out. I like the way I feel and look at my current weight—so I continue to make those little modifications every day that add up to keeping my weight about the same—give or take a piece of cake.

I Changed My Thinking

Today I think of diet as my usual food and drink consumed. I enjoy food, as most people do. But I accepted that my overweight was inevitable unless I changed the food I ate and learned to enjoy food differently.

My experience includes examining my attitudes toward food—and overweight. Overweight can happen even if your diet is healthy. When I eat too many calories, no matter if the food is healthful, I gain weight.

I had to learn to eat differently and create a new way of eating, and now my usual diet is the one I use to stay naturally thin. But naturally thin isn't natural to me—it's deliberate. What keeps my weight stable is what has become *second nature* to me. My natural lifestyle means eating good foods in the portion size that serves to fuel my activity. That's my diet.

It would be *unnatural* for me to eat fatty, fast food or drink sugary soda. I left those habits in my past and will never go back.

What I Do To Stay Thin, Naturally

1. **Diet:** Instead of snacking on refined carbs all day, I now eat either small snacks or small, balanced meals every few hours.

2. **Activity:** I make a point of walking, biking, or using an aerobic machine every morning for at least 30 minutes. If I feel I need to lose a few pounds, I increase my activity at least 20 minutes daily until I lose the weight.

3. **Stress:** I used to start snacking after dinner, but by planning a sweet, low calorie evening snack, I relax instead of overeat. My favorite is a cup of sugar-free hot chocolate and a crisp green apple.

4. **Journaling:** For the first six months of my weight loss program, I wrote in my journal each evening—but made it easy because I used a pre-made meal and activity log, and checked off what I ate and drank—all I had to do was add in any extras. The same for my activity—I had a pre-planned exercise schedule, and noted any additional deliberate activities. Each evening I reviewed my next day's schedule.

The weight loss diet that I used to lose weight wasn't mysterious, didn't exclude any food groups, and didn't include any products or supplements. It was very basic, and took the guesswork out of eating. I imposed structure on my eating—I was ready for it and found that knowing what I was going to eat, and how much, relieved a lot of the anxiety about eating for the first few weeks. Gradually, I incorporated portion control into eating wherever I went.

My goals were to eat differently, increase my activity, replace some habits with healthier habits, and reduce my stress. Oh, and I wrote it down every day. Writing down the goals for the day and logging what I ate produced the record of action that allowed me to set my goal for the next day.

Know More—Weigh Less

I enjoy food and make it a habit to learn more about foods all the time. As I deliberately learned more about food, calories, nutrients, and recipe modification, I began to think differently about my eating, and my healthy living behaviors became second nature. Then, I made food and nutrition my vocation. My usual diet is a healthy one—with the right calories for me to maintain my weight. I don't count calories, but I do stay mindful of portions—and because this has become second nature to me, I mentally—almost unconsciously—understand how many calories I'm consuming without counting them.

I'm Not Lucky—I'm Determined

I may be lean, but I'm not "lucky." If you saw my family, you'd know that I come from the same genes as the general population. I was a thin kid because my parents encouraged us to get outside and play. But, once I entered my teen years, I began to struggle with my weight. At the age of 16, I lost about 40 pounds and went from "soft body" to anorexic. But, by the time I graduated, I weighed 25 pounds more than I do now! And, there were a lot of diets in between.

Everything changed in my mid-20s. I was a researcher in a migraine study, and we found that eating six small meals a day would help decrease migraine intensity and frequency. Although this wasn't a weight loss study, my participants kept telling me that not only were they not "hungry," they were losing weight and feeling great! That's when I started eating six times a day and I haven't skipped a meal since. I found that eating every two and a half or three hours, even if I wasn't hungry, helped me stop overeating and my weight slowly began to drop and then stabilize to the weight I am today (for 25 years and counting).

Dr. Jo Lichten, "Dr. Jo," PhD, RD
Author of *Dining Lean* –
How to eat healthy when you're not at home
www.drjo.com

What's the Best Diet?

Claims of "miraculous" results—overnight, in your sleep, without exercise—are everywhere. Just type *diet* into your Web browser or pick up a newspaper or turn on a shopping channel. Today I heard an advertisement on the radio for the "Amazing new breakthrough in weight loss." "Lose all the weight you want," the women said, "and eat when you want and how much you want of pizza and hamburgers, too."

It is amazing that so many people buy these unproven products that are often very hard on the pocketbook. But it's difficult for some to face the prospect of eating differently, often because overeating helps them deal with stress or anxiety.

The nonprofit Calorie Control Council reported that 33 percent of Americans, or 71 million people, are currently on a diet—the highest number of dieters in the past 15 years. I'm frequently asked, "What do you think about the (fill in the blank) Diet?" Strangers, when finding out that I'm a registered dietitian, will ask me about the latest book, product, or celebrity diet program. My answer? Well, if you follow the program and you exercise, you'll probably lose weight. Diet products and programs that "guarantee" weight loss usually include a statement of default, usually in tiny letters at the bottom of the page, or chanted unintelligibly at the end of the advertisement, *"This program requires you follow a reduced calorie meal plan and incorporate exercise into the program."*

When you reduce calories and exercise—with or without the supplement or equipment, won't you lose weight anyway?

A study published in the March 6, 2007, issue of the Journal of the American Medical Association compared four popular diets: Atkins (very low carbohydrate); Zone (moderate unrefined carbohydrate with a higher ratio of protein and fat); Ornish (very low fat with unrefined carbohydrate); and LEARN-Lifestyle, Exercise, Attitudes, Relationships, and Nutrition (calorie-controlled; low in fat, high in carbohydrate, based on national guidelines) to see which produced the most weight loss and to measure the effect on certain metabolic indicators[1].

And what happened? *All* participants lost weight; the very low carb plan produced—as expected—the most initial weight loss and all the diets showed improved blood lipids, even the high fat Atkins plan. On the Atkins diet, carbohydrates are dramatically restricted for at least the first two weeks, and people lose a lot of "weight," including a lot of fluid. After one year, the very same low carb group that had lost the most gained the most weight back.

So, no surprise there! They proved it again! All diets work. For most people, a "Diet" means changing what you usually eat and eating fewer calories. Low carb works, low fat works, and very low fat works; but no diet works permanently without permanent lifestyle change. By the end of this study, all the participants had started to regain the weight. In fact, there hasn't been one study that demonstrates that any particular *weight loss diet program* is *better* at keeping weight off long-term.

The glycemic index diet is a good example of how some authors focus on nutrients instead of nutrition. The glycemic index is assessed by having one or more people eat a specific amount of a single food—usually 50 grams of digestible carbohydrate, or total carbohydrate minus the fiber. Changes in blood sugar levels are then measured and compared with levels after eating a control food (usually white bread or glucose) containing the same amount of digestible carbohydrate. What results is a single number that represents the average change in blood sugar levels over a set period of time relative to the levels after consumption of the control food. Sounds complicated? Unnecessarily so!

The glycemic index doesn't consider portion size or fiber—two important factors that influence the food's impact on blood glucose. To focus on individual foods, and look up a "value" and make a decision about eating a food based on that number is unrealistic and misses the point.

In general, high glycemic index foods are highly processed—breads, cereals, mashed potatoes, and white rice. Lower glycemic index foods are generally "whole" foods—vegetables, fruits, legumes, unprocessed grains including oatmeal and long-grain brown rice, dairy, and meat. However, baked potatoes and corn flakes have higher glycemic indices than jelly beans and soft drinks—but does that make candy and soda "better"? The glycemic index of carrots is 49, but a Snicker's bar is only 40. While a candy bar might be OK for the (very) occasional treat, carrots are dandy...daily.

Some other considerations for the glycemic index include:

- A person's blood sugar response to eating a food can vary from day to day.

- How the food is prepared can affect blood glucose response.

- The ripeness of the food, as in the case of bananas, can affect the glycemic index (the more ripe the banana, the higher its glycemic index).

- Once a food is combined with other foods (such as cereal and milk or peanut butter and bread), the glycemic index of the meal will be very different from that of either food alone.

- The amount of food eaten to measure the glycemic index is often different from the amount of food eaten in a typical serving.

Balance Is Best

The best advice from the American Dietetic Association and the American Diabetes Association is to enjoy a balanced meal plan, with an emphasis on unrefined carbohydrate foods—including whole grains and whole grain breads and cereals—and whole servings of fruit (instead of juice).

The skin of fruits and vegetables contain healthy fiber, too, so scrub and eat! "Whole" should precede the grain listed in packaged cereals and breads—whole wheat, whole oats, whole corn or any other grain.

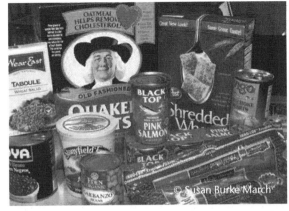

Stock up on healthy staples: nonfat yogurt, canned beans and salmon, whole grains and whole wheat pasta.

Top Naturally Thin Weight Management Tips

Make it Second Nature

My second nature behaviors make weight maintenance feel natural.

1. **Re-define Diet**: Using *diet* as a verb is passé. I dumped that definition and redefined my goals. Most people go on a diet and lose weight, then go off the diet and usually return to the old attitudes and habits that made them overweight. I made my diet healthy and balanced and filled up on lower calorie fruits and vegetables, but included most foods in the right portion size. And, voila! You can, too…stay healthy and at your goal weight. How, you ask? Read on…

2. **It's Never, Ever Too Late!:** Even if you have a "bad day" and overeat, the rule is, don't give up. Get right back to your plan tomorrow. One day won't kill your progress…it may slow it, but you can overcome by adding 30 minutes of power-walking for five days and burn off the extra calories.

3. **Be Accountable:** A very important component of change is staying accountable to your behavior—that means, checking in consistently to communicate your progress, your challenges, and your accomplishments. The best is a one-on-one meeting with a caring professional—a registered dietitian with weight management experience or a group like Weight Watchers that has face to face meetings. They also have e-Tools so you can stay ultra-connected and an online program that calls for weekly (or more) logging in. Stay connected and stay on course.

4. **Don't Demonize Food:** There are no "good" or "bad" foods. Food doesn't have human qualities, but food does have content characteristics, such as high fat, low sugar, high fiber, and high calorie. Everyone likes a treat now and then, and that's OK, as long as it's occasional. The rule is to balance out the high calorie treat by making the rest of the day healthy.

5. **Stick With It:** My friend Glenn lost 35 pounds with a high fiber, low fat diet program. He eliminated all processed foods, but especially soda and white flour. Now it's water or flavored carbonated soda (no-cal), and he sticks to whole grains. Just by cutting out one 20-ounce bottle of soda (approximately 200 calories!) every day, you can lose up to 10 pounds yearly—without doing anything else.

Weight Loss Myths Continued...

There's no "magic" in weight loss. If it sounds too good to be true, it is. Watch infomercials if you want to get a laugh—they advertise "miraculous," "effortless" weight loss gimmicks. But no potion, powder, or pill produces automatic weight loss. Weight loss is a numbers game…but not a gamble. There is a payoff when you pay attention.

Don't "go on" a diet, adopt YOUR new way of eating, and include daily activity. Make small changes—embrace them, stay with them—and the weight loss will stay with you. Small changes pay off, big time. Consistency pays off in pounds of weight lost. You may "wish" you were thinner, fitter, stronger…even taller, but there's no magic in weight control. Even a marathon runner or a professional athlete or a dancer or someone who does manual labor for a living can't eat injudiciously. Even very active people ultimately need to control their diet—if they're constantly eating too much for their needs, no matter how great their calorie requirements are, they're bound to gain unwanted pounds. I need to constantly be aware of the calories going in and the calories I burn—daily.

Please notice: I didn't say, "Make small changes temporarily." Nope. These small changes need to be adopted for your very own. And when you do adopt them, you'll achieve permanent weight loss. Make a few key modifications to your usual diet and exercise habits—make new habits second nature.

It's the small stuff that adds up. By changing what you eat, you can lose weight and maintain the loss, and stay satisfied and energized. When I accepted that I had to make *changes* to my *usual* diet and lifestyle—the *old way*, when I stayed in *action* mode and worked the changes, I became thin, naturally.

I made it my job to make it happen. I had a goal—a time frame—and a framework for calories and exercise, and I got the job done.

Taking Charge

It started out innocently. I tried on a dress I hadn't worn in a while. I put it over my head, pulled it down and realized I was sucking in my breath—then I had to move the zipper side to side. I could barely get it over my breasts, and no further. It didn't fit.

How did that happen? What the hell! Did the dress shrink?

Of course not. I just gained some weight.

I was not going to throw away all my clothes because I had gained some weight. At first, I didn't know how much weight, but it didn't matter. I was determined to get back into shape.

I cut down on refined starches and sugar, stopped drinking juice and eating pasta, potatoes and rice. I never even looked at chips—of any kind, baked or fried—which I used to grab to have with a soda if I skipped lunch. I switched to salads for lunch, making them different every day so I wouldn't get bored. I stuck with grilled chicken or fish and veggies—as much as I felt like eating—and started meals with a tossed salad. I drank at least four glasses of water a day and cut back alcohol to one or, at most, two glasses of red wine with dinner.

The most important change was my exercise—and that's permanent. I walk or run on a regular basis. No excuses for weather, or if I feel tired, or cranky. I found that walking or running gave me a second wind after work and let me indulge in movies, some television or reading at night. And exercise helps me sleep like a log!

All these changes helped, and gradually I lost the weight, and my clothes look great. Today, my diet is mostly fresh fish and salads with a baked potato or a cup of rice with vegetables—still as many veggies as I want to eat. Food is no longer a reward for a long day at work—occasionally I indulge in a nonfat, sugar-free frozen yogurt with about 45 calories.

Charlotte Tomic,
Tomic Communications

SMALL CHANGES BECOME SECOND NATURE—STAY THIN *NATURALLY*			
Old Way Old Calories	New Second Nature Choices	Calorie Differential	Potential for Weight Loss
Add butter and sour cream to your baked potato means 100 extra calories per tablespoon	Add 2 Tbsp of tomato salsa to your baked potato	Reduce each meal by 75-150 calories	Calories saved add up to 8 to 10 pounds so have your baked potato and enjoy it, too.
Order an entrée of fettuccine Alfredo (pasta and cream sauce)—may contain 1200 calories per serving!	Broiled fish and broccoli—about 400 calories	Reduce by 800 calories: replace just 1 meal per week	About 12 pounds worth of calories per year, and more lean protein, less saturated fat and refined carbs
Eat a BIG bran muffin—can have more than 600 calories and huge amount of sugar and fat	Crunchy, low sugar cereal, nonfat milk, and a cup of berries only 300-400 calories	Reduce by 200 calories per day—a deficit of 1,400 per week.	Ditch what is, essentially, a huge pastry: lower the fat and sugar and increase the nutrition and protein—the calorie difference is huge! More than 20 pounds worth.
One 12-oz can of regular soda per day (or cup of juice) has about 150 calories	Skip the sweet stuff! Drink water or switch to diet soda—0 calories	Reduce by 150 calories (at least!) per day. Drink water and save dollars, too	Create a 16-pound calorie deficit by eliminating soft drinks. I stopped drinking all diet soda—better for my teeth and pocketbook.
2 beers daily has about 250 calories	A glass of dry white or red wine (3-4 ounces) with dinner	Reduce by 100-150 calories per day	Create a yearly 10-15 pound calorie deficit by decreasing alcohol consumption; may replace with sparkling water too.
A handful of shelled and roasted peanuts is a quick way to get more than 500 calories	A cup of peanuts in the shell ~200 calories	Reduce by about 300 calories	Nuts add up fast! Save more than 20 pounds a year and "earn" your snacks by shelling your own nuts.

Can Vegetarian Diets Make You Fat?

Americans make up only five percent of the world's population (USDA Economic Research Service) but eat a disproportionate amount of beef. As Mark Bittman wrote in the *New York Times* (February 4, 2008), in America we "process" almost 10 billion animals yearly, more than 15 percent of the world's total.

Although small portions of lean meat may be fine, advertisers will have you think that "real Americans" enjoy "big meat" No paltry 3-ounce steak, as recommended by the USDA's MyPyramid.gov. No, we're chowin' down on 16-ounce, 24-ounce, and all-you-can-eat portions. When you add dairy and eggs to the meat equation, it adds up. The total amount of American meat consumption (red meat, poultry, and fish) amounted to 200 pounds per person, 22 pounds above the level in 1970.

More than 80 percent of corn grown in American goes to feed cows, and some studies link diets high in red meat with some cancers. Americans consume nearly double the protein they need to be healthy, more than 100 grams on average. Calculate approximately how much you need by multiplying your weight in pounds by 0.4. For instance, a moderately active man who weighs 180 pounds needs about 72 grams of protein daily to stay healthy.

Protein is present in nearly *all foods*, except fat. Even fruit has a small amount of protein.

I weigh about 128 pounds, I'm moderately active, and eat approximately 1800 – 2000 calories daily. I aim for approximately 25% of my calories from protein (450 – 500 calories), divided by 4 calories per gram, so I aim for approximately 113 - 125 grams of protein daily.

My breakfast has good protein:

- One cup of my favorite Kashi GoLean cereal (13 grams)

- One cup of blueberries (1 gram)

- One cup of nonfat milk or unsweetened soy milk (8 grams)

This adds up to 22 grams. I can boost the protein by adding a scant handful of almonds (6 grams of protein). Even if you don't eat animal products, there's plentiful protein in nuts, dark green leafy vegetables, legumes, lentils and whole grains—all these foods are especially nutritious and tasty—and rich in protein, important nutrients, including fiber, and have wonderful flavor.

ONLINE CALCULATORS

Want a cool tool to determine how many grams of protein will keep you healthy? How many calories do you burn daily (your basil calorie expenditure) and how many should you aim for to lose weight (calories for weight loss)? How many minutes of walking will it take to burn off that extra pat of butter? Online health calculators take your personal information (age, weight, activity level) and displays your unique evaluation. (Online calculators are not a substitute for your physician's advice).

Calorie Control Council:
http://www.caloriecontrol.org

Your Total Health, from iVillage.com:
http://www.ivillage.com/diet/healthcalc

University of Maryland Medical Center:
http://www.umm.edu/healthcalculators

HealthStatus Health Risk Assessments:
  http://www.healthstatus.com/calculators

I was 19 years old when I read a book titled *Diet for a Small Planet (Frances Moore Lappé)* and first realized the connection between the costs of commercial production of meat and poultry and the negative impact on our environment--I was deeply affected by use of important food resources that could be benefiting humans, especially in third-world countries. Factory farms are unnatural—the animals are raised in pens and fattened for slaughter, often fed antibiotics that wind up ingested by humans. Workers too suffer—huge manure lagoons emit noxious gasses; repetitive motion injuries are common in processing plants. It made sense to me to give up meat, and I think that eating "lower on the food chain" and avoiding meat and poultry raised in feedlots makes more sense than ever. What began as a moral and ethical issue became a health issue, too, and by avoiding commercially raised meat and poultry, I lower the risk of consuming antibiotics or growth hormones.

But at 19, I was impatient and careless. Although I was significantly impressed to swear off all meat, poultry and fish, I was also ignorant and immature—and didn't take the time to learn about different grains and sources of amino acids, and I didn't practice the food-combining regimen the author recommended, to consume a sufficient balance of essential amino acids from various plant sources. I did what many people today still do when they decide to "go off" meat. I ate cheese. A LOT of cheese. I ate whole-milk mozzarella cheese in equal amounts to the meat that I had banished from my diet.

In only three months, I had gained 15 pounds, without doing anything else but substituting cheese for meat in every meal.

My good friend writer John McGran once told me about a visit to a famous and venerable pizzeria in Greenwich Village. He decided on a vegetarian slice of pizza, thinking that it would be better than his usual pepperoni. But when it was delivered, he knew he was in trouble.

"It had an inch of white cheese on it," John complained, knowing that he'd been scammed. It was the word *vegetarian* that fooled him—and that's how vegetarian diets can make you fat.

Just because it's vegetarian doesn't make it healthy. Even though it's meat-free, if it's loaded with fatty cheese, then it may be higher in calories and fat than the meat-laden pizza.

Choosing Cheese to Gain Weight

	1 pound broiled Sirloin Steak	1 pound Mozzarella cheese (whole-milk)	1 pound broiled Red Snapper
Calories	1134	1361	547
Fat grams	70	101	8
Saturated fat grams	28	60	2
Cholesterol milligrams	408	368	213
Protein grams	126	100	119

Hands down, fish has the best nutritional profile—with more protein and a fraction of the fat, saturated fat, and cholesterol, as compared with sirloin steak and, especially, cheese.

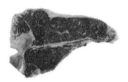 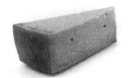 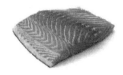

In updated versions of *Diet for a Small Planet,* Lappé' writes that food-combining to achieve a "complete protein" for every meal isn't required, but it is important is to eat a variety of foods—from beans, legumes, nuts, grains, vegetables, fruits, and seeds—over a one to two day period—and that will provide all nutrition necessary for good health.

All these years later, I still like cheese, but I respect it as a source of concentrated calories and practice portion control. A worthwhile indulgence is fresh mozzarella—especially homemade mozzarella—with fresh basil and tomatoes, known in Italian as *insalata caprese.* I love it.

I have never returned to eating red meat. I usually eat fish once or twice weekly and enjoy eggs and egg whites, but I now buy them pastured, and budget for the more expensive eggs. I'll eat turkey at least once a year when I'm at our friend's house for Thanksgiving dinner.

Replacing meat with beans and legumes—not with cheese—will dramatically decrease the amount of saturated fat and cholesterol in the diet, and that's a payoff in a reduction of risk for heart disease, type 2 diabetes, Alzheimer's, and various cancers such as colorectal, prostate, breast, and pancreatic cancer.

If you're going vegetarian, vary your diet and don't eat the same foods day after day—mix it up. Include different grains, nuts, seeds, and legumes so that you get all the important nutrients—vitamins, minerals and antioxidants—you need to keep you healthy.

SUSTAINABLE TABLE

For those who want to continue eating meat, the organization Sustainable Table provides information about health and environmental issues connected to factory farming. The website contains well-researched information about sustainable agriculture, but also provides useful information and realistic behaviors that you can adopt improve your diet, your environment and your community. Their mission is to promote "a way of growing food that is healthy, does not harm the environment, respects workers, is humane to animals, provides a fair wage to the farmer, and supports farming communities. Characteristics of *sustainable* agriculture include: conservation and preservation, biodiversity, animal welfare, economic viability and socially just." To learn more about Sustainable Agriculture, log on to www. sustainabletable.org. To locate markets, stores and restaurants that offer fresh local, sustainable food in the USA and Canada, log on to www.eatwellguide.org.

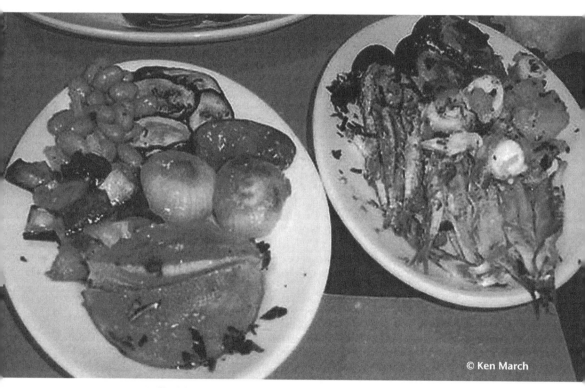

© Ken March

Grilled fish and fresh vegetables, Mediterranean living

Start off by eating less meat—substitute fish a few times a week. Try to vary your fish, however, and avoid fish known to be high in mercury, such as swordfish, king mackerel, and tile fish. Use meat, poultry, and fish more as a condiment, or ingredient, in your diet. I include dairy daily (nonfat or low fat) and eggs, usually a couple of times weekly, for adequate iron, selenium, vitamin B-12, zinc, and calcium.

Soy Sense

Soy foods—not soy isolates or pill supplements—make good nutritional sense. Soybeans contain a complete complement of essential amino acids-- that is, amino acids that humans must get from food in order to synthesize protein. Buy soy that's fortified with calcium and vitamin D, a healthy food that's good for your bones and helps prevent osteoporosis.

Scientists and health professionals emphasize that there are probably hundreds of protective compounds in soy foods, so it's best to enjoy the benefits of soy from food or soy protein powder, not pills. Soy is a good food, but just as no single food causes disease, no one food will cure you.

Vegetarians: Focus on Nutrients

Most people think of vegetarian as someone who eats a plant-based diet. I don't eat meat or poultry, but I do drink milk, and eat fish. A vegan strictly avoids animal products or by-products, including honey (from bees), eggs and milk, or anything made from milk such as cheese, yogurt or other. Vegans also avoid wearing leather, wool, or silk.

A vegetarian may also include:

Lacto-Vegetarian: Lacto (dairy): add dairy

Ovo-Vegetarian: Ovo (eggs): add eggs

Lacto-ovo Vegetarian: Plant-based diet including eggs and dairy

Pesce-Vegetarian: Pesce (fish): add fish

Visit **www.MyPyramid.gov**, and choose the Vegetarian Resources page to learn to eat healthy without eating meat.

Nutrient	Body Needs	Vegetarian Sources	Other Information	Daily Recommendation
Protein: Most people think protein is only found in animal sources, but other foods are rich in essential amino acids, the "building blocks of protein."	Essential for growth, maintenance.	Beans, nuts, peas, and legumes, including soy: tofu, tempeh, and textured vegetable protein.	For Lacto-ovo vegetarians, milk and eggs are good sources of protein.	Most people need about 0.8 grams of protein per kilogram of weight. Multiply your weight in pounds by 0.4 for an approximation. For example, 150 pounds x 0.4 = 60 grams of protein daily.
Iron: Although animal protein is rich in easily absorbable "heme iron," iron is also found in many plant sources.	Necessary for oxygen transport to muscles.	Iron-fortified cereals; spinach and turnip greens; molasses; whole wheat breads; dried apricots; prunes; raisins; black-eyed peas; kidney beans; and lentils.	People at higher risk for iron deficiency anemia include dieters (because of lower calorie intake); pregnant and menstruating women; vegetarians (less iron is absorbed from plant sources compared to meat sources) and frequent blood donors.	Most women need approximately 15 mg of iron daily; men need about 10 mg. Include a source of vitamin C in your meatless meal for better iron absorption: for example, lightly sauté some broccoli rabe and spinach in a tsp. of olive oil in a cast-iron pan and finish with a squeeze of fresh lemon juice.

Nutrient	Body Needs	Vegetarian Sources	Other Information	Daily Recommendation
Calcium: Although many think that dairy is the best source of calcium, many plant and fortified foods are good sources, too.	For strong bones and teeth; may help with weight loss; helps with blood pressure control.	Fortified soy products and soymilk; fortified breakfast cereals; calcium-fortified orange juice; and dark green leafy vegetables (collard greens, turnip greens, bok choy, mustard greens).	Lacto-vegetarians can boost calcium consumption with yogurt and dairy products. Osteoporosis affects more than 44 million men and women and is a silent disease—often, the first sign is fracture. Eating a diet with adequate calcium and doing weight bearing exercises regularly can help ward off osteoporosis.	The National Institute of Health recommends approximately 1000–1500mg daily—more for young teens and older adults.
Zinc: A little is necessary, but more is not better. Animal protein is rich in zinc, but plant foods provide plenty.	Necessary for a healthy immune system; also for cell division and muscle growth and maintenance.	Dried beans including white, kidney, and chickpeas; zinc-fortified breakfast cereals; wheat germ; almonds; pumpkin seeds; and brewer's yeast	Excessive zinc can weaken immunity rather than strengthen it. Lacto-vegetarians : milk and dairy	The Daily Reference Intake for zinc is 8-11mg per day.

Nutrient	Body Needs	Vegetarian Sources	Other Information	Daily Recommendation
Vitamin B12: According to the Vegetarian Resource Group, animals become a source of B12 from eating foods that have been bacterially contaminated with B12; therefore, vegans need to eat B12-fortified plant foods.	Necessary for red blood cell manufacture and maintenance: involved with energy and metabolism.	Fortified breakfast cereals; fortified soy-based beverages; veggie burgers; and nutritional yeast.	Lacto-ovo vegetarians: milk and eggs. With age, there's a decrease in production of a stomach enzyme necessary for B12 absorption from food.	The DRI is 2.6 micrograms (mcg) for women/2.8 for men. Some health experts advise vegans to consider a daily vitamin B12 supplement of 5-10mcg or a weekly vitamin B12 supplement of 2000mcg.

(USDA Center for Nutrition Policy and Promotion n.d.c)
(Vegetarian Resource Group)

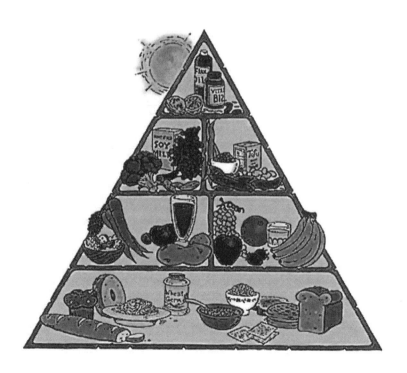

Vegetarian Food Guide Pyramid

Naturally Thin Vegetarian Eating

It's quite simple to stay healthy and meat-free

- **Dairy substitutes:** Find them right next to conventional dairy in your grocer's aisles; natural foods stores and larger chains offer dairy substitutes, including soy milk and soy yogurt. Others: Almond milk; rice milk; oat milk. Read labels and choose low-sugar brands.

- **Plant proteins:** Naturally low in fat and high in fiber: especially dried beans, soybeans, lentils, peas, and brown rice.

- **Grains:** Whole grain pasta, fortified with protein and fiber. Strict vegans: read the label, as some protein-added pasta is fortified with eggs.

- **Pairings:** Pasta with legumes provides enhanced protein complement: add a can of chickpeas or black beans (drained) to drained pasta, then some virgin olive oil and fresh or dried herbs.

- **Nuts and Seeds:** Add raw or roasted walnuts, pine nuts, and sunflower and sesame seeds to mixed grain casseroles, salads, and cereals to boost protein and fiber and to add texture and crunch.

- **"Meat":** Vegetarian meat substitutes such as veggie burgers, tofu hot dogs, and "meat crumbles" are OK—occasionally, but they are often loaded with sodium. Read labels and avoid HVP, or hydrolyzed vegetable protein, which contains a lot of monosodium glutamate (MSG). The FDA's position on MSG is that it's safe, with caveats that some people may be sensitive to it and suffer headaches, chest pain, nausea, and other "MSG Syndrome" symptoms. The Food and Drug Administration requires that labels list MSG in its "pure" form, but not when it is an ingredient in other ingredients, such as hydrolyzed protein. I rarely eat processed foods because they are likely to contain MSG (unless they are labeled "does not contain MSG").

- **Tofu:** Comes in different textures for use in different menus and recipes. I like firm for stir-fry dishes, silken for cream-cheese substitute and dips, and extra firm for grilling.

- **Tempeh:** Versatile and meat-like, tempeh is a chewy cultured soybean cake. Grill kabobs: thread marinated (light soy sauce; lemon juice and a little olive oil) chunks of tempeh and vegetables on skewers .

- **Bean burgers:** High in protein and fiber, veggie burgers are generally low in saturated fat and cholesterol (read labels).

- **Cheese substitutes**: Vegans should read labels. *Casein* and *rennin* are coagulants made from dairy.

My Favorite Foods
The Beauty of the Mediterranean

Fresh fish from the sea, olive oil, pasta, cous cous, and some local wine with dinner—when I *think* Mediterranean I just *feel* better. Unfortunately, like so many European Union countries who have adopted unhealthy behaviors, the countries bordering the Mediterranean don't adhere to their traditionally healthy foods or portions, but we can try! I love all the foods from that region—the way they're cooked, the freshness and flavor of the foods. The traditional Mediterranean eating plan focuses on healthy fats from olives and olive oil, fatty fish, and nuts and seeds. You won't find white flour, white rice, or refined carbohydrates—instead, the menu includes unprocessed, fiber-rich foods, including fruits and vegetables of all kinds.

Unlike calorie-restricted or nutrient-specific diets, the Mediterranean Diet promotes healthy immunity and may lower risk for inflammation and heart disease, and deliciously features monounsaturated fats and omega-3 fatty acids from olive oil, nuts, seeds and fatty fish and eschews refined carbohydrates and processed and fast food. In a Mediterranean-type meal plan, red meat is eaten occasionally, but the portion size is much smaller than what Americans typically consider a "small" steak (which is usually seven or eight ounces, at least 56 grams of protein, plus at least 10 grams of saturated fat and 135 milligrams of dietary cholesterol!). Enjoy eggs, and dairy including whole milk goat's or sheep cheese or yogurt—also lower calorie 1% or nonfat dairy.

As with all meal plans, pay attention to portion size, because calories count—even "good" calories. Since the traditional Mediterranean diet plan includes foods naturally high in fat, learn the portion size that best fits your menu and needs. For example, olive oil, with its favorable ratio of "good" monounsaturated fat to "bad" unsaturated fat, is certainly heart-healthy but will not, in itself, prevent disease. A single food won't kill you nor cure you, and habitually dipping bread into oil just adds hundreds of calories to your diet.

A Mediterranean *lifestyle* means enjoying delicious meals with friends and relatives, staying active, not smoking (Even Italy and France have banned smoking—we're waiting on Greece!), and reducing stress.

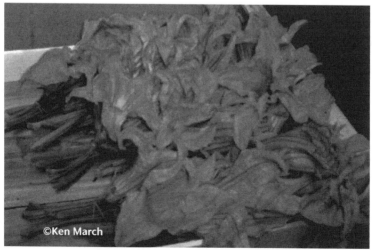
©Ken March

Squash blossoms - Italian market

The Oldways Mediterranean Diet Pyramid[2]

Log on to Oldways, a nonprofit advocates for the "gold standard" in nutrition and health programs, the science and culture of healthy lifestyle, sustainable food choices, and preservation of traditional foods. **www.oldwayspt.org**

They created the Mediterranean Diet Pyramid as a response to the prevalence of 'no fat' diets in the early 90's. Instead of "no-fat" diets, the Mediterranean Diet Pyramid graphically depicts a delicious, plant-based diet, including "good" fats from mono and polyunsaturated oils, such as olive oil, nuts and seeds, fatty fish and avocado. The aim of Oldways is to promote foods that are satisfying—and includes promoting a healthy lifestyle, sharing food socially, while respecting your body and your environment. Oldways says, *"eating healthy is about management, not banishment"*.

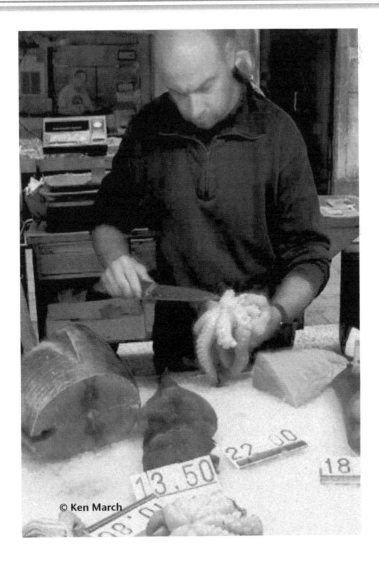

© Ken March

Mercury

In terms of mercury content, here are the best fish—and worst fish—to eat, according to the Environmental Protection Agency (EPA). In addition, the EPA recommends not eating Chilean Sea bass, Bluefin tuna, and Grouper due to over-fishing—an environmental hazard in itself. Local fisheries may be contaminated with mercury, PCBs, and other chemicals—so, it's important to check with your local health department before eating any fish caught locally.

BEST	WORST
Salmon: wild (Alaska), canned pink sockeye	**King mackerel**
Mahi Mahi	**Salmon** (farmed—negative ecological impact)
Sardines	**Shrimp and prawns** (imported from Southeast Asia and Latin America)
Mussels, oysters, and clams (U.S. farmed)	**Shark**
Mackerel (Atlantic)	**Tilefish**
Sablefish/black cod (Alaska)	**Swordfish**
Shrimp: farmed (U.S.); northern (Canada)	**Canned albacore tuna**
Anchovies	**Locally-caught fish,** unless first checking with the local authorities: go to **www.epa.gov**
Pacific Halibut	**http://www.epa.gov/ waterscience/fish**: click on "advisory report" and then your state to see all advisories[3]

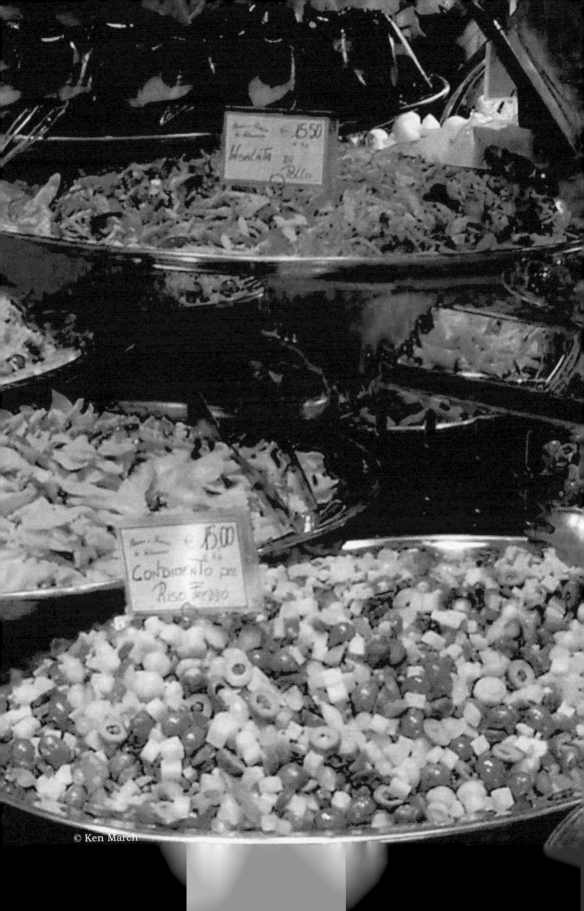

Chapter 7

Your Naturally Thin Diet
Make Smart Eating Second Nature

Success is nothing more than a few simple disciplines, practiced every day,
while failure is simply a few errors in judgment, repeated every day.
—Jim Rohn

I like to think about words and how they change over time. The word *diet* used to provoke fear and loathing—to me, *diet* meant hunger, deprivation, boredom, and failure. Today, I define *diet* differently; I focus on *eating*, not *dieting*.

The true meaning of the word *diet* is quite different than how most people use the word in everyday language. People commonly use *diet* as a verb—an action word—as in "to diet" or to "go on a weight loss diet."

I dug a little deeper, sought out the dictionary definition, and discovered that the Latin root of *diet* is from the Greek *diaita*; to live one's life.

I like that! To live! The Greeks had it right—what you choose to nourish your body with, *your natural diet*, is what gives you life. Your diet gives you health.

DEFINITION

Diet

—adjective

1. Having relatively few calories; "diet cola"; "light (or lite) beer"; "lite (or light) mayonnaise"; "a low-cal diet."

—noun

1. The usual food and drink consumed
2. The act of restricting your food intake (or your intake of particular foods)

—verb

1. To follow a specific eating plan, as for health reasons.
2. To eat sparingly, for health reasons or to lose weight.

Old days, Bad ways

Do you think of *diet* as a verb? The definition, *the act of restricting your food intake (or your intake of particular food),* translates to what most people think the word "diet" signifies—something you "go on"—namely, a weight loss diet—when you take in fewer calories than you normally do by eating *differently* from your *usual diet.*

Most would think that "going on" a *diet* means changing what you *usually* eat to a prescribed meal plan.

That's not necessarily a bad thing—especially at the beginning, when you're in "weight loss mode" and learning about food. Especially when, perhaps like I used to do, you eat without thinking, and you're overeating constantly. A structured weight loss plan worked for me: I used a portion-controlled program, learned to reduce my calories by making better choices, lost weight, and learned that by making better everyday choices I could keep the weight off. I kept it off for about five years by continuing to exercise, but then I began to backslide, and using the social excuses so common to newlyweds (married for the first time)—eating out often, entertaining—and I found myself up about 10 pounds. Hmm...I had slipped back into portion distortion. I was living in Manhattan and working in Queens, New York, and each neighborhood's Italian restaurants are fabulous. I was loving my pasta—far too much!

Although I'd learned that all calories count, I had stopped paying attention to portion size. Although I wasn't eating "bad" food—I still avoided fried foods and rarely ate desserts—I was eating larger portions than I could handle and had to get back to basics. I *knew* what worked—I had to eat less pasta and more crunchy vegetables—I had to replace those "calorie-dense" foods with high fiber, "low energy-density" foods. I upped my activity—I walked for an hour every morning and went to the gym at least three times a week, and I gradually got back to my comfortable size.

I can attest to this—after the "diet" it's time to "live it." If you "go off" that weight loss diet and return to the habits that made you fat to begin with—well—most likely you will return to the pre-weight-loss-diet weight. Most dieters know this—they know that studies show that they will likely lose from five to ten percent of their body weight on a weight loss diet, then gain it back (plus more!)[1].

Instead of dieting, I changed the way I live. I associate the word *diet* with what I usually eat, not as a prescribed eating plan to lose weight. That works! I can remain thin *naturally* by changing my thinking and my choices.

Now, that doesn't mean I stay exactly at the same weight every day—day after day. No. There are leaner months and fatter months, depending on what type of social activities are going on and how much activity I've been doing. Sometimes I'm experimenting with new pizza recipes, and I hit on one that's especially good. I know I shouldn't eat that third slice, but I can't resist my own homemade pizza! So, if my jeans get too tight, it's back on the road, adding 15 minutes of aerobic activity every day to my usual 40-50 minutes—and I can lose the extra couple of pounds in a couple of weeks just by making modifications to *my* diet, not going on someone else's diet.

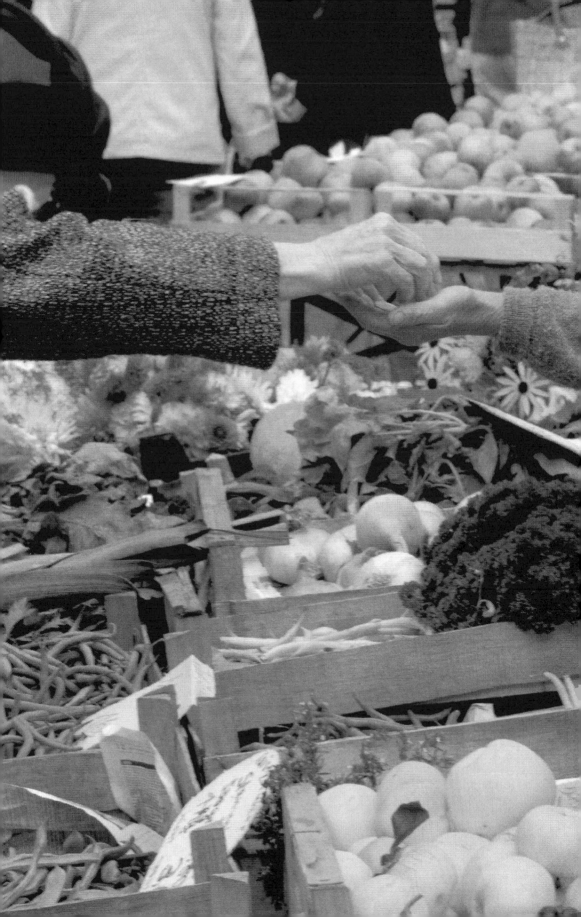

My Food Buckets

Counting portions is now something I do mentally as I go throughout my day. I read labels to learn about foods—but don't count every calorie. I mentally tally my portions—if I haven't had two fruits by mid-afternoon, I'll opt for a piece of fruit as a snack or dessert. If I've already had four servings of cereal/bread by dinner, then I'll opt for a bigger salad or cup of cooked vegetables and skip the starch.

Here's how I do it. I know what I'm supposed to be eating daily to maintain good health, and I mentally organize my planned foods into different "buckets."

Fruit Bucket: Two to three servings of whole fruit like berries, melon, and small pieces of fruit: I don't use juice because it's too easy going down (just a half-cup counts as one whole fruit, and has no fiber to fill you up)

Dairy Bucket: Two to three single-cup servings (I like nonfat milk and yogurt)

Protein Bucket: About six or seven ounces: usually fish, low fat cheese, tofu, or eggs

Starch Bucket: About six servings of whole grain cereal, bread, crackers, and starchy veggies. Fat Bucket: About two or three servings—a handful of nuts; a couple of tablespoons of olive oil or avocado on my salad

Vegetable Bucket: Full! I don't put a limit on crunchy vegetables, such as carrots, broccoli, and squash.

"Treats" Bucket: A glass of wine, some olive oil and some nuts.

Each day, I automatically think about what I will eat that day *before* I eat it. Hmm...how many servings of starch do I need today? Ah...yes...for weight maintenance, I need about six servings. I want cereal for breakfast (OK, I put cereal into the bucket), and that leaves me with five more. I put a cup of milk into my dairy bucket (OK, that leaves me with one or two more). I have a cup of berries (that goes into my fruit bucket) and think, I have two more to go! I may get hungry for a snack at about 10:00 a.m. (OK, I'll grab that other fruit—one apple or orange. Maybe I'll have a handful of almonds, too (as a snack, they go into the fat bucket). Lunch may be a big salad with a small, 3.5 ounce can of salmon (that goes into the protein bucket). Suppose I want pizza for dinner—then I'll skip bread for lunch and have two or three small slices of my homemade pizza. I visualize two more servings of starch in my bucket, the cheese goes into the fat, the shrimp goes into the protein bucket, and the wine goes into the treats bucket.

I'm not counting calories—I'm counting down portions, and try to fill each food-type bucket with what I need. At the end of the day, I usually get it right.

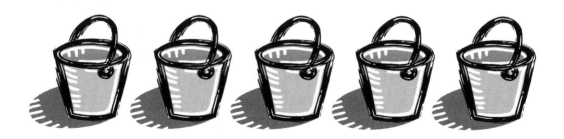

Naturally Thin vs. Dieting

Before you go on a weight loss diet, be prepared to adopt a *naturally thin* lifestyle

Take this survey to assess your eating style:

1	How often do you eat out? a. Occasionally—I usually cook for myself and my family b. More than once a week c. At least once day d. More than once a day e. Never	6	When do you eat? a. Usually when I'm hungry, and I try to stop when I'm full b. When it's time to eat c. When I'm depressed, anxious, or tired d. When my spouse, friend, or someone else urges me to	
2	Do you order food in? a. Never—I can make it faster and better than the delivered stuff b. Only occasionally—sometimes I'm caught unprepared c. At least once a week—I look forward to delivery service d. At least once a day e. More than once a day	7	How much activity do you usually do? a. At least 30 minutes or more of deliberate activity every day b. I walk the dog—sometimes c. I'm a weekend-warrior, but not every weekend d. I'm not active right now	
3	Do you eat deep-fried fast food? a. Never b. Only occasionally c. At least once a week d. At least once a day e. More than once a day	8	How many fruits do you usually eat daily? a. At least two or three—always one or two with breakfast, then one as a snack or dessert b. One or two, usually c. One at most d. Sometimes none	
4	Do you eat breakfast? a. Every day—I eat high fiber, low sugar cereal; nonfat milk; fresh or frozen fruit; and sometimes nonfat plain or flavored sugar-free yogurt b. Most days—but not always c. Only occasionally—sometimes I grab a muffin or bagel d. Never—I either skip breakfast or just have a cup of coffee	9	How many servings of vegetables do you usually eat daily? a. Always at least three or four—I try to have a salad with dinner, add lettuce and tomato to any wrap or sandwich, and snack on veggies b. At least one or two, usually c. One at most d. Sometimes none	
5	Do you buy lunch during the work week? a. Almost never—I usually pack my lunch b. A couple of times weekly c. Once a week d. Every day	10	Do you think you can go off your diet after you lose weight? a. I think my diet is the way I eat—I eat to live, and enjoy a variety of foods, but sometimes I have to watch it! b. I go on a diet every few months, because I find the weight comes back c. I'm getting ready to go on a diet—I just haven't found the right one yet	

What Did You Answer?

As you probably guessed, choosing the first answer "a" for each of the questions shows you have a *naturally thin* lifestyle. These choices have become *second nature* to me—and I can eat whatever I like, but I discriminate. I have developed a taste for whole foods, and my palate rejects greasy, fried foods loaded with sodium or artificially sweetened, overly sweet foods. I don't let life get in the way of activity—it's critical, since I will regain just as quickly as the next person if I don't burn calories consistently. I save calories, boost nutrition and bank the dollars that I'd spend dining out too frequently, and since I happen to like remaining thin—these behaviors work perfectly.

Prioritizing Your Life

I was sitting in a restaurant with my old friend, "Alicia." As we sat down, she stated that she was heavier than she'd been since her college days...the days when she used to "party" a lot and drink a lot of beer. Those days were long gone, but although Alicia wasn't eating more than usual, her life had changed. She said that she wanted to lose weight, but she didn't have time for much of anything except work and commuting—she felt like she was busier than ever, but she was also more sedentary. Her full-time job (that began at 7:30 in the morning) required her to get started at 5:30 a.m. with a traffic-snarled commute, and said that just sitting in the car stressed her out. Her weekend seemed devoted to housecleaning. So her time was not her own, and she was challenged! As she reached for the second pat of butter on her bread, I suggested she could start by not putting butter on her bread, because each pat of butter adds up so quickly, pointing out that she'd just added 200 calories without even thinking about it.

She said, "But I like it."

I realized that she was *not* in "preparation" stage. Maybe she was contemplating change, but she wasn't ready to change. I decided to mirror her concerns and agreed. "Yes, butter tastes so good and it's so easy to get used to eating it, without realizing how quickly it adds calories to your day."

YOUR Guide to Naturally Thin

Let's Get Started

When I was overweight, I tried a number of different plans, and guess what? They all worked—temporarily. But since I was using someone else's diet to lose weight, as soon as I went off the program, I regained the weight—and sometimes more than I had lost.

Going on a diet doesn't have to mean avoiding one food group entirely—or eating foods in prescribed combinations. But it does mean changing from what you usually eat to eating differently.

One of the most common misconceptions associated with dieting is that doing something short-term will have long-term results. Unfortunately, without permanent lifestyle change, going on diets means weight loss is temporary, and most people regain all the weight they lost within a few years. Even gastric bypass surgery isn't a guarantee of permanent weight loss. Evidence shows that, after a few years, many patients begin to regain.

I was ready to make significant changes in my diet and lifestyle, and I lost the weight and have kept it off for more than 25 years.

The Best Diet is *Your* Diet

What worked for me was simplicity and structure. I worked with my weight loss counselor to determine how many calories I needed for weight loss, and then I started to learn about food. This proved very important—as I learned about food, I began to respect it more. I learned how to translate a "menu" into actual food choices—I learned that I was eating many more calories than I realized. For instance, when I poured a bowl of cereal, I was serving myself more than two cups, and I at the same time, I poured at least two cups of milk on top of my cereal. That glass of juice? It was a big tumbler, and when I poured it back into the measuring cup to see what I was drinking, I was surprised to see that I usually drank about 12 ounces—three servings of juice! Weighing and measuring what *I usually* ate was certainly a revelation—without it, I would have never known how much I was overeating.

Track your usual diet for the first week and then you can make adjustments where they are needed. Then, you may want to try pre-planned menus—I think that they are very helpful, especially at the start. My motto is, "Prepare to succeed." When you know in advance what you can eat—and follow your plan—you don't end up stuck in front of a vending machine late in the afternoon, famished, with chips or candy bars your only choices.

Know Your Portions, and Stay on Track to Permanent Weight Control

There is no single diet plan that's right for everyone, and that's why *your diet* should consist of the foods that you prefer most. Don't forget to respect your preferred eating pattern. If you absolutely hate to eat first thing in the morning, then don't feel forced to eat "breakfast," instead try a mid-morning snack and use your portion guide to strategize your personal plan. As far as nutrient percentages, it should be flexible. A low carb approach makes sense for people who feel more satisfied with lean meat and poultry. However, some feel deprived if they can't eat pasta every once in a while; if they choose a strict low-carb meal plan, it will backfire. It's also fine to use meal replacements—they are proven to work, and help take the stress out of planning. Portion-controlled meal plans are smart strategies for those who don't have the desire, time, or inclination to cook, or for those who may do well with structure and convenience. Some products are better, healthier choices than others: watch the sodium in frozen entrees—aim for 800 milligrams of sodium or less per serving. You can switch from convenience meals to recipes, as long as your portions are consistent. And if your budget can handle meal delivery, there are many options that can work well—just remember that once you lose the weight you want, it's still important to maintain portion control.

And pay attention to what is happening to your body. For example, if you choose a 1200 calorie portion plan and you lose more than two or three pounds a week, you're likely not eating enough to fuel your body, and you need to adjust the portions upward. A "weight loss diet" is, by definition, not set in stone. It has to be fluid, and you can adjust the portions if you need more fuel and still continue to lose weight gradually without compromising your nutrition and your energy.

Lifestyle and Experience

I lost weight by a combination of eating *more* foods that didn't contain a lot of calories and making high calorie foods an occasional treat. When I was overweight, I had no idea that I was eating so many calories for breakfast, and just by changing that meal, I started to tip the scale in my favor.

With a little effort, you can eat healthfully without spending a lot of time. The secret is in simplicity, and buying in bulk when possible. When I was "in weight loss mode" I set aside an hour on late Sunday afternoons to prep my dinners for the week. Wrap chicken breasts or turkey cutlets—topped with fresh lemon slices, a dash of herbal seasonings, and a splash of teriyaki sauce—in plastic wrap or foil, and freeze. For dinner, just unwrap and pop into a pyrex dish, and microwave for a few minutes. Take advantage of pre-washed, pre-cut vegetables and salads—another quick favorite is salad with canned sardines or salmon, with low calorie salad dressing such as Walden Farms'. Try quick-cooking brown rice and cous cous with some grilled chicken, or microwave a sweet potato and stuff it with a mixture of low fat cottage cheese and diced tomatoes or tomato salsa.

One of the most common complaints about diets is that diet food is boring. The solution is to never "diet" again! Instead, enjoy your usual recipes and cut the fat and sugar without sacrificing flavor. Cut the calories consistently, and you can maintain your weight without trying. Tell your family and friends that you are shopping and cooking smart. Instead of full-fat mayonnaise, reach for fat-free or light; nonfat or 1% milk is what's in your refrigerator; you buy low fat and nonfat salad dressings, and you pack a lunch most of the time.

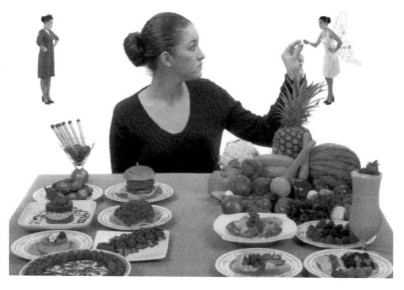

How To Make It Better, Naturally

Cooking is really not difficult, but being prepared makes it easier to make it right.

- **Unleash Your Inner Artist**: Cooking can be a relaxing outlet for your creative talents. Planning a menu and bringing it to the table brings a feeling of accomplishment, a truly artistic endeavor. Invite your neighbors, family and friends to share.

- **Nonstick:** Stock up on nonstick pans for baking, grilling, sautéing—even for soup. Nonstick is one of life's little pleasures—no oil means naturally fewer calories—don't skimp on flavor by using use a little cooking spray, or wine, water, or juice to start the cooking process.

- **Method:** Bake, broil, grill, poach, or sauté foods instead of deep-frying. Check out the "Better-Than-Fried Chicken" recipe below…you will be amazed by the flavor.

- **Reduce:** Simply reduce the amount of fat and/or sugar in your recipes. For example, replace half the oil with applesauce or fruit puree for an equally moist muffin or cake; use one-third less sugar in cakes or cookies and use dried fruit in place of sugar, and sweeten naturally. Experiment with sucralose (Splenda) for baking: Try some of the excellent sugar-free syrups and low-calorie pudding mixes.

- **Baste:** Instead of basting the turkey with butter or margarine, cut the saturated and (especially) trans fat by basting with flavorful vegetable broth, white wine, or orange juice (my personal favorite!).

- **Lean:** Buy the leanest cuts of meat and trim all visible fat before cooking. Buy ground meat 95% lean. Try turkey burgers for a change, or replace a third of your ground beef with ground turkey breast, not just "ground turkey" which is usually fairly high in saturated fat, similar to ground beef, because it contains turkey skin and dark meat.

- **Dairy:** Whole milk contains 1 gram of saturated fat per ounce. Pediatricians recommend switching normal-growth kids to 1% or nonfat dairy by age two (lower in saturated fat and cholesterol compared to whole milk). Buy low-fat or nonfat milk, sour cream, yogurt, and cheese. Low-fat buttermilk makes a good substitute for whole milk in many of your favorite recipes. Nonfat evaporated milk has a "creamy" consistency and substitutes well in sauces, pies, ice cream, and, of course, in tea and coffee. Choose evaporated milk instead of condensed milk, which is heavily sweetened with sugar.

- **Eggs:** Substitute two egg whites for one whole egg and reduce fat, cholesterol, and calories

- **Crumbs:** Instead of commercial bread crumbs—usually full of oil and trans fat—use crunchy, lower-sugar breakfast cereal such as a 'nugget' cereal or Nature's Path FlaxPlus Flakes as the coating for fish or chicken (dip into a mixture of egg whites and low-fat buttermilk.)

- **Cut:** The average American suffers from "portion distortion." Bigger doesn't mean better, it just means more calories than you need! Use smaller plates and bowls—slice that cake to serve 12 instead of eight.

Let's Start with the Top Things to Know About Choosing a Smart Diet

Here are some ideas that will help you learn what *you* need in order to lose, maintain, or even gain weight. Choose one that suits your lifestyle and food preferences.

1. **Food Preferences**: Choose a program that features the foods you enjoy. If you feel deprived, you won't stick with it over the long haul. It's all about modification. If you love cereal and grains, a low carb approach is not the best way to get started on your weight loss program. Portion control is the secret to weight loss and maintenance.

2. **Adequate calories:** Most women need a minimum of 1300-1400 calories—and men approximately 1600—just to cover their basic metabolic functions, and more when you incorporate more activity and muscle building exercises. Avoid very low calorie diets...you may experience quick weight loss, but experts say that the quicker you lose it, the quicker you put it back on. Slow, gradual weight reduction—about one to two pounds a week—is likely to be permanent.

3. **Fads:** Avoid programs that require eating certain foods with other foods, such as, "Only eat fruit after meals, never with protein," or other such unscientific recommendations. Very low carb diets produce quick and dramatic weight loss, but, for example, the Atkins program asks you to consistently change from very low carb to a more balanced plan and are not meant to be that low carb permanently. If you choose a "branded" diet, *read the book* and follow the instructions. Eating a variety of foods is the *natural* way to permanent weight loss.

4. **Meal patterns and mealtimes:** How do *you* like to eat? I prefer to eat every few hours, because I don't like a large meal mid-day. I prefer a smaller lunch with a snack a couple of hours later; that way, I am not famished, and it's easier to control my portions when I eat dinner with my husband. I always eat a small breakfast. I like a cup of cereal and milk, then a snack of some nuts and fruit or a nonfat yogurt at about 10:00 a.m. when my energy levels are low.

5. **Preparation:** Dieting is hard enough. Don't choose a recipe plan if you don't have time to cook. The right plan suits your lifestyle. Meal replacements are ideal for portion control, and many successful weight maintainers use them consistently. Use quick cereals, individual portions of yogurt, and frozen entrees—they're balanced and nutritious and don't require too much planning or prep.

6. **Balanced nutrition:** Choose a program that includes a variety of foods so you don't become bored and lose your motivation to continue. High fiber vegetables, whole grains, lean protein, and healthy, monounsaturated fat (from olive oil and fatty fish) are the ingredients of a healthy diet that you can maintain permanently.

7. **Budget:** An important consideration, because some plans are very economical and others are more expensive to maintain. The most flexible and frugal is the recipe-type plan. Learn all you can about nutrition and replace any item in your menu with one that's on sale. Economize by purchasing large-sized portions of fish, vegetables, chicken, or fruit. Pre-portioned prepared foods are more expensive, but for some, it's worth the price to enjoy the convenience and portion control.

8. **Support:** Support helps keep you on track and motivates you to reach your weight goal. Commit to meeting with an expert, a coach, a group, or a friend—especially at the beginning of your behavioral change. Support may be face-to-face, or sign up for a free or fee-based online program. It's BEST to commit to a scheduled meeting time or, better yet, a program that lasts at least 12 weeks with a continuing maintenance program. A face-to-face consultation with a registered dietitian who will stay in touch by phone or email is the best game plan.

9. **Maintenance:** Once you're at your goal, it's ideal to stay with the program you used for a year, modifying it to add variety so you may fully adopt your new healthy behaviors. The best program transitions to a maintenance program once you reach your weight goal.

Living It Every Day

I think that people automatically assume that I am 'naturally thin', but I watch what I eat and incorporate exercise into my day -- every day! If I didn't do both of those things, I would definitely have a "weight problem." Maybe there are some people who are "naturally thin," for whom the scale doesn't budge no matter what they eat and whether or not they exercise. I exercise every day, walking around the block or going to the park with my husband, a terrific way to catch up with the other on the day's events. Most days I also hit the treadmill or lift light weights. I can't say I really like strenuous exercise, but I always feel so much better afterwards. The exercise 'high' keeps me going and allows for some indulgence in my weakness, sweets. On a daily basis, I satisfy carbohydrate cravings with whole grain cold cereal with soy milk, raisins, and nuts (thanks, Trader Joe's), and often add carob powder. On the weekend, my husband and I often share a "real" dessert at a restaurant. I "got" early on that depriving myself of foods I like would only backfire. Fortunately, I genuinely enjoy many healthful foods -- fruits and vegetables, whole grains, and fish. My balancing act of exercise, judicious (though enjoyable, for me) eating, with occasional splurges, is comfortable and has enabled me to stay within a five- to eight-pound healthy weight range for decades.

**Erica Bohm, M.S. - Vice President and Director
of Strategic Partnerships,
HealthyDiningFinder.com**

What Are YOUR Needs?

Your current weight, your age, your body type, your daily activity, and your goals all influence your unique calorie needs.

This is a guide—a starting off position—to structure your meals and make it simple. Eating *naturally* means creating *your natural diet* using the guide to healthy eating. It's not *a diet* in the sense of a temporary fix for weight loss. It's a guide to healthy eating and to eating well *naturally*.

By learning all you can about food and approximate calories per serving, it's easier to make smart choices wherever you go. I started by eating about 1600 calories daily and completing at least an hour of aerobic activity. As you become more fit and, perhaps, challenge yourself by joining a karate class or biking tour, you'll pay attention to healthy snacking—so you can fuel your fitness!

Set a lifetime goal for daily walking, plus at least three days a week where you exert extra effort; for example, join a dance class, or self-defense, or roller-blade for 30 minutes, or use a DVD in your own home.

When eating for weight loss, it's important to include all the nutrients necessary for good health and fitness—"dieting" needn't mean losing energy. Even if you are small in stature, your body needs calories, especially when you're burning calories with exercise—you can't run on "empty". Your body needs clean fuel to run efficiently, and think of junk food as "dirty fuel" that gunks up your engine. Fill up on crunchy vegetables and lots of water—if you're not used to eating a lot of fibrous foods, start with two cups daily and then add more. Don't worry—your system will gradually get used to the fiber.

If you're losing more than two pounds a week or if you're hungry, add healthy 100-calorie snacks, such as two cups of baby carrots with some nonfat salsa, or a large apple with a 1/2 cup of nonfat yogurt—if you wish, add a drop of vanilla and a packet of no-calorie sweetener or teaspoon of honey (24 calories). Eating too few calories can backfire and slow or even stop weight loss. If you're exercising more than an hour a day and you're not losing weight, gradually increase your protein or legumes by about 100 calories per day (an additional one to two ounces of lean protein or ½ cup of dried beans/legumes).

The same holds true once you reach a point that you want to maintain. Naturally thin eating means allowing for variety in your diet, and as long as you understand your approximate portion needs, you can choose more freely.

Dieting Online—Personalizing a Meal Plan

When I joined the online weight loss company eDiets.com in January 2000, I remember "googling" the word *diet* and getting nine million hits—astounding to me then, but almost inconsequential today when more than a billion people worldwide use the Internet. I recently repeated that experiment, and this time, *diet* revealed more than 330 million hits.

I learned a lot about different diets while leading development of eDiets.com's weight management plans. In my first year with eDiets, there was only one basic meal plan and seven years later, we had more than 22 programs. We digitized some of the best—and some of the most controversial—diets. "Members" self-reported success on all of the diets offered, including our Heart Smart, Living with Diabetes, Mediterranean, Glycemic Impact, Low Fat, Lactose-Free, and Vegetarian and on all the branded diets, including the Atkins, Zone, Perricone, and others.

Choose from dozens—maybe hundreds—of online diet programs. The best ones come with a variety of online "eTools" to quickly assess and personalize your program to your unique food and lifestyle preferences. Online food databases make it easy to track your meals and number of calories you burn, and

You can't 'click' away the weight--but online is a great place for information and support.

with a "click" you can produce graphs and reports and see your progress. Costs range from free websites to more pricey customized programs with professional coaching and expert advice.

Online may be effective for exactly the reasons you'd expect—certainly for accessibility and convenience, and for some the anonymity is attractive—they'd rather go online rather than show up for a face-to-face meeting, however, the most often-heard criticism is that accountability is missing with the online model.

It's certainly true that many people who go online for a diet are similar to those who buy diet books without thinking about the process of change. Yes, they want to lose weight! And, with the best intentions, they purchase that diet book, or they type "diet" into their web browser and click on a website and key in their credit card.

But, do they return to the website and start using the calculators—do they read the articles or take the eating evaluation? Just like people who buy diet books, many never get past the first chapter. Even if their credit card is charged monthly, they may never return. Maybe they're having a "click" moment—similar to impulse buying. Maybe they have moved from contemplation to preparation—but the "click" to join doesn't mean they are ready to do the work. Not necessarily.

Programs That Work—But You Have To USE It—to LOSE It

A structured program is helpful because by following it, you learn what you need to eat to lose weight, and how to modify it when you want to maintain your weight loss. First learn about what you're eating—practice label reading; know what a portion of fish, or cereal or a glass of wine looks like, and the calories behind the portion.

The best weight loss programs focus on behavioral change, provide accountability, ideally last at least six months, and usually involve weekly visits—either to a clinic or a registered dietitian.

Program components should include:

Self monitoring: The act of writing down or logging your diet, activities and thoughts about your progress helps you stay aware—and pinpoint any areas where you may be having difficulties to plan for change. You can share your logs with your diet coach, either face-to-face or online. Learn about calories in food and how your activities burn calories by logging on to a web-based program.

Cognitive restructuring: Dump "negative self-talk"—instead of striving for "skinny" or a certain number on the scale, strive for following the program, and improving your weight and fitness. Replace with positive affirmations, such as "I will walk every day for 30 minutes and stretch afterwards" or "when I go out to eat, I'll order grilled, baked or broiled, and not fried food." Abandon the "all or nothing" attitude that gets in the way of healthy lifestyles, and refocus from "weight" to "living well."

Stimulus Control: So, do you find yourself in front of the vending machine when you get hungry in the afternoon? Bring that healthy snack with you, and put the change in a jar on your desk where you can see it fill up, evidence of your new behaviors. Do you put off exercise until after work, but never seem to get to it? Schedule activity earlier in the day, and log it.

Stress management and problem solving: You dread going to that barbeque—you always overeat. Or you have a big presentation due, and you have to work overtime and always overeat when you're tired. What really works is to plan in advance what you're going to eat—have a healthy snack before you go; be prepared to stay fueled over that long workday keeps you motivated. Controlling stress can help control weight, especially when overeating is used to assuage a stressful situation.

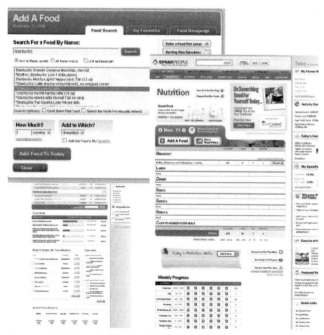

Log your foods, activities, and create your own logs and reports.
(www.sparkpeople.com)

Physical activity: It's important to start slowly, and enjoy your activities—that's what is going to keep you on track to permanent weight control. Choose activities you enjoy! "Exercise" means doing anything that gets your heart rate up—including dancing, or biking or just walking—briskly.

Relapse prevention: have strategies in place to prevent weight gain—if you regain a few pounds, then returning to a structured menu and increasing your activities[2].

Online may be a good solution for those who find the "gold standard" face-to-face programs out of reach financially and/ or geographically. A program that replicates a meeting room

GO ONLINE FOR CONTROL

Online programs are ideal for time-challenged consumers who appreciate the convenience, personalization, and economy of the Internet. And the online tools offer a lot of information—just by logging your foods you can learn a lot about your usual diet, and what changes you can make to improve your habits. Most importantly, get support online. Join a meeting, log on to a chat (sign up for a membership with a monitored website).

- Create your own meal plans by entering everything you eat and drink into an online food database. Then you can "click" to see what you're eating and "click" again to see what happens if you substitute better choices.

- Some make specific suggestions—instead of this food, try that food—to lower calories, grams of fat, or sugar.

- Assess your current weight and find how many calories you need for weight loss, then your personalized menu translates calories into portions per meal

- Get a meal plan with recipes for one—or for two or more

- Buy a food delivery service and have a portion-controlled meal plan sent to your home.

- Choose an online program that provides a printable shopping list listing everything you need to buy

- for a week's worth of meals. View online cooking demonstrations...not only will you learn, but be prepared to be entertained!

- Get a fitness plan: view videos and learn proper techniques

- Get a buddy, get involved with a "challenge" to drink water, eat healthfully, step daily, log weight lost

online and holds scheduled online meetings weekly does better than a program that's strictly self-help[3].

Having someone or something responding intelligently to your concerns or successes may help make permanent the new thoughts and behaviors you're incorporating into your lifestyle[4]. Online programs that use targeted email to enhance their diet plan increase the likelihood of successful weight loss and maintenance[5]. Other subscription-based programs offer more comprehensive structure, and personalized support such as dietitians or personal trainers

If you don't have the financial or time resources to work one-on-one with a registered dietitian, or join a commercial weight loss program, there are other options for learning your nutritional needs for weight loss. You can use the guide I have provided or log on to one of the free online programs that I've referenced in the Resources section. Web-sites such as www.MyPyramid.gov, www.SparkPeople.com, or www.FitDay.com are examples of free programs that make online food tracking a lot of fun.

If It Costs More, Will You Use It?

Some people are motivated to log on more frequently or be sure to return to the nutritionist if they make a financial investment. Online is the same. If you don't use it, it won't work. If you join a program and that's where it ends, don't be surprised if the scale doesn't move.

Online programs offer opportunities for people stay connected in a safe and monitored environment, for example, SparkPeople's community boards and "SparkTeams". Connect with someone or a team to identify goals for change, and celebrate achievements together. Of course, to thine ownself be true, and if you feel that "free" isn't going to bring you back as consistently, then invest in a program that connects you with a registered dietitian or fitness expert. If you're so motivated, bank the dollars and reward yourself with a living thin naturally treadmill or fitness vacation.

Track It!

Whether you're trying to lose weight or just improve the way you eat, it's going to be helpful to take a close look at what you usually eat, so you can make changes going forward.

For your first week, use your log sheets to journal what you eat—how much you eat, when you eat, and how you feel. Are you eating because you're hungry? Are you eating because it's time to eat? Are you eating because you're bored or tired? An example of online technology is at www.myPyramid.com.

Log in your vital statistics and it will display your Body Mass Index (BMI) (if you are muscular, pregnant, or over age 65, BMI isn't used to assess your risk for diseases associated with being overweight). You can create a meal plan with calories to *maintain* your weight or gradually *lose weight* toward a healthier weight (weight loss plan). The next page displays the recommended number of servings from each nutrient category—grains, vegetables, fruits, milk, meat, and beans—and details about how much physical activity to aim for, depending on your weight goal.

Next, you can click on each food category for information—what to choose and in what amounts. For example, if you click on grains, it takes you to a screen that shows the new pyramid; click again, and MORE information about all different types of grains and cereals; click AGAIN, and SEE a picture of what a serving of cereal looks like. It's genius!

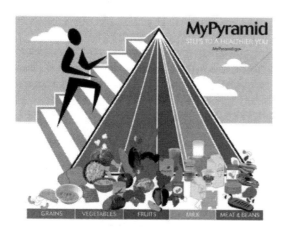

Track your foods and activities www.MyPyramid.gov

Next, go to your Tracker www. MyPyramidTracker.gov. Use this program every evening—before you go to sleep—and anticipate what you're going to eat the next day. Then the following evening, compare what you logged to the recommended intake for important nutrients.

The software is great, as long as you remember the GIGO principle—*garbage in, garbage out*. Be HONEST—if you log in what you are eating, you may be surprised to see that you underestimate how much you eat and overestimate how much you exercise. Most people do.

Use the trackers—and all online tools—to understand your usual habits and learn about nutrition. It's not a contest to see how thin you can get—the number on the scale is never as important as the way you feel, how strong you are, how you are eating, and how active you are. I don't obsess about calories—I focus on portions and activities[6].

What Does *Serving Size* Mean?

What's a serving size, and how does it translate into practical terms?

Serving Size: Portion Distortion!

Start by comparing food to everyday objects, such as a tennis ball or your hand. For example, a 3-ounce portion of cooked meat is what health experts consider normal, and it's about the size and thickness of your palm. Here are other comparisons, but remember, they are approximate. Take the time to measure and weigh your food for at least a few days—it's going to be an education!

A serving (cup) of cold cereal	*looks like*	A clenched fist	
A serving of hot cereal, oatmeal, or cooked grain (½ cup)	*looks like*	Half a tennis ball	
A piece of bread	*looks like*	A computer disc	
A serving of fruit (medium-sized piece)	*looks like*	A baseball	
A serving of dried fruit, such as raisins or dried cranberries (¼ cup)	*looks like*	A large egg	
3 ounces of meat or poultry	*looks like*	A deck of cards	
4 ounces of fish	*looks like*	A checkbook	
1 cup of cooked pasta, rice, or mashed potato	*looks like*	A tennis ball	
½ cup of cooked vegetables	*looks like*	Who cares...eat all you like!	
1 cup of raw vegetables	*looks like*	Same for raw veggies...the more the merrier!	
1 ounce of shelled nuts	*looks like*	A small handful that fits into a closed fist	
½ cup of ice cream	*looks like*	A tennis ball sliced in half	
1.5 ounces of hard cheese (such as Cheddar or Swiss)	*looks like*	2 playing dice, stacked,	
1 tablespoon of butter	*looks like*	The tip of your thumb	
2 tablespoons of peanut butter	*looks like*	Your thumb-tip plus first joint	

Food Groups: What Does a Serving Look Like?

The Starch Group: Keep the Starch Group Interesting

Try an interesting starchy substitute at breakfast. Instead of breakfast cereal, try 7-grain Kashi pilaf. The FDA advises making at least half your grains whole grains but I think eating more is even better! Whole wheat pasta is better than white; whole wheat bread is whole grain and includes the benefits of nutrients from the kernel—but a product labeled "wheat bread" may just have a small amount of whole wheat flour. Whole grains and starches provide filling fiber—great for your digestion and your heart; high fiber diets may lower LDL (bad) cholesterol and raise healthy HDL cholesterol.

Starch Group: each serving means

Breads:
1 slice whole-wheat bread

Crackers:
4-7 per 1-ounce serving (depending on product)

Cereals:
1 cup flaked cereal; 1.5 cups puffed cereal; ½ cup hot cereal (cooked)

Starchy Vegetables (including potatoes):
½ cup cooked; small baked potato or sweet potato

Grains and Legumes:
½ cup (cooked)

Pasta, Rice:
½ cup cooked (note: most people are used to eating big bowls of pasta; a half-cup serving of rice is best served with lots of vegetables)

Nutrition per serving:
approximately 100 calories
15g carbohydrate
3g protein
Trace-1g fat

You Choose: Bread

The shorter the ingredient list, the better. Whole wheat should be the first ingredient.
- Bread
- Pita bread
- English muffins
- Wraps
- Mini-bagels
- Tortillas

Genius Selections

First ingredient should be 100% whole grain, such as
100% Whole wheat
100% Whole rye
100% Whole oats

You Choose: Crackers

Crackers are good snacks; however, beware of trans fat: the ingredient label should not contain hydrogenated oils; trans fat should read "0." Choose "whole wheat" whenever possible. Although the front of the package may say "whole wheat," always read the ingredient list first. Example: some Whole Wheat crackers contain only 1g of fiber per serving. If the first ingredient is "enriched flour," not "whole wheat flour," look elsewhere.

Genius Selections

The first ingredient is "Whole wheat" or other whole grain:
at the very least, 2 grams of fiber per serving.

You Choose: Grains, Rice, Pasta, Other

As with cereal, bread, and crackers, whole grain rules! Many whole grains are now available in "quick cooking" varieties.

Genius Selections

Whole oats
Brown rice: can buy it "quick" cooked, but the pre-cooked rice has oil and preservatives
Kasha (buckwheat groats)
Barley: pearled barley is high in fiber and great added to soups
Bulgur wheat (cracked whole wheat that doesn't require cooking)
Millet: very digestible and nutrient-rich
Quinoa (a high protein grain that's translucent when cooked and is great in cold salads)
Wild rice (actually a grass, higher in protein than rice)

Dairy Group: You Choose:

I eat dairy because it's rich in protein, minerals (including calcium and potassium), and vitamins D and A. I usually choose low or nonfat dairy, including yogurt and cheese, but occasionally indulge in whole-milk feta or goat's milk cheese. If you don't like dairy, substitute calcium and vitamin D-fortified soy milk and soy yogurt (watch out for added sugar in many soy milk products), and boost calcium by eating fortified products, including cereals, orange juice, and dark green leafy vegetables. Use nonfat evaporated milk in place of cream for any recipe—it makes soups 'creamy' without the fat and calories.

Dairy Group: each serving means

Occasionally: 1 cup pudding made with nonfat milk or ½ cup low fat frozen yogurt	Here's where I put what the MyPyramid.gov people call "discretionary" calories: 1 serving has approximately 200 calories 46g carbs 7g protein 0g fat
¾ cup nonfat or low fat cottage cheese	Approximately 120 calories 2-5g carbs 20-21g protein 0.5-2g fat
1/3 cup dry milk	80 calories 8g carbs 8g protein <0 g fat
1.5 ounces natural cheese (low or reduced fat); 2 slices (¾ ounce each) hard Swiss or 1/3 cup shredded; 1/3 cup low fat Cheddar	146 calories 2g carbs 21g protein 6g fat
1 cup low fat or nonfat milk or yogurt; 1 cup fortified low fat or nonfat soy milk or yogurt	Nutrition per serving: 80-120 calories (average 100 calories per serving) 12g carbohydrate 8g protein 0-3g fat

How to Choose: Dairy

Calcium is the main mineral that strengthens bones, and most of the stored calcium for bone strength is laid down by age 17. Adults need adequate calcium to prevent bone loss.

If you have kids at home, pediatricians advise that all children past age two enjoy low fat and fat-free dairy products.

Kids and parents can enjoy a variety of milk, cheese, and yogurt daily. Children age four should have 2 cups or equivalent daily; ages nine to 18 should aim for 3 cups daily.

The USDA 2005 guidelines advise adults to aim for 3 cups daily, but depending on your calorie needs, that may be excessive. Aim for at least 2 cups, low fat or fat-free.

"Just OK" Selections

2% cottage cheese

Make nonfat more "creamy" by mixing 1 cup nonfat dry milk into a quart of nonfat milk and refrigerate.

I'm not a fan of chocolate milk, unless it's for dessert. Adding hundreds of calories weekly to your diet from sugar-sweetened milk is not a good idea.

Genius Selections

Milk: Fat-free, skim milk or 1% low fat milk

Cottage cheese: Low fat (1%) or fat-free cottage cheese

Yogurt: *Careful of the "fruit on the bottom" yogurts—unless the label reads "sugar free," it can contain up to 6 added teaspoons per 6-oz container.* Choose low fat or fat-free (plain) yogurt

Cheese: Low fat and reduced fat cheeses

Control the Cheese

Since full-fat dairy and cheese are so calorie-dense, choose low or nonfat—occasionally, I indulge in full-fat cheese, but because it has full flavor, I can use less. Use cheese as a condiment rather than a protein source; a flavor-enhancer, not the focus of the meal.

- Slice it thin—unlike lean meat, whole-milk cheese is full-fat. Try a thin slice with two medium slices of lean meat.

- Hard cheeses such as Cheddar and Parmesan have more calcium and fewer calories per ounce compared to soft brie or camembert.

- A soft goat's milk cheese is a healthy and lower calorie choice compared to other soft cheeses.

- Try a "lighter" touch—or use less. A 2-ounce (¼ cup) serving of whole milk ricotta has 8g fat and 5g saturated fat. Switch to light: only 3g fat, 2g saturated fat, and half the calories.

- Try "light" versions of Swiss, Cheddar, Mozzarella (also "part skim"), cream cheese, cottage cheese, and ricotta cheese—even "cheese food" comes in light varieties.

- When dining out, say "Light on the cheese, please," to your server.

- Grate: A very fine grate of full-flavored Parmesan cheese enhances food without adding a lot of fat and calories—one tablespoon has 1.5g fat and 1g saturated fat.

- "Cheese food" isn't real cheese, but may be made from cheese. It comes in individually-wrapped slices, bricks, jarred spreads, and even in aerosol cans. It's made from milk or reprocessed cheese and contains additional ingredients, including emulsifiers, stabilizing agents, flavorings, and colorings. Two tablespoons of processed cheese spread has 90 calories, 7g fat, and 5g saturated fat.

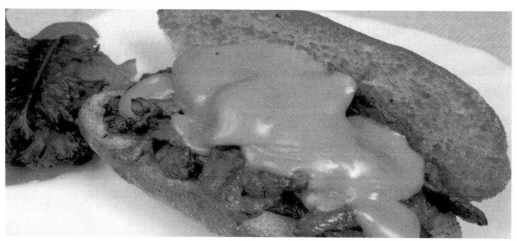

Philly Cheese Steak with more cheese!

Meats and Meat Substitutes: You Choose

Vegans (they eat no animal products) can stay healthy, too, since all the amino acids (building blocks of protein) are found in plant foods, especially dried beans and legumes.

Fish: All fish are great, including shellfish. Lean cuts of beef, pork, and skinless poultry fit.

Avoid fatty meats, and remove skin from poultry before eating.

I think of eggs as perfectly complete "vehicles" for good nutrition—and only 70-80 calories each. One egg has about 6 grams of protein (including all "essential" amino acids), and generous amounts of vitamins and minerals, notably vitamins A, D and E, selenium, iodine, riboflavin, choline, and lutein, found mostly in the yolk (80% of calories come from the yolk; 20% from egg white). Eggs yolks contain about 200 milligrams of dietary cholesterol, however, most experts advise that people on a low-fat diet can eat one - two eggs a day without an increase in "bad" LDL cholesterol. Eggs are naturally very low in saturated fat, so keep them healthy and calorie-friendly by boiling or cooking in a nonstick pan...don't fry. Eggs are not just for breakfast—they're also great for entrees. I cook great frittatas (open-faced omelets) with tons of vegetables—easy, inexpensive, and very tasty. Buy organic eggs if possible—the chickens enjoy cage-free living with access to outdoors.

Plant proteins are genius choices. Dry beans and lentils are full of protein and fiber. They're especially good when combined with all types of vegetables—in stews, soups, and cold in salads.

Protein Group: each serving means

3 ounces cooked lean meat; 3 ounces skinless poultry; 4 ounces cooked fish or shellfish	2-3 whole eggs; 4-6 egg whites; ¾ cup egg substitute	3 ounces tofu or 1 veggie burger	½ cup cooked dry beans, peas, or lentils

Nutrition per serving (approximate):

Meats range from 105 calories / 0-3g fat (very lean) to 200 calories / 8g fat (high fat)

21g protein (½ cup cooked dried beans are very lean and have about 4g of protein)

How to Choose: Meat, Chicken, Fish, Eggs

Americans love their protein, but often eat more than they need—up to double the amount necessary for good health. Recommendations range from 15% to 30% of calories daily. (For someone following an 1800-calorie meal plan, that's 68 – 135 grams). Animal protein contains all "essential" amino acids—the building blocks of protein—besides other nutrients, but some animal proteins are very high in saturated fat and cholesterol, which contributes to heart disease and obesity. So choose smart: lean and skinless, and remember, portion size counts. You can eat no animal products, and still stay healthy.

"Just OK" Selections

Burgers:

Beef: All hamburger isn't equally lean—skip the fast food burgers and cook your own from 95% lean beef.

Turkey: Remember, unless it says "turkey breast burgers," the meat will probably contain as much fat as beef.

Dark meat poultry contains more saturated fat and cholesterol and about 30 more calories per ounce than white meat, but it's also more flavorful.

Whole eggs: As long as you're not worried about high cholesterol, eggs can be eaten daily, say health experts. To lower the calories in a recipe or meal, substitute 2 egg whites for 1 whole egg. Omelets are great for dinner, but cook without added fat in a nonstick pan sprayed with cooking spray.

Meat substitutes: Soy dogs; "Boca Burgers"; soy crumbles add taste, texture, and protein to casseroles and salads. Read the labels—some soy products are high in fat and often contain cheese.

Genius Selections:

Beef: Lean cuts such as sirloin, bottom or top round, or brisket;

Poultry: All poultry is lean, as long as you leave the skin on the plate. The skin contains most of the bird's saturated fat and cholesterol. You can cook the bird with the skin on, but remove it before eating. Turkey breast burgers are great, but avoid "turkey burgers," as they usually contain the skin and other parts of the bird and are usually not low fat.

Fish: Fish, including shell fish, are very low in saturated fat and are good sources of protein. Fatty fish are rich in omega-3 fatty acids, especially salmon, sardines, mackerel, and tuna. The only problem with tuna is that it's a deep water fish and can accumulate contaminants, so vary your diet. Eat tuna one day, salmon the next, shrimp the next, and so on. All these lean protein choices are great, but preparation method is very important.

Eggs: boiled; scrambled in a non-stick pan; in an omelet or frittata. Eggs are little nuggets of good nutrition—the preparation method makes them healthy or not. Since all the fat and cholesterol is in the yolk, substitute 2 egg whites for 1 whole egg if you're counting calories.

The Vegetable Group You Choose

My naturally thin secret is really a well-known fact. Vegetables have more water and fiber than any other food—and eating more crunchy (not starchy) veggies means you can fill up without adding excess calories. When I want a quick snack, I just microwave a couple of cups of frozen crunchy veggies such as broccoli florets or green beans—only 50 calories per cooked cup. You can't eat too many vegetables! Go for rich colors—deep green, red, purple, and orange—the deeper the color, the richer the antioxidant nutrition. I *eat* fruits and veggies instead of drinking them, because juice doesn't have the fiber of the unprocessed produce.

Vegetables Group: each serving means

1 cup raw leafy greens	1 cup crunchy vegetables	½ cup cooked crunchy vegetables	6 ounces 100% vegetable juice (don't forget—you miss out on filling fiber unless you choose fiber-added juices)

Nutrition per serving (approximate):
25 calories
5g carbohydrate
2g protein
0g fat
2g or MORE **fiber** per serving, depending on your selection

The Fruit Group: You Choose:

All fruits are great sources of natural nutrition, but portion size counts. Fruit is sweet because of natural fruit sugar, or fructose, and that's why it's best to eat fruit, instead of squeezing the fructose into a glass. Depending on your needs, aim for at least three servings daily.

Fruit Group: each serving means

1 small-medium piece of fruit	1 cup melon or berries; 12-15 grapes; cherries	½ cup applesauce or fruit puree	6 ounces 100% fruit juice *(Note: juice has the same calories per ounce as soda—that's because most of the fiber is removed, and you're left with fructose—fruit sugar—in water. Make juice an occasional thing.)*

Nutrition per serving (approximate):
60 calories
15g carbohydrate
0g protein
0g fat
2g or MORE fiber per serving, depending on your selection

How to Choose: Fruits and Vegetables

It's just about impossible to make a bad choice in the produce department. All fruits and veggies fit into a healthy diet, and although starchy veggies—such as potatoes and peas—need to be treated more like grains due to their high amount of starch, they are appropriate in the right portion size. As with proteins, the way you prepare and serve your veggies makes the difference. If you deep-fry vegetables or potatoes, they become vehicles for fat. Steam, sauté, stir-fry, bake, or broil your vegetables for great nutrition and few calories. A vast array of antioxidant vitamins and minerals in fruits and vegetables promotes heart health and guards against cancer; fruits and veggies contain beneficial soluble and insoluble fiber.

Genius Selections

All varieties of fruit and vegetables are great: in fact, to achieve the widest spectrum of nutrition, variety should be your goal. Each fruit and vegetable contains different nutrients in differing amounts, so aim for at least 3 servings of fruit and 5 servings of vegetables daily.

Whole: Scrub the skin and eat the entire fruit. The fiber in fruit is heart-protective and helps fill you up.

SERVING SIZE:

   Fresh: 1 medium-size apple, orange, pear, peach, nectarine, or plum; 1 small banana or ½ medium banana

Serving Suggestions:

   **Add fruit to smoothies with nonfat milk and yogurt.

   **A cup of berries adds sweetness and fiber to breakfast cereal without adding lots of calories or sugar.

   Vegetables: Think color! The deepest greens, brightest reds—orange and yellow fruits and vegetables rule! Include at least three...even five servings daily. It's easy!

SERVING SIZE:

Salad greens: 1 cup

Cooked vegetables: ½ cup

Have a big green salad every evening before dinner: buy pre-washed greens for convenience; throw in crunchy broccoli, snap peas, tomatoes, and cucumber:

Snack on baby carrots, radishes, and mushrooms.

Buy a bag of pre-washed, stir-fry vegetables and microwave or steam—serve with tomato salsa.

"Just OK" Selections

   100% fruit juice: 1 serving is 4-6 ounces. The first ingredient must be 100% fruit juice. Stay away from "fruit drinks" and those with added sweeteners, including "fruit juice concentrate."

   Dried fruit: (serving size—¼ cup) raisins, dates, apricots, prunes, and dried apples (higher in sugar and calories). Brush your teeth or chew sugarless gum after eating.

   Canned or bottled fruit: (serving size—½ cup) OK in a hurry—best in 100% fruit juice or water, not in "syrup."
Vegetable juice: opt for the "low sodium" variety.

Natural Snacking: You Choose

Would you be surprised if I told you that snacking is good? When it comes to snacking, people are confused. Instead of raiding the vending machine for candy bars, I use my daily menu and modify my meals into smaller, "mini-meals"—what some think of as snacks.

I found that the old "three squares a day" didn't help me at all. I don't like a big breakfast—cooked food doesn't appeal to me in the morning. Eating smaller meals more frequently helps me maintain energy and motivation, especially when I am watching my calories. But that's what is natural for me. For you, it may be different. That's why I showed you how to choose according to your appetite and habits. At the end of the day, the total calories that you eat should total up to what's right for your needs.

Snacking on the right foods keeps you fueled and energized, and snacking is a proven strategy that motivated me when I was losing weight—and it keeps me naturally thin. By eating smaller meals more frequently, I don't get too hungry, and I don't feel deprived. Weight loss should not mean deprivation: you're taking good care of yourself, and the results will be fantastic!

How to Choose: Snacks

Veggie Dips: Healthy and tasty avocado dip (guacamole), chickpea dip (hummus), or tomato salsa. Smart dips: Nonfat mayo mixed with nonfat yogurt and onion soup mix; nonfat sour cream mixed with chives.

Nuts: Super-nutritious, cholesterol-free; instead of oiled nuts already shelled (too easy to overeat), roasted peanuts in the shell are portable and fun.

All Fruit: Berries, melon, apples, oranges, and grapefruit have the most fiber and fewest grams of carbohydrate per serving.

For quick snacks, stock up on single servings of:

- fat-free yogurt
- cottage cheese
- sugar-free nonfat pudding

Cereal: Who says cereal is just for breakfast? Individual servings of hot cereal—stir a cup of low sugar 100% whole grain cereal into a cup of nonfat yogurt and go.

Produce: Grocery stores carry pre-washed, ready-to-serve bags of crunchy, dip-ready veggies. Baby carrots, celery, and sugar-snap peas are great dippers.

Genius Selections

Be a genius and keep junk out of the house. That includes fried chips, crackers made with trans fat, and full-fat cheese. Instead, stock up on healthy snacks.

Popcorn: Air-popped popcorn sprayed with olive oil and tossed with a tablespoon of Parmesan cheese.

Smoothies: Fresh or frozen fruit blended with ½ cup nonfat yogurt.

Sandwiches and Wraps: Smart snacking means eating smaller meals more frequently. One half of a sandwich means 1 slice of whole grain bread with 1 slice of lean meat: add veggies and moisten with mustard or nonfat mayo.

Mini-pizza: Whole-wheat pita split open, spread with tomato sauce; sprinkle on tablespoon of low fat mozzarella cheese and Italian herbs. Broil until cheese is just melted.

Mix cottage cheese or yogurt with salad herbs or black pepper for added flavor.

Soup: Make a big pot on Sunday and freeze in smaller, single-sized microwave cups; single-serving canned soup (lower sodium and add your own pepper and spices).

The Fat Group
All liquid fat contains approximately 50 calories per teaspoon, but that's where the similarity ends. Some fats are healthy—such as monounsaturated fat from olives, olive and canola oils, nuts, seeds, avocado, and fatty fish. Avoid trans fat (hydrogenated fat) in margarine and shortening entirely. And butter? The fat in whole-milk cheese? Occasionally, for a treat.
Nutrition per serving: 1 teaspoon oil or butter (a pat)—50 calories 1 tablespoon mayonnaise or oil—approximately 100 calories 1 tablespoon nut butter—approximately 100 calories

How to Choose	Genius Selections
Read food labels and choose foods with less than 5% of the Daily Value for saturated fat. Avoid foods with hydrogenated fat. Choose grilled or broiled fast foods to avoid (hydrogenated) trans fat. Choose commercial salad dressings made with mono-unsaturated olive, canola, or flaxseed oils.	Both walnuts and flaxseed (best from cold-pressed oil) contain healthy omega-3 fatty acids: add to casseroles and salad dressings. Olives and sliced avocado (½ cup each—120 calories). Almond and cashew butter are nice alternatives to peanut butter. One serving of almonds (or walnuts, cashews, or pecans) is about 12-20 small nuts (approximately 150 calories). All nuts are rich in polyunsaturated fat and fiber. Sauté and cook with a nonstick pan and a quick shot of cooking spray.

Can You Drink and Stay Thin, Naturally?

Food without wine is a corpse;
wine without food is a ghost;
united and well matched they are as body and soul, living partners.

—Andre Simon (1877-1970)
http://www.foodreference.com/html/qfood.html

Diets and Drinking

When I started my new program, my goal was for weight loss and increased fitness and stopped drinking. Calories aside, since alcohol relaxes you, it may interfere with your resolve to stick to your plan. Yes, it's possible to drink and diet, but since I had to be frugal with my calories, I decided to forego alcohol for the first three months of my weight loss lifestyle—along with dining out. I couldn't believe how much easier it was to lose weight. In my formerly fat days, I didn't count alcohol calories—I had no idea how much I was imbibing. Just by cutting out the alcohol, I figure I lost seven pounds—without doing anything else.

Once I got to the weight where I felt comfortable—energetic and healthy—I chose to drink responsibly. If *you* choose to drink, strategize the extra calories by increasing your exercise to keep the scale balanced in your favor. A single glass of wine, a vodka and soda, and one "light" beer all have about 100 calories. Don't replace good nutrition with alcohol—living thin naturally means alcohol is secondary to smart eating.

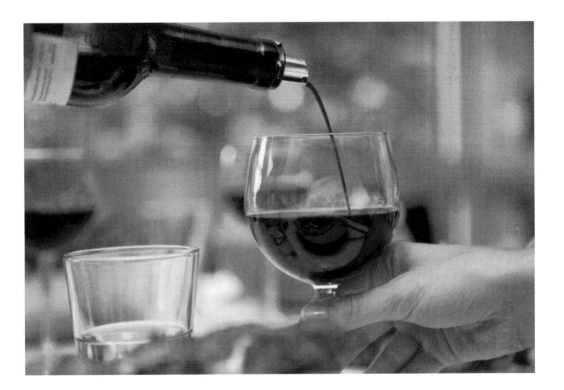

Alcohol—Health Pros and Cons: [7,8]

Alcohol—Health Pros and Cons: Some studies show that moderate amounts of alcohol can help raise healthy HDL cholesterol and also lower your risk for stroke. But excessive alcohol consumption has the opposite effect.		
Pros	**Cons**	
MAY reduce risk of heart disease and stroke (in moderate amounts: one drink per day for women, two for men). A serving of alcohol is one 5-ounce glass of wine, a 12-ounce beer, or 1 ½ ounces of spirits—calories range from 80-100 (dry white wine or "light" beer) to 150 calories (regular beer).	Alcohol has seven calories per gram and adds up quickly—and as you drink, you may lose your motivation to stay with the program. Excess calories lead to weight gain, obesity, and increased risk for diabetes.	
Although some studies point toward the health benefits of moderate alcohol, the AHA says that eating a healthy diet and exercising—and not smoking—will produce similar benefits.	Can interfere with weight loss: the body utilizes alcohol for energy before fat.	
	Studies link alcohol to increased risk for breast cancer in women.	
	Can decrease levels of vitamin B12 in women.	
	Drinking too much can raise triglycerides and increase blood pressure. Binge drinking can lead to stroke.	

Advocates of Mediterranean diets cite red wine and olive oil as dietary factors contributing to a lower risk for heart disease and stroke. But if you don't currently drink, experts advise you not to start—the health benefits associated with alcohol are easily obtainable by eating a diet high in fruits and vegetables, eliminating trans fat, and not smoking—exercising regularly and reducing stress are also important. Enjoying wine with dinner is OK, but if you drink to change your mood—perhaps overdoing it—all bets are off.

Just as refined carbohydrates are less nutritious than whole grains, and just as trans fats are unhealthy compared to monounsaturated fats, there are "good" drinks, and there are some very, very "bad" drinks. Some drinks are more like dessert—with hundreds of calories—that slide down way too easily.

So, are there health benefits associated with drinking alcohol? And if so, which should be your drink of choice?

Health experts continue to weigh in annually: some say red wine is best; others say the alcohol—not the grapes—is what lowers blood pressure and may reduce heart disease. But the jury is still out, and the American Heart Association says that any known benefits are equally accessible through healthy diet and exercise.

Some people shouldn't drink at all. Pregnant women or those who have certain medical conditions or prescribed medications that prohibit alcohol consumption should not drink. If you're unsure if you fall into one of these categories, speak with your physician.

Alcohol reduces the amount of fat the body burns for energy. Only a small portion of the alcohol consumed is converted into fat; the rest is converted by the liver into acetate, which replaces fat as a source of fuel[9].

To maintain my weight, I stay away from sweet mixers, regular soda, or juices—they all add sugar and calories. No "umbrella drinks" for me—they're just like dessert, and I've put them in the "been there, done that" column, along with adding fat to my food (spreading butter on bread or dipping into olive oil) and eating deep-fried foods.

Some Smart Strategies

I hear "You must be naturally thin" all the time! Well, yes, I'm thin, but it's because of what I eat and how much I exercise.

Like most people, I am pressed for time! Most weeknights my husband and I don't even get home until 7 or 8 p.m. How do I handle this? I cook ahead and use convenience items, avoid complicated recipes and make one-pot meals that I can double or triple and pop in the fridge. Most of these go well with a salad.

I may use healthy frozen foods, and I just can't feel guilty about it—they are my saving grace. That said, I am careful to choose healthier products—I read the labels and select those with fiber, protein, and are low or moderate in fat and low sodium. Fiber and protein help me feel fuller—another good strategy for watching my calories.

I buy some organic products, like veggie chili and salt-free canned soups which. I quickly pair with frozen veggies (just pop into the microwave) and bagged salads. Don't be afraid to add extra canned beans or frozen vegetables to bulk up soups. I add a bit of dried fruit, flavorful cheese and olive oil to salads—a little bit goes along way in terms of boosting flavor and texture.

I eat a lot of calorie-dense foods—nuts, cheese and oil but I watch portions and find that they help me feel satisfied, and that helps keep calories in a healthy range.

By the way, none of this feels like much of an effort for me. I like being healthy and fit and I don't feel deprived because I let myself splurge every now and then—a special dinner out or on vacations—sometimes a really wonderful food feels like a real treat. I never say never!

Linda P MS, RD
Des Moines, IA

5 Best Naturally Thin Drinks (When You're Trying to Cut Calories)

Type of beverage	Amount	Calories per serving	Recommendations & Comments
Wine: red or white	5 ounces	100 calories	Stay dry for fewest calories
Beer	12 ounces	Regular-150 Light-100	"Low carb" beer does not mean "low calorie"
Liquor: Vodka, rum, whiskey, gin, or bourbon	1 shot, 1 ounce	100 calories	Avoid sweet mixes, sugary soda, and juice—even 100% juice—adds calories and sugar. Best with club soda and lime or diet soda
Vegetable juice cocktail	6 ounces	Approximately 40 calories	Mix 1-ounce vodka with 4 ounces vegetable juice; pour over ice. (Watching your sodium? Buy low sodium variety)
Club soda with fresh lime or lemon	Unlimited!	Zero calories	Serve with a splash of orange juice or squeeze of lemon or lime. Refreshing, hydrating, delicious!

Drink To Your Health

Are you hungry—or just thirsty? When I was in weight loss mode, I found that drinking a few ounces of water every half-hour was helpful, and continue to deliberately drink water and decaffeinated teas.

- **Water.**
  - **For your body:** Calorie-free, refreshing, hydrating and thirst-quenching, water is my number one drink. More than half the weight of the human body is water, and water is the basis of all body fluids, including digestive juices, blood, urine, lymph, and perspiration. Water is necessary for digestion (for elimination and to prevent constipation) and for regulating your body temperature by distributing heat and cooling the body via perspiration. How many glasses a day? That depends on a number of different personal factors, including your weight, age and activity. The old "8 x 8" rule (eight 8-ounce glasses) is a good one, but if you're exercising and perspiring, especially in a dry climate, then more is called for. Over-hydration can lead to a dangerous electrolyte imbalance, so in this case, stay hydrated, not soaked.

  - **For the environment:** Water has no calories or artificial sweeteners or flavors. My municipal water company produces a high quality product at an inexpensive price, so I don't buy bottled water—which is less problematic for the environment and my budget! Regulations on tap water are more stringent than bottled water, and since it's "free," it's better than paying a premium. The carbon-footprint associated with bottled water should be considered too—especially for imported water in glass bottles.

  - **For your weight:** Drinking water will not cause you to lose weight, but drinking water between meals can help curb your appetite—and so will snacking on water-filled fresh vegetables and fruit.

- **Milk. Nonfat** vitamin D and calcium-fortified milk has all the protein and minerals of whole milk, without the artery-clogging saturated fat.
  - **Low fat or nonfat fortified soy, rice, or almond milk products are alternatives to cow's milk but often contain too much added sugar. Buy unsweetened and add your own honey if you prefer a slightly sweet taste.**

  - Buttermilk is cultured low fat milk and is more easily digested than regular milk—with a tangy, delicious taste. I add buttermilk to my egg white omelet, and when I'm baking, I substitute low or nonfat buttermilk in place of regular milk.

  - I like to whip up a smoothie with a cup of nonfat milk, a ½ cup of nonfat yogurt, and a cup of berries and pour it over my breakfast cereal.

- **Tea.** Black, green, and white teas contain antioxidants and health benefits. The processing of the tea influences the color—green is the least processed. Green and black tea contain about the same amount of caffeine...about 30mg per cup (half that of coffee). Further research is needed, but studies point toward lower rates of heart disease and cancer in populations of heavy tea-drinkers. However, these populations may also be slimmer, have less stress, and eat more fruits and vegetables—healthy habits that keep people healthy, too.

- **Coffee.** In moderation, coffee may help boost your immunity because it contains healthy antioxidants. Studies show that a cup of java in the morning helps get you going. But coffees injected with heavy cream or flavored syrups or topped with whipped cream are out of my diet. You might opt for a "skinny latte" made with nonfat milk—but don't overdo the brew, because too much caffeine can cause insomnia and the jitters.

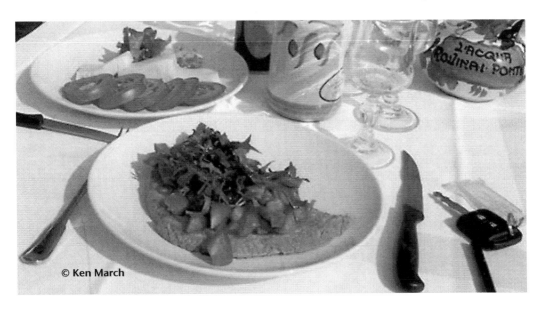

© Ken March

- **Juice**. Occasionally. I'm NOT a fan of juice, and juice was a food I eliminated from my diet because I wanted to feel fuller while consuming fewer calories. However, if you're maintaining your weight, 100% fresh juice is a great treat. One way to enjoy juice without so many calories is to mix one part fresh fruit juice to two parts cool or sparkling water. Juice is best when it's fresh...fruit and vegetable juices contain vitamins and minerals. An 8-ounce glass of fruit juice has approximately 120 calories and goes down awfully easy. Don't fall for the marketing claim that "you could have had" a glass of vegetable juice instead of eating your veggies. There's 880 milligrams of sodium in one 12-ounce serving, and you lose out on the fiber in fresh, whole vegetables.

- **Sparkling water.** Sometimes a glass of sparkling, fizzy water can satisfy your urge for something higher in calories. Your grocery store offers many different varieties of club soda, seltzer, and flavored sparkling waters—some with artificial sweeteners, some without. Consider sparkling water without sodium, if you really dislike water. Add a splash of fruit juice to sparkling water—drink it as a cocktail in a wine glass.

The way I controlled my calories was by aiming for a certain number of portions from each food group daily, and using a nutrition guide to plan my menus. It's so easy to do this today by utilizing the online program. If you want to do it the "old fashioned" way, here is a simplified guide.

Calories Equal Food: What to Eat
How Many Servings Do You Need?

Make Your Menus

Second Nature Eating		
Eating smaller meals more frequently works ideally for me: I translate this eating pattern into portions: for example,		
	1300-1400 calories	1500-1600 calories
Breakfast	~250	~300
Lunch	~400	~500
Dinner	~400-500	~500
Snack	~100	~100-150
Snack	~100	~100-150
Snack	[if you need a third snack, make it crunchy vegetables—unlimited]	[if you need a third snack, make it crunchy vegetables—unlimited]

What To Eat?	1300-1400	1500-1600
Starches: grains, breads, legumes, starchy vegetables	4	5
Meats and meat substitutes: *Non-meat eaters, estimate ¼ cup cooked dry beans, 1 egg, 1 tablespoon of peanut butter, or ½ ounce of nuts or seeds can be considered as 1 ounce of meat*	4-5	6-7
Dairy and Dairy Substitutes: unsweetened soy milk or soy yogurt.	2	2
Crunchy Vegetables	At least 4-more is fine	At least 4-more is fine
Fruits	2+	2+
Added fats and oils (light spreads, avocado, olive or canola oil-based salad dressing)	1-2	3+ added
Other treats, such as wine or chocolate, depending on your activities!	A glass of wine has about 100 calories	2 miniature bars of dark chocolate have about 100 calories

Sample Menu	1300-1400
Breakfast: ~250 calories 1 milk 1 fruit 1 starch	1 cup nonfat milk: 1 milk—**80** calories 1 cup berries: 1 fruit—60 calories 1 cup Kashi cereal: 1 starch—approximately 100 calories Total: ~240 calories
Snack: ~100 calories 1 milk	1 6-ounce cup yogurt: 1 milk—100 calories
Lunch: ~400 calories 2 meat 2 starches Veggies	2 slices whole grain bread: 2 starch—200 calories 2 ounces turkey: 2 protein/meat—200 calories Mustard Carrots and cucumbers—free
Snack: ~100 calories 1 fat	1 small handful almonds (24): 1 fat—approximately 100 calories
Dinner: ~400 3 meat 1 starches 2 veggies 2 fat	3 ounces broiled snapper: 3 lean protein—210 calories 1 small baked potato with salsa: 1 starch—100 calories Broccoli and tomatoes, sautéed in nonstick pan with ½ tsp olive oil and herbs: free veggies plus 1 fat—50 calories Tossed salad with vinegar, lemon, and ½ tsp olive oil—50 calories
Snack ~100 1 fruit 1 milk	Sugar-free hot chocolate—60 calories ½ Granny smith apple, sliced thin—40 calories

Sample Menu	1500-1600
Breakfast: ~300 calories 1 milk 1 fruit 1-2 starch	1 Cup of nonfat milk: 1 milk—80 calories 1 cup berries: 1fruit—60 calories 1-1.5 cups Kashi cereal: 1-2 starch—approximately 150 calories
Snack: ~150 calories 1 milk 1 fruit	1 6-ounce cup yogurt: 1 milk—100 calories 1 orange: 1 fruit—60 calories
Lunch: ~500 calories 3 meat 2 starch 1-2 fat vegetables	Large tossed salad: free vegetables 3 ounces canned salmon: 3 meat Whole wheat pita bread: 2 starch 1 tablespoon nonfat salad dressing: 1 fat

Sample Menu	1500-1600
Snack: ~100 calories 1 milk ½ starch	1 nonfat yogurt: 1 milk 2 tablespoons nugget cereal: ½ starch
Dinner: ~500-600 3 meat 1-2 starch 1 fat	*Shrimp with broccoli* 4 ounces medium-sized shrimp sautéed with 1 teaspoon olive oil; garlic, tomatoes, red peppers, and snow peas: 3-4 lean protein, 1 fat — approximately 300 calories Tossed salad with vinegar, lemon, and ½ tsp olive oil — 50 calories ½- 1 cup brown rice: 1-2 starch—100-200 calories
Snack ~100 1 milk 1 fruit	Sugar-free hot chocolate—60 calories ½ Granny smith apple, sliced thin—40 calories
Total: about 1500-1600 calories	Add a glass of red wine or a square of dark chocolate—approximately 100 calories

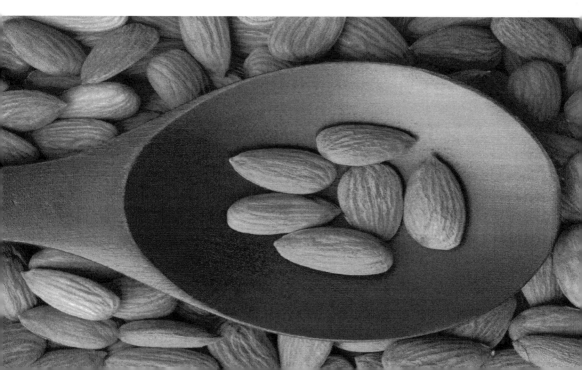

Sample Simple Menu

- Breakfast
    - Fruit
    - Whole-grain cereal
    - Nonfat milk
- Lunch
    - 2 cups fresh spinach salad
    - 2 ounces grilled fish
    - 2 Tbs olive oil vinaigrette
    - 1 small whole-wheat pita or ½ cup whole grain cous cous
    - Wedge of melon or piece of fruit
- Dinner
    - 5 ounces broiled fish or chicken with grilled onions and tomatoes
    - 1 small sweet potato or 1 cup brown rice pilaf
    - Sautéed spinach (1 Tbs olive oil) with garlic
    - Glass of red wine
    - 3 fresh figs and decaf espresso
- Mid-morning snack: 1 cup of plain low or nonfat yogurt with 1 tsp honey
- Mid-afternoon: 1 small handful of almonds, peanuts, pecans, or walnuts
- All day long, whenever I may feel hungry: crunchy vegetables
- Water: 8 ounces each
    - in the morning before I walk
    - if I'm working out
    - after the workout or walk or bike ride
    - mid morning
    - mid afternoon
    - with dinner

Sample Menu	1300-1400
Breakfast: ~250 calories 1 milk 1 fruit 1 starch	
Snack: ~100 calories 1 milk	
Lunch: ~400 calories 2 meat 2 starches Veggies	
Snack: ~100 calories	
Dinner: ~400 3 meat 1 starches 2 veggies 2 fat	
Snack ~100 1 fruit 1 milk	

Sample Menu	1500-1600
Breakfast: ~300 calories 1 milk 1 fruit 1-2 starch	
Snack: ~150 calories 1 milk 1 fruit	
Lunch: ~500 calories 3 meat 1-2 starch 1-2 fat vegetables	
Snack: ~100 calories	

Sample Menu	1500-1600
Dinner: ~500 3 meat 2 starch 1 fat	
Snack ~100 1 milk 1 fruit	
Total: about 1500-1600 calories	If you include a glass of red wine or a square of dark chocolate—approximately 100 calories

Inspired Foods: I could easily expand this list to 25—or 50!—foods that inspire me. Here are some inspiring foods and food groups that have extra-special nutritional value and are easy to incorporate into your naturally thin diet.

1. Nuts: Don't be afraid to eat nuts—just eat them wisely. Nuts contain a combination of healthy monounsaturated and polyunsaturated fats—yes, fat—good fat! They're also full of fiber, protein, iron, and magnesium. I pass on nuts in jars that have been processed with oil and salt. I say, "Yes!" to roasted peanuts (did you know that peanuts are legumes?) in the shell or crack a few walnuts or almonds. I buy raw almonds, walnuts, and pecans in bulk and toast them in the oven at 250 degrees F for about 20 minutes. One 22-nut serving of roasted almonds has about 160 calories.

Shop Smart: Top Shopping Tips

- Shop with a list: A list helps you structure your shopping and avoid impulsive buys that can wreck your progress. Create your own Staples List and make copies to shop from weekly.

- Cruise the OUTSIDE aisles first: The freshest food items—produce and dairy, fish and other perishables are located on the perimeter walls of the grocery store.

- Start in the produce aisle, and think variety—here you can be flexible—if green beans are on your list this week but the leeks look interesting, try something new!

- Find your dairy, eggs, and tofu in the dairy aisle.

- Next, head to fresh meats, fish, and poultry.

- Finally, venture into the middle of the store, but stick to the list. This should be a short trip, because you know what you want—and you're on guard for hype—a label showing waving wheat doesn't make it "whole wheat"; colorful fruits and vegetables doesn't always mean there's good stuff in the package.

Label Reading: Back to Front

Common claims: The Center for Food Safety and Applied Nutrition under the US Food and Drug Administration governs the claims that manufacturers are permitted to print on the labels of packaged foods[10].

Read the ingredient list first! Pay no attention to the advertising or pretty pictures on the front of the package. Remember, there is no fruit in Froot Loops—just fruit flavors.

- Low calorie: 40 calories or less per serving
- Fat-free: less than 0.5g fat per serving
- Low fat: 3g fat or less per serving
- Reduced fat: 25 percent fewer calories from fat per serving compared to reference food (does NOT necessarily mean low fat!)
- Low saturated fat: 1g fat or less per serving
- Lean: fewer than 10g fat, 4.5g saturated fat, and 95mg cholesterol per serving
- Extra Lean: fewer than 5g fat, 2g saturated fat, and 95mg cholesterol per serving
- Trans fat-free: less than 0.5g trans fat per serving (may include hydrogenated fat in the ingredients)
- Low cholesterol: 20mg or less cholesterol and 2g or less saturated fat per serving
- Cholesterol-free: 2mg or less cholesterol and 2g or less saturated fat per serving
- Less cholesterol: 25 percent fewer milligrams cholesterol per serving compared to reference food; 2g or less saturated fat per serving

Sample Label for
Macaroni and Cheese

Start Here

Nutrition Facts

Serving Size 1 cup (228g)
Servings Per Container 2

Amount Per Serving

Check Calories | **Calories** 250 | Calories from Fat 110

	% Daily Value*
Total Fat 12g	18%
Saturated Fat 3g	15%
Trans Fat 3g	
Cholesterol 30mg	10%
Sodium 470mg	20%
Total Carbohydrate 31g	10%
Dietary Fiber 0g	0%
Sugars 5g	
Protein 5g	

Vitamin A	4%
Vitamin C	2%
Calcium	20%
Iron	4%

Limit These Nutrients

Get Enough of These Nutrients

* Percent Daily Values are based on a 2,000 calorie diet. Your Daily Values may be higher or lower depending on your calorie needs.

Footnote

	Calories:	2,000	2,500
Total Fat	Less than	65g	80g
Sat Fat	Less than	20g	25g
Cholesterol	Less than	300mg	300mg
Sodium	Less than	2,400mg	2,400mg
Total Carbohydrate		300g	375g
Dietary Fiber		25g	30g

Quick Guide to DV

5% or less is Low

20% or more is High

Learn more about the Nutrition Facts Label online at: http://www.cfsan.fda.gov/~dms/foodlab.html

2. Seeds: Flaxseed is but one of the seeds I include in my naturally thin diet. Flax has become popular of late because it's rich in alpha linolenic acid, a type of heart-healthy omega-3 fatty acid. Other nutrient-rich seeds include pumpkin (zinc), sunflower (B-vitamins), and sesame seeds (calcium). Like nuts, the calories from seeds are derived mostly from fat—but the fat is unsaturated and healthy. Lately, I've been adding a tablespoon of organic ground flaxseed to my morning smoothie (I pour it over my high fiber cereal). I mix raw sunflower seeds into my salads; tahini in hummus is delicious.

3. Deep Colors: Break out of your rut and try some new fruits. The richer the color, the better the nutrition. I live in a tropical climate and have seasonal access to different fruits including fresh guava and pomegranate, high in vitamins C and A, potassium, niacin, and fiber, but frozen fruit is fine—sometimes more nutritious than fresh if the fresh stuff has been sitting in the store for too long. If you drink juice, choose 100% juice, and ignore juice drinks, usually sweetened with sugar or high fructose corn syrup, and high in calories.

4. Coffee and Chocolate: Women who drink coffee have a lower risk for diabetes; dark chocolate has similar antioxidants as heart-healthy tea, red wine, and some fruits and vegetables. Real cocoa powder is richest in antioxidant flavonoids—milk chocolate barely counts, and most commercial candy bars offer only excess calories. The secret to success with these foods is in how you eat and drink them—how often and in what quantity. I love my coffee black—without added fat and calories from cream and sugar, and enjoy an ounce of really good dark chocolate as a treat.

5. Dairy or Dairy Substitutes: Nonfat or low fat dairy has all the protein and calcium of regular, whole milk dairy without the saturated fat and cholesterol—and extra calories. For example, a cup of nonfat, unsweetened yogurt has about 30 percent of your Daily Value for calcium and 12g of protein—all for about 100 calories. If you choose soy dairy substitutes, buy calcium and vitamin D-fortified unsweetened or just lightly sweetened (limit to four to six grams of sugar per serving). Organic soy or dairy are produced without antibiotics, growth hormones, or pesticides.

6. Pasture-raised: The term "free-range" means little, but "pasture-raised" means just that—uncaged animals, and by most accounts will produce healthier animals and eggs. Organic products are produced from animals raised without additives and antibiotics.

7. Fish: Many types of fish contain a balance of nutrition with heart-healthy benefits. Fish contain monounsaturated and polyunsaturated oils and little saturated fat and are low in calories when baked, broiled, grilled, or poached—without fatty sauces. Lean, white fish such as haddock provides only about 100 calories and less than 1g fat per 3-ounce (or 100 gram) serving, and fatty fish such as salmon, mackerel and tuna, contain omega-3 polyunsaturated fatty acids—which lower triglycerides and cholesterol in the blood. A 3-ounce serving of salmon contains 168 calories and 7g of mainly healthy, unsaturated fat.

8. Garlic and cruciferous: Think crunchy, think garlic—think perfect packages of flavor and phenomenal nutrition. Vegetables in the brassica family, including broccoli, cauliflower, Brussels sprouts, and all of those deep green greens—arugula, kale, collards, and more—are packed with antioxidant phytochemicals. Garlic, onions, leeks, and others in the allium family offer immune-boosting properties.

Too Much Salt!

The NHLBI recommends less than 2,400 milligrams of sodium daily, about the amount in one teaspoon of salt. This doesn't mean "added salt", it means ALL sodium and salt consumed daily. High sodium diets are linked to higher risk for stroke and heart disease, and people diagnosed with high blood pressure or pre-hypertension should aim for less than 1,500 milligrams daily. Stick to fresh foods, especially fruits and vegetables, which are good sources of potassium, a good balance for healthy hearts. You absolutely cannot lower your dietary sodium if you frequent fast food or eat a lot of packaged foods. For example, just one grilled chicken sandwich contains more than 1,200 milligrams of sodium.

Read the nutrition facts labels—or go online to determine the sodium content of your favorite packaged and fast foods. http://www.nhlbi.nih.gov/hbp/prevent/sodium/sodium.htm

How Sweet it Is?

Artificial sweeteners have been around for more than 100 years—dating back to the discovery of saccharine in 1879. There are many options for those who want to indulge without damaging their diet, including five no-calorie sweeteners approved by the Food and Drug Administration, who regulate them as food additives: Saccharin (Sweet 'N Low), aspartame (NutraSweet), acesulfame potassium (acesulfame K), sucralose (Splenda), and most recently, neotame. Other sweeteners include sugar alcohols—mannitol, sorbitol, xylitol, lactitol, isomalt, maltitol, and hydrogenated starch hydrolysates (HSH)—which occur naturally in foods and come from plant products such as fruits and berries. They are not no-calorie but have less than one-third to one-half the calories of sugar.

Those with *phenylketonuria*, a very rare (1 in 15,000) inherited disease, should not consume aspartame.

When I was in "weight loss mode" I scheduled my daily "sweet treats," a cup of sugar-free gelatin and especially my evening sugar-free hot chocolate, and they helped me feel satisfied and never deprived.

Remember, just because it's labeled sugar-free doesn't make it calorie-free. Read food labels and be aware of how many calories are in each serving. Some sugar-free (and fat-free, for that matter) food varieties have the same—or even more—calories as the original.

Some people consume too many artificially sweetened foods. Everything shouldn't be sweet—or salty. Overly processed foods are often overloaded with seemingly conflicting hidden ingredients such as salt, high fructose corn syrup, and other flavor enhancers, and if you're constantly overwhelming your taste buds with these artificial flavors, you lose your taste for the real thing. I've spoken to many clients who say that they don't "like" water. They expect all beverages to be sweet and find water unappealing. Everything begins to taste the same, so they eat more processed foods to get the taste they want, and then natural foods aren't satisfying.

Make Label Reading Second Nature

When I stopped eating meat, before learning about health, I thought "healthy" meant "low calorie." I heard about carob, a "natural" chocolate substitute, and made the same mistake as I did with cheese.

My thought process went like this—

> *Carob = vegetarian = healthy!*

Uninformed reasoning, since carob is sweetened with sugar (or honey or some other sweetener), and it still has calories just like any candy. I still didn't have a clue about nutrition—still thought that foods labeled "healthy" meant "eat all you want."

I thought, *Meat is bad, ergo, cheese is good. Therefore, eat all the cheese you want.*

Uninformed reasoning—cheese put the pounds on faster than anything I'd ever eaten.

It took a while, but I learned. I learned to read all labels from back to front.

I read:

◊ Serving size first.

◊ Then number of servings in the package.

◊ Then the calories per serving.

Think: how many servings am I going to eat? That's MY portion.

◊ Then I calculate how many calories are in my portion.

What's a gram? [11]

Confused in the Kitchen? Although the Nutrition Facts Label lists measurements in metric, if you don't use it, you don't learn it.

Log on to StartCooking.com for measuring instructions and how-to-cook videos.

WEIGHT

2 teaspoons = 10g

1/3 ounce = 10g

1 ounce = 28g

1 pound = 450g

1 cup butter or margarine = 210g

VOLUME

1 teaspoon = 1/3 tablespoon = 5ml (ml stands for milliliter, one thousandth of a liter)

1 tablespoon = ½ fluid ounce = approximately 15ml

1 cup = 8 fl oz = approximately 250ml

1 pint = 2 cups = 16 ounces = approximately 500ml (½ liter)

1 quart = 2 pints = approximately 1 liter

1 gallon = 4 quarts = approximately 4 liters

LENGTH

1 inch = 2.5 centimeters

Converting American Measurements to Metric

Volume Measures

- 1/5 teaspoon = 1ml
- 1 teaspoon = 5ml
- 1 tablespoon = 15ml
- 1 fluid ounce = 30ml
- 1/5 cup = 50ml
- 1 cup = 240ml
- 2 cups (1 pint) = 470ml
- 4 cups (1 quart) = .95 liter
- 4 quarts (1 gal) = 3.8 liters

Weight Measures

- 1 ounce = 28g
- 1 pound = 454g

Converting Metric Measurements to U.S.

Here is a guide for converting from Metric to U.S. measures

Volume Measures

- 1ml = 1/5 teaspoon
- 5ml = 1 teaspoon
- 15ml = 1 tablespoon
- 30ml = 1 fluid ounce
- 100ml = 3.4 fluid ounces
- 240ml = 1 cup
- 1 liter = 34 fluid ounces
- 1 liter = 4.2 cups
- 1 liter = 2.1 pints
- 1 liter = 1.06 quarts
- 1 liter = .26 gallon

Weight Measures

- 1g = .035 ounce
- 100g = 3.5 ounces
- 500g = 1.10 pounds
- 1kg = 2.205 pounds
- 1kg = 35 ounces

And finally, a dash is a scant sixteenth of a teaspoon.

A pinch is a little larger—about an eighth of a teaspoon.

LOG IT — My Second Nature Eating Diary

Monday Date: 04/27/08	
My Breakfast	Mini-wheat bagel with 1% cottage cheese and wedge of melon Tomorrow, I'm going to remember the lemon for the melon! 2 cups of black coffee
My Lunch	Healthy Choice frozen entrée (at work) and club soda
My Dinner	Broiled chicken (breast); baked potato with salsa; big salad with diet dressing and some walnuts sprinkled on top; 4-ounce glass of red wine
My Snacks	10 AM: apple (at work) Lots of water today—I think I drank at least 3 half-liter bottles (about 51 ounces!) 4 PM: 100-calorie bag of microwave popcorn (at work) 9 PM: 1 cup sugar-free 50-calorie hot chocolate
My Activity	6–6:25 AM: Walked the dog: moderate pace (ran/walked/ran/walked—25 minutes) 6:45–7:15 AM: dance video tape (workout pace—30 minutes) 12 PM: walked at work (30 minutes) 6 PM: walked the dog (20 minutes)
My Feelings	It's hard getting started sometimes, but after just a few minutes, I feel so great...I have to get up earlier so I can go a little longer tomorrow. Man—dancing is FUN! Salsa moves—want to do this tape again! It's still hot outside—I'm looking forward to November! Glad I have those towelettes in my desk drawer. Glad I have those towelettes in my desk drawer. This isn't too strenuous—she stopped at every mailbox to sniff—glad I got my aerobics in the morning. A very good day—feel good, feelin' strong!

LOG IT — LOG IT — Your Second Nature LIVING Diary:
Copy this diary and log your foods, activities and feelings

Monday	Tuesday	Wednesday	Thursday	Friday	Saturday	Sunday
My Breakfast	My Breakfast	My Breakfast	My Breakfast	My Breakfast	My Breakfast	My Breakfast
My Lunch	My Lunch	My Lunch	My Lunch	My Lunch	My Lunch	My Lunch
My Dinner	My Dinner	My Dinner	My Dinner	My Dinner	My Dinner	My Dinner
My Snacks	My Snacks	My Snacks	My Snacks	My Snacks	My Snacks	My Snacks
My Activity	My Activity	My Activity	My Activity	My Activity	My Activity	My Activity
My Feelings	My Feelings	My Feelings	My Feelings	My Feelings	My Feelings	My Feelings

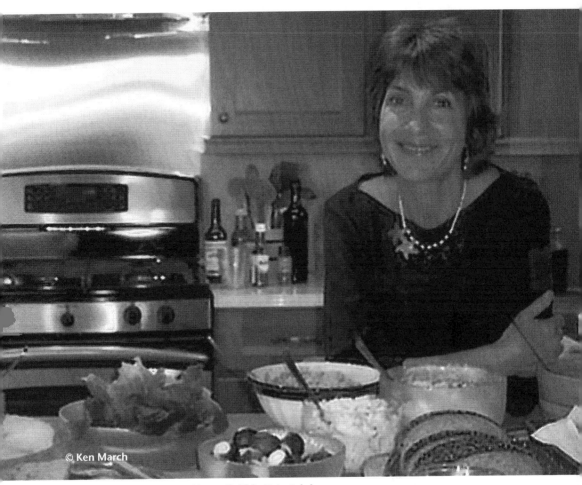

© Ken March

Naturally Thin Entertaining

"Living Thin Naturally" Kitchen Equipment

You don't have to buy all this equipment at once, but I suggest buying the starred items first.

Plates and Bowls: Size Counts: Oversized bowls and plates encourage overeating. Are your dishes gigantic? Use smaller-sized plates and bowls. Studies prove that the more you're served, the more you eat, and if you're always eating out of oversized dishes, you learn to eat more. Most people eat with their eyes instead of their stomach!

Hardware
- Nonstick pans:
    - *Saucepan
    - *Baking pans
    - Wok
    - Pizza pan
    - Grill pan
- Tea kettle
- Mixing bowls with lids
- *Pyrex bowls with lids (for microwaving, re-heating and cooking; can double as mixing bowls)

Electronic Kitchen
- Microwave oven
- *Blender: full sized
    - Optional: Mini-blender (portable, for quick smoothies on-the-go); hand blender (great for soups and sauces)
- Crock pot
- Countertop grill
- *Hot air popcorn maker
- *Food scale (if it's in your budget, electronic scales are great)
- Standing mixer with attachments, including dough hook
- Rice steamer
- Coffee pot

Utensils and Such
- Skewers for kabobs
- *Spatula for nonstick pan
- *Wooden mixing spoon
- *Good chef's knife
- *Paring knife
- *Serrated knife
- Garlic press
- *Kitchen shears

Miscellaneous
- *Measuring cups and spoons
- Ice cube trays (for frozen fruit treats)
- *Salad spinner (the insert can double as a colander)
- Colander
- Vegetable steamer (may skip and use Pyrex bowls with covers in the microwave)
- *Plastic containers: Serving-size (small and medium) plastic containers with lids that go from freezer to microwave
- *Marking pens
- *Plastic storage bags: Gallon, quart, and sandwich-sized plastic re-sealable bags
- *Flexible cutting boards (use dedicated cutting board for chicken to keep kitchen safe: disinfect in dishwasher after use)

Main Dishes

Better-Than-Fried Chicken (or Turkey or Fish or Tofu): After you've tasted this recipe, you'll never miss fried chicken again.	Serves 6 253 calories, 2g fat, 0.5g saturated fat, 21g protein
Ingredients: • 1 cup fat-free ranch dressing • ½ cup nonfat milk • 1 cup branflakes or cornflakes, crushed • ½ cup wheat germ (toasted, no sugar added) • 1 tsp dried Italian herbs • ¼ teaspoon cayenne pepper (optional) • Salt and pepper to taste • 6 chicken breasts (or turkey breasts or firm fish or extra firm tofu): approximately 3-4 ounces per person. If using chicken, choose skinless and boneless breasts (about 1-1.5 lbs)	Directions: • Preheat oven to 350 degrees F. • Spray a glass baking dish with cooking spray. • In a shallow bowl, whisk milk and dressing until smooth. • Mix cereals and seasonings in second shallow bowl. • Coat protein with dressing, then coat with cereal mixture and place in single layer into baking dish. • Chicken or turkey: bake until done (no longer pink) about 45-50 minutes. Fish or tofu: cut cooking time to about 20-30 minutes.

Asian Salmon Salad On Roll: Use the recipe as a guide for good eating. Think of all the substitutes for fish—chicken, tofu, turkey—you can use in this flavorful salad.	Serves 4 283 calories, 9g fat, 1.3g saturated fat, 11mg cholesterol, 575mg sodium, 11g protein
Ingredients: • 1.5 cups canned salmon, drained and flaked (also, diced, cooked chicken breast or canned chicken breast is ultra-easy; or microwave and dice 2 skinless, boneless chicken breasts) • 1 kiwi, peeled and diced • ¼ cup diced celery • ¼ cup diced red bell pepper • ¼ cup reduced-fat mayonnaise (or 2 Tbsp nonfat mayonnaise and 2 Tbsp nonfat plain yogurt) • 1 Tbsp toasted, chopped walnuts or almonds • 4 whole grain rolls	Directions • Combine salmon, kiwi, celery, bell pepper, mayonnaise, and nuts together in a medium bowl and mix • Mound onto sliced roll halves • Top each with shredded lettuce More Options Instead of chicken, substitute: • Turkey breast • Canned tuna • Canned salmon • 4 hardboiled eggs • 5 ounces firm tofu, mashed

Buffalo Chicken Wraps: Have fun with some "bar food" without all the calories and fat of traditional fried wings. Be creative and feel free to substitute what's on sale (turkey instead of chicken; grilled fish instead of fowl; add more veggies as desired).

Serves 4
190 calories, 2g fat, 487mg sodium, 4g fiber, 28g protein

Ingredients:

- 2 cups shredded, cooked chicken-breast meat (about 2 chicken breasts) or quickly grill or broil firm fish fillets
- 2 Tbsp hot-pepper sauce
- ½ cup fat-free blue cheese dressing
- 4 10-inch wheat tortillas
- 2 cups shredded romaine lettuce
- 1 cup diced celery
- 1 cup peeled, seeded, and diced cucumber
- 1 cup peeled, shredded carrots

Directions:

- Combine the chicken or fish and hot-pepper sauce in a small bowl.
- Spread 2 Tbsp of fat-free blue-cheese dressing over each tortilla.
- Arrange ½ cup lettuce from the top down in the middle of each tortilla.
- Top each with ½ cup chicken, ¼ cup celery, ¼ cup cucumber, and ¼ cup carrots.
- Fold each side of the tortilla toward the center, then roll up tightly from the bottom to the top.

Best Black Bean Burgers: Who needs beef!

Serves 4: approximately 200 calories per burger: 11 g protein, 10 g fiber, 35 g carbohydrate, 3 g fat per serving

Ingredients

- 1 (16 ounce) can black beans
- 2 green onions, diced
- ½ red bell pepper, diced
- 2 cloves garlic, smashed
- 1 egg or 2 egg whites
- 1 tablespoon chili powder
- ½ teaspoon cumin
- ½ teaspoon hot sauce (more to taste)
- ½ cup of whole wheat bread crumbs
- 1 large tomato
- 1 medium red onion

Directions
Grill on oiled baking sheet, or bake in preheated oven at 375 degrees F.
or grill bean burgers:

- Drain and rinse beans: transfer to medium bowl and mash thoroughly.
- Finely dice onions, pepper and garlic; stir into beans
- Add egg whites and seasonings and mix well; then just incorporate breadcrumbs---don't over mix; mixture should hold together.
- Using your hands, form into four patties: slick tomato (thick) and red onion (thin).
- Place on greased baking sheet, and bake approximately 16-20 minutes, turning once.
- Serve with mustard, on whole-wheat buns, with thick slices of tomato and thin slices of red onion.

Cool Chili: The simplest of recipes— make it ahead of time and freeze.	Serves 7 345 calories, 3.4g fat, 28mg cholesterol, 13g fiber, 24g protein
Ingredients: • 1 pound 97% lean ground beef or turkey or firm tofu, drained • 1 onion, diced • 2 cloves garlic, minced • 1 green pepper, seeded and diced • 1 tsp olive oil • 1 28-ounce can tomato puree (no salt added) • 1 15-ounce can *each* kidney beans, white beans, and pinto beans— rinsed and drained • 3 small-medium baking potatoes, scrubbed and cubed • 2 Tbsp chili powder • ¼ tsp salt • 1 tsp cumin • 2 cups water	Directions: • In a large, nonstick saucepan over low-medium high heat, heat olive oil. Add garlic and cook until just softened. Add the onion and pepper and cook 2 more minutes; then add the ground meat or crumble in the tofu: cook about 5 minutes. • Drain off fat if using meat; add pureed tomatoes, canned beans, potatoes, seasonings, and water. • Reduce heat to low and simmer, covered, for approximately 30 minutes or until potatoes are tender. • For thinner chili, add a cup of broth, wine or water. • Serve with a tossed salad.

Country-Style Crock Pot Chicken: Crock pots are perfect for convenient but healthy meals. Substitute any of your favorite meats, vegetables, and flavorings to make it your own.	Serves 4 209 calories, 5g fat, 30g protein, 1.75g fiber
Ingredients: • 1 cup baby carrots, diced • 1 cup celery, diced • 1 cup white onion, diced • 2 cloves garlic, crushed • 4 chicken breasts, chunked pieces • 1 can (10-3/4 oz) low fat cream of celery soup, undiluted • 1 envelope dry onion soup mix • 1 Tbsp Italian dry herbs • ½ cup chicken broth	Directions: • Dice vegetables and place in crock pot with chicken broth. • Place chunked chicken on vegetables. • Spread undiluted soup over chicken and sprinkle with dry onion soup mix and herbs. Do not add any water. • Cook on low for 7-8 hours or on high 4 hours, or until chicken is done (meat thermometer reads 170 degrees F).

Substitutions and Additions:	Substitutions and Additions:
For Chicken:	For Chicken:
• Pot roast	• Pot roast
• Turkey cutlets	• Turkey cutlets
For Vegetables:	For Vegetables:
• Green beans	• Green beans
• Brussels sprouts	• Brussels sprouts
• Mushrooms	• Mushrooms
• Sugar snap peas	• Sugar snap peas
• Zucchini	• Zucchini
• Okra	• Okra
	For low fat cream of celery soup:
	• Low fat cream of mushroom soup
	• Low fat cream of broccoli soup

Dips

Great Guacamole: Avocado fits well into healthy diets; it's the perfect source of mono-unsaturated fat (the heart-healthy kind) and is naturally creamy without the saturated fat and cholesterol of mayonnaise.	Serves 16 (2 Tbsp each) about 50 calories, 4g fat, 0mg cholesterol, 1.6g fiber, 295mg sodium, 0.7g protein
Ingredients: • 2 medium avocados, peeled, pitted, and diced • 1 tsp sea salt • 1 large tomato, seeded and diced • ½ red onion, diced • 1 jalapeno pepper, chopped • 1 Tbsp chopped fresh cilantro • 2 Tbsp fresh lime juice • ½ tsp hot sauce (optional)	Directions: • In a medium bowl, mash the avocados and stir in salt. • Mix in diced vegetables, cilantro, and lime juice. • Cover and chill in the refrigerator at least 30 minutes before serving.

"Creamy" Dip: Substitute nonfat dairy products and never miss the saturated fat and cholesterol.	Serves 16 (1 Tbsp each) 17 calories, 167mg sodium
Ingredients: 2 Tbsp fat-free mayonnaise 1 container (8 oz) fat-free plain yogurt 1 package onion soup mix	Instead of mayonnaise, substitute nonfat plain yogurt and nonfat mayonnaise; mix with envelope of dry onion soup mix.

Snacks

Fruity Gelatin Delight: Make this with your favorite flavor gelatin; serve with nondairy whipped topping.	~60 calories per serving
Ingredients: • 1 package sugar-free fruit flavored gelatin (my favorite is raspberry) • 1 cup boiling water • ½ cup peeled and diced Granny Smith apple (about ½ medium apple) • ½ cup peeled and diced pear (about ½ medium pear) • 1 cup fresh (not from concentrate) orange juice • ½ cup chopped walnuts (1/4 cup for fewer calories)	Directions: • In a large glass bowl, dissolve gelatin in hot water. Add orange juice and refrigerate until partially firm (about 1 hour; you can speed it up by putting it in the freezer for 20 minutes). • Stir in fruit and nuts and refrigerate until set, about 1 hour.
Options: – Substitute or add: Can of mandarin oranges, drained Diced celery	Can of crushed pineapple: drained Cup of small grapes: halved

Smoothies & Frosty

Strawberry-Banana Tofu Smoothie	Serves 4 150 calories, 2.6g fat, 0g cholesterol, 8.3g protein, 3.3g fiber
Ingredients: • 1 (12 oz) package silken tofu • 1 cup nonfat milk or soy milk (unsweetened) • 1 banana, peeled, chunked, and frozen • ¼ cup frozen orange juice concentrate	Directions: • Blend ingredients at high speed until smooth. • Serve in a frosted glass with a sprig of fresh mint. • Optional: Add non-nutritive sweetener of choice or a tsp of honey (20 calories).

Chocolate Banana Frosty	Serves 2 165 calories, >1g fat, 5g protein
Ingredients: • 1 medium banana • 1 cup nonfat milk or soy milk (unsweetened) • 1 cup crushed ice • 1 "squeeze" chocolate syrup	Directions: • Blend ingredients at high speed until smooth. • Serve in frosted glass.

Orange-Mango Delight	Serves 2 125 calories, >1g fat, 5.5g protein
Ingredients: • 1 cup fresh orange juice • 1/3 cup diced mango (available frozen and unsweetened) or other fresh fruit, such as peach, nectarine, or cantaloupe • 1 cup nonfat sugar-free plain or vanilla yogurt • 1 cup crushed ice	Directions: • Blend ingredients at high speed until smooth. • Serve in frosted glass, garnished with fresh mint or an orange slice.

Smart Snack Strategies

Crunchy Yogurt: Mix a ½ cup low sugar/high fiber cereal such as Kashi GoLean into a 6-oz container of nonfat plain or sugar-free yogurt (186 calories)	**Nut Butter and Crackers:** Almond butter (2 Tbsp) and 5-6 whole grain crackers—trans fat-free, of course! (202 calories)
Berry Yogurt: Mix a 6-oz container of nonfat plain or sugar-free yogurt with 1 cup seasonal berries (189 calories)	**Power Cottage Cheese:** ¼ cup low fat cottage cheese mixed with 1 oz roasted shelled peanuts (220 calories)
Popcorn: Air popped (3 cups/90 calories), or 100-calorie pack low fat microwave (1 package/100 calories)	**Veggie burger:** Microwave a veggie burger; eat with whole wheat tortilla and 1 Tbsp ketchup (230 calories)
Oatmeal to Go: Microwave package of oatmeal with 1 cup nonfat milk or soymilk and ¼ cup raisins (243 calories)	**Peanut Power:** Mix 1 oz dry roasted peanuts and ¼ cup raisins (242 calories)
Fruit and Nut Fun: Slice a medium Granny Smith apple into quarters and spread with 1 Tbsp unsweetened cashew nut butter (172 calories)	**Avocado Dip:** Mix ½ cup diced avocado with 2 Tbsp fat-free thousand island dressing—eat with baby carrots (205 calories)
Turkey Roll-Up: Layer 1 slice turkey breast and ¼ cup cucumber slices on a whole-wheat tortilla; top with 1 tsp each nonfat mayo and mustard (175 calories)	**Nut and Raisin Energy Mix:** 1 oz *each* dry roasted almonds, chopped walnuts, and pecans, plus ½ cup raisins—mix and separate into 4 baggies (202 calories per serving)
Soup Stop: Microwaveable soups are perfect snacks—favorites are bean, vegetarian, and chicken with veggies (approximately 150-200 calories per serving)	**Quick Veggies:** Microwave 4 cups frozen crunchy veggies (broccoli, cauliflower, green beans); drain, sprinkle with Butter Buds (100 calories)
Pear and Cheddar: 1 oz low fat Cheddar and 1 medium pear (130 calories)	**Portable Protein:** 2 hard-boiled eggs (160 calories)
String Cheese: 2 oz reduced fat Mozzarella (160 calories)	**Cereal bar (uncoated):** Whole grain, low sugar, at least 2g fiber (approximately 150-200 calories)
Middle Eastern: 3 Tbsp hummus and 1 cup baby carrots (170 calories)	**Waffle Walk:** 1 whole wheat toaster waffle spread with 1 Tbsp peanut butter (180 calories)

Sandwiches

How to Make: Sandwiches

Talk about portable nutrition! But when does a sandwich become a diet buster? When it's overstuffed. Get creative with sandwich fillings, but watch your portion size. Stuff with all kinds of veggies, but stay lean on the meat and fillings that are higher in fat, such as nut butters and cheese.

Genius Selections	"OK" Selections
Start with 100% Whole grain: • Bread, wraps, tortillas, English muffin, mini-bagels Fill with: • Skinless turkey or chicken breast; canned tuna, salmon, sardines, or mackerel, and sliced avocado and tomato	Luncheon meats: Choose low fat and low sodium varieties; lean roast beef; low fat cheeses; lean ham; no-sugar-added nut butter
	Mayo vs. Mustard: Each tablespoon of mayonnaise adds 100+ calories. Mix 1 tsp of mustard with 2 tsp of nonfat mayo for a creamy Dijon-type spread that's yummy.

Desserts

Peach Melba Light: Instead of full-fat ice cream, substitute nonfat vanilla frozen yogurt. Top with sugar-free strawberry syrup and sliced peaches.	168 calories, 4g fat, 2g saturated fat, 19g sugar
Ingredients: • 1 cup light vanilla ice cream, about 100 calories per serving • ½ cup sliced peaches in juice • 3 Tbsp sugar-free raspberry syrup	Directions: Scoop ice cream into parfait glass. Top with sliced peaches and syrup. Garnish with a sprig of fresh mint.

Chocolate Pudding: Enjoy a sweet treat and strengthen your bones by making this dish with protein- and calcium-rich nonfat evaporated milk.	80 calories, 0g fat, 0g saturated fat, 0g cholesterol
Prepare instant sugar free pudding as directed, substituting nonfat evaporated milk for a creamier pudding.	

Heavenly Bread Pudding: Ethereally light because I substituted nonfat evaporated milk and reduced the sugar to only ½ cup. The raisins make it sweet and add fiber.	Serves about 8 Approximately 234 calories, 3g fat, 0.5g saturated fat, 1.5g fiber
Ingredients: • 2 cups nonfat evaporated milk • 1 cup low-fat buttermilk • 2 cups egg substitute • ½ cup sugar • ¼ tsp vanilla • 4-5 slices whole wheat bread • ½ tsp cinnamon • 1 tsp sugar • ½ cup raisins	Directions: • Preheat oven to 400 degrees. Lightly spray a 10"x12" baking pan with cooking spray. • In medium bowl, combine evaporated milk, buttermilk, egg substitute, ½ cup sugar, and vanilla. • Layer bread on the bottom of baking pan; pour milk mixture over bread. • Mix cinnamon with 1 tsp sugar and sprinkle over everything. Spread raisins evenly on top. • Cover with foil and place pan in a larger pan; fill smaller pan with hot water about halfway up the sides. • Bake 75-90 minutes or until set. Remove and let cool slightly before serving, or refrigerate.

When in Rome—or Milan, Venice, or Bologna—do as the Italians do and eat pizza. In Roman times, pizza was simply baked bread with herbs and olive oil, known as foccacia. Then in the 1600s, with the discovery of tomatoes in the New World, peasants from Naples began topping foccacia with tomatoes and cheese and baking *pizza* in lava-lined ovens. In the late 1800s, the *Margherita Pizza* was created for the (then) Queen of Italy. This most traditional of pizzas incorporates the colors of the Italian flag—red for tomatoes, green for fresh basil, and white for the mozzarella cheese.

Our latest trip to Italy was in search of the perfect pizza. We sampled pizza in six different cities: Venice (five times), Milan (four times), and once each in Bologna, Parma, and the northern, lakeside cities of Stresa and Tremesso. We found many "perfect" pizzas. They were all perfectly delicious! My favorite pizza on this gastronomic tour was in Milan. We dined outside, in a sidewalk *osterie*—a bar with a kitchen—and enjoyed a pizza topped with *Gaeta* olives (small, black olives), capers, fresh chopped tomatoes *rocket (*what the Italians call arugula), and shaved Parmesan cheese.

Susan's Pizza

Depending upon weather conditions and where you live (high humidity, altitude, etc.), you may need more or less flour, so go slowly.

I use a Kitchen Aid Mixmaster with a dough hook attachment. I've had this model for more than 12 years and it still works perfectly, but any stand mixer with a bread hook will do. By the way, since the dough needs to be kneaded, a blender won't do. You can also make the dough the old-fashioned way and burn some calories at the same time. Add flour to the yeast mixture slowly, a ½ cup at a time, mixing well with a wooden spoon until dough can be turned out onto a floured (preferably cool) surface. Then, knead for at least five minutes (adding remaining flour), until dough is elastic.

Pizza Dough

1 cup warm, not scalding, water
1 packet or 2 Tbsp active, dry yeast
1 tsp honey
½ cup whole wheat flour
approximately 3-5 cups unbleached bread flour

Directions:

1. Place warm water, yeast, and honey in the bowl of the mixer. Stir to dissolve yeast, add ½ cup of whole wheat flour, stir until incorporated, and wait about 15 minutes, until it gets a bit bubbly.
2. Using the dough hook attachment on slow speed, add bread flour in about 1/3 cup at a time (about 3 cups—or more as needed) and then increase speed and knead until dough comes together and doesn't stick to the mixer bowl. You should be able to stick your index finger into it and leave a slight impression— it shouldn't be too sticky to handle.
3. Coat a large bowl with cooking spray, place the ball of dough in the bowl, turn once to coat, then cover with plastic wrap or your bowl's cover. Let sit for 30 minutes until the dough approximately doubles. Now you're ready for pizza!
4. Punch down and follow directions for pizza below.

This recipe makes enough for two thin-crusted pizzas. You can also refrigerate dough in a large zip-lock bag—just shoot a quick spray of cooking spray inside—for about two days

Pizza Topping
Cooking spray
⅛ tsp red pepper flakes (optional)
1 small red onion, diced (about 1 cup)
1-3 garlic cloves, as preferred, crushed
1 package (10 oz) pre-washed spinach (or collard greens or kale)
2 cups sliced mushrooms—I like Portobello, but any will do!
large seeded and chopped tomato
1/3 cup chopped fresh basil (optional) or 2 Tbsp dried Italian herbs
½ to 1 cup shredded part-skim mozzarella cheese—or reduced fat mixed cheese, such as Cheddar and Jack

Before making the topping, "stage" your dough. Roll out or spread in a nonstick pizza pan or rectangular pan that's been sprayed with cooking spray and cover with a dishtowel—let rise a second time, at least 45 minutes.   Do this so the dough has a chance to raise again—it makes the crust good and chewy.

1. Coat a nonstick sauté pan with a quick spray of cooking oil and heat over medium heat.
2. Sauté red pepper flakes over medium heat for 1 minute.
3. Add red onion and garlic; stir and cook for 2 minutes.
4. Add spinach or other greens; cover and cook 3 minutes; uncover, stir, cover, and cook for another minute or so, until wilted.
5. Stir in mushrooms and continue to cook, covered, for about 5 more minutes; uncover and cook for 2 minutes until all liquid is evaporated.

6. Let cool about 15 minutes, and then spread over the dough.

7. Lay on chopped tomato and basil, and then sprinkle on cheese.

8. Bake in the middle of the oven at 435 degrees for about 20 minutes, until cheese is browned.

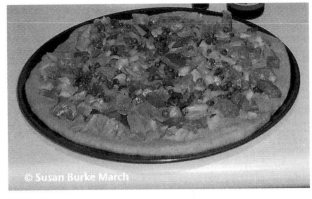

My homemade pizza fits perfectly into my natural 'diet'

Optional additions:

Medium shrimp: I buy frozen, pre-cooked medium-sized shrimp; rinse, drain, and place on pizza before the cheese.

Sardines: Rinse and drain a small can of sardines and place on pizza before cheese.

Makes 8 slices

Nutritional information, approximately

Calories 207

Fat 2-3g

Saturated fat 1g

Trans fat 0g
Cholesterol 4mg

Fiber 5g

Sodium 70mg

Protein 8-10g (depending if you add fish or tofu)

Carbohydrate 5g

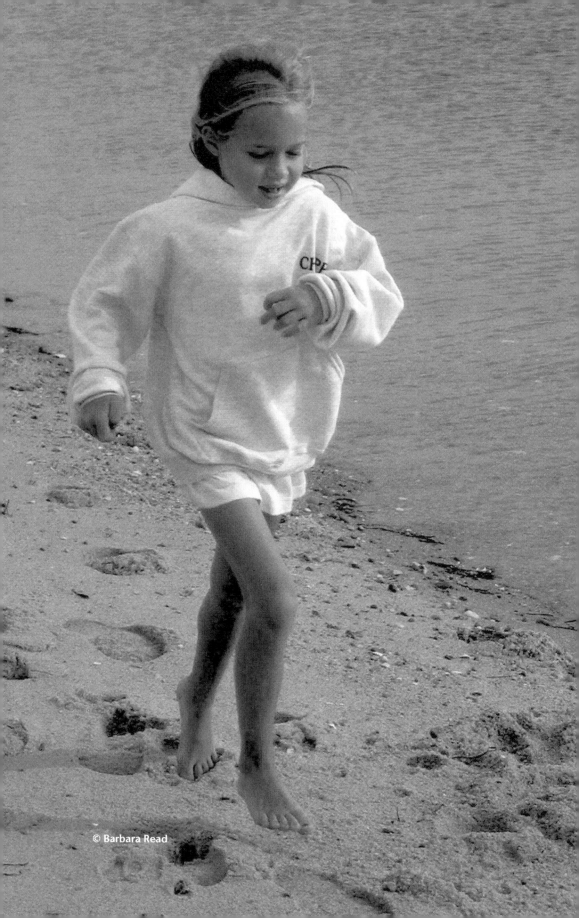

Chapter 8

Simple Steps to Natural Fitness Cement the Path to Permanent Weight Loss by Making Activity Second Nature

*A man too busy to take care of his health
is like a mechanic too busy to take care of his tools.*
—Spanish Proverb

As in previous chapters, I began by examining a word or term that we use in conversation—words that have become second nature to the way we think. We use words to define how we live, and it's always fun and valuable to *think about how we think*. That's how I learned to think differently—and translated my thoughts into new habits.

Almost 25 years ago, I thought about how my daily habits are enhanced when I think about what I do *every day*. Splitting the word into two doubles the impact.

By changing the way I use this common term and applying *every* and *day* to describe how I think about the food I eat and the activity that I schedule for myself, I've transformed my thoughts about the way I live.

DEFINITION

Everyday

—adjective

1. A routine event, in the ordinary course of events
2. Familiar and commonplace, "I make my walk an everyday habit"

Deliberate

—adjective

1. Something done with careful consideration and planning, "a deliberate decision."

—verb

1. to with careful thought and conversation reflect upon and discuss an issue—considering both sides, "they deliberated before deciding to buy the new treadmill."

Making a healthy lifestyle *second nature* takes effort—real effort. My transformation from *overweight* to *in control* took place one thought at a time—and one day at a time. *Naturally thin* people will tell you that they do something aerobic most every single day; it's become routine, a natural part of their daily lifestyle, and somehow, every day, they find time to "do" something deliberate. I re-thought my attitudes about exercise. I continue to mentally monitor how I think about my lifestyle.

Living Day By Day

I used to think that *diet* meant a weight loss diet. I now think that *diet* describes my natural way of eating. My diet is what I eat to stay naturally thin.

I use the words *every* and *day* as component parts of the internal scripts that I think about when I may feel lazy or tired, and I remind myself to think these words when making routine daily choices.

I visualize the dictionary definitions—when I think about activity, I can see the words **every day** as two distinct words. I rarely miss a day of doing at least 30 minutes of deliberate activity—first thing in the morning—and this habit is part of my *natural* life. That means it has become *second nature* for me to do **something** everyday that deliberately gets my heart rate up.

It would be **unnatural** for me to ride when I can walk or to take the elevator if there are stairs I can climb. If my stop is not too far up, I will naturally climb the stairs. If my stop is too far to walk, I'll take the elevator to a floor below my stop and walk up.

Of course, sometimes this is inconvenient, but convenience is fattening and I've got to work those strategies into my life in that way I make my life work for me. Isn't life grand!

Activity Strategies

Dietitians know about the many little strategies people can do to add activity minutes to their day—every day. For example, I try to incorporate some stretching into dusting, and—I'm sure you've heard this one, but I really do it—I park at the far end of the parking lot and walk. If I'm stuck in traffic, I tighten my butt—hold—and release. On an airplane, I always choose the aisle seat—in advance—and walk up and down the aisle when I get the opportunity. I take the stairs whenever possible—both up and down.

These are just additions to my **deliberate** daily aerobic activity—aerobic means "requiring air," as in activities that make your heart work harder, such as dancing, running, or walking fast enough to break a sweat.

Every day activities are like breathing—they're automatic—I just do them without thinking about it. But in addition to the everyday activity, I do some type of **deliberate** exercise, something more challenging that will make me breathe more deeply, and I try to do this type of activity every day.

This is what keeps my body happy and my weight under control. I don't stay active every other day or every third day. I stay active everyday. **Every day.**

Some days I do more deliberate activity—I may take a longer bike ride—and I go to the gym for 30 minutes of weight training three or four times weekly. Some days I do less, but I do something **every day.**

My Working for Fitness

Fitness doesn't happen automatically just because you want it. Just joining a gym doesn't create muscle. January is a very busy month at the gym—many people have resolved to lose 20 pounds, and the gym is buzzing with newly committed members, with wonderful intentions.

I Fell in Love with Fitness

Ironically, even if I can't see my clients, I get that 'naturally thin' comment. I consult with my clients mainly by phone or email, but not in person, so I do not know what my clients look like nor have they seen me. One day while consulting with a client on the phone, she said to me that she could just picture me sitting there all pretty and thin without having to worry about my weight.

I have to say, I am fortunate, but not because I do not have to worry about my weight. I am fortunate to have fallen in love—with fitness! It has been 25 years since I fell in love with movie Flash Dance and I got involved with the Jane Fonda aerobics craze. I am also fortunate to have been raised with parents who, although having been overweight most of their adult lives, are not obese. My parents always believed in eating home cooked meals and we rarely ate out. Today, my husband and daughter and I continue to follow this healthy tradition.

My staying slim is due to my healthy behaviors. Even though my parents were not raised with fitness conscious parents, they did not have to worry about fast food—it just wasn't an option when they were growing up. They gained weight over the years due to lack of exercise and overindulgence.

So, yes, I am "sitting pretty and thin," but it took a lifetime of work to build this machine, and having started early gives me a huge advantage because my body works more efficiently. Hence, it is true that you don't gain weight overnight, and taking it off is a process which requires patience, persistence and perseverance.

Renee Brunetti, LD, CPT
Coconut Creek, FL

But by February, the attendance drops off. The gym relies on this phenomenon; they couldn't possibly accommodate all the new members they enrolled in January—they'd have to build a new facility. They know that while most people have great intentions, many won't follow through. Of course, they want to be fit—they joined the gym, didn't they? But they skip the most important next step. They don't schedule an appointment with the personal trainer to set up a fitness program. Or they join a gym that's too far away from their house. Or their plan is to do it themselves, and they buy a piece of fitness equipment that's either too cheap to be effective or too complicated to use. Instead of putting it right up front in the living room, in front of the television where they will see it, maybe they place it down in the cold basement or on a hot back porch—somewhere they don't really want to hang out. Or it serves as a clothes hanger in the bedroom!

When you're ready for a fitness plan, make it as easy as possible to do it every day. And fitness happens every day—just like a diet; fitness is what you usually do, every day, to bring activity to your body.

Activity is a three-part affair, and these parts are synergistically effective—that is, they all enhance the others. First, it should be aerobic—get that heart rate up. Second, make your muscles work—that helps build strength and increases your metabolic rate. Third, be flexible—stretch your tendons and muscles gently, but regularly, to avoid injury. Using an online diary makes it easy to plan your week—you can type in what type of cardio you plan to do daily—walking, biking, swimming, dancing; and schedule 2-3 days of weight training or resistance band workouts.

As *diet* means what you *usually* eat—your *usual* choices for breakfast, lunch, and dinner—so does *fitness* mean how much of your time is devoted to deliberate activity. Deliberate activity is scheduled and is designed to build endurance and burn fat.

From Fat to Fit

Before I took control, I thought of fitness as a foreign land, a place where I'd never reside. Just like I used to think that I'd never break myself of the overeating habit, I also couldn't imagine finding time or motivation to be fit.

In 1976, I was 22, and I was in big trouble. I was overweight, smoking cigarettes, and binged on food about once a week. I was drinking a lot, and was out of control of my health—both physically and mentally. In September of that year, I ran into "William"; he was 20 years older than me and in great shape, having just completed a cross-country bike ride from Seattle to Washington, DC. He was in Florida to buy a sailboat to sail to Australia, and I was very impressed by all of his dreams and accomplishments—the fact that he was old enough to be my father was also a significant part of the (mutual) attraction.

One day he said, "Let's go jogging."

Uh-oh, I thought, *this isn't going to be fun. Can't we go to the beach?*

We drove to the local high school, where I sat in the bleachers as he ran his laps around the track. Each time he passed, I felt worse about myself. I could barely walk around the track—never mind jog. My old scripts played in my head, "Why can't I do this? Why am I so out of shape? He must really think I'm lazy. How does he keep going? Why can't I even start?"

The longer he ran, the more embarrassed I felt. He seemed to be running on autopilot, almost without thinking, although it was obvious from his perspiration that he was making an effort. I'd never seen anyone "in the zone" before, and I didn't understand why—although I was admiring his endurance—it was somehow making me feel bad about myself. He ran for about an hour, then finally slowed to a walk, and finished with stretches on the bleachers.

As I followed him back to the car he said, "Running keeps me fit. You should do it, too."

That did it. I felt even worse about myself and so embarrassed that I was so out of shape. Looking back, I realized that I had given up before I could even get started. I compared myself to him, and lacking in ability, I didn't even try to walk around the track. I just sat there, defeated.

Two years later, nothing had changed. Taking just enough credits to keep me in school, I clerked evenings in a convenience store, stuffing myself with pretzels and crackers. Refined carbs were still my drug of choice, snack foods that I craved. I now know these foods were sending my blood glucose levels soaring, forcing my body to produce more insulin to counteract the effect—leaving me feeling low and anxious. The vicious cycle of overeating and mentally castigating myself was accompanied by purging—and in that way, I kept my weight from ballooning even higher.

I struck up a friendship with a tall, slim woman who, like me, was taking an evening class to fulfill requirements for graduation, but unlike me, was on a defined path to a career, finishing up her MBA with a promise of a position in her family business. But she was very helpful, and I soon learned that she lived in an apartment near the beach and ran every morning—*every morning...for five miles...on the sand.*

I was astounded. I had never met a woman who ran regularly, let alone for that significant distance. And I soon learned that she traveled frequently, and in every city she visited, she ran. She had run in Paris, New York City, Melbourne, and London. Every single day, she ran—**every day. Daily** activity was a part of her life.

But it wasn't until I was back in New York, on that cool March evening, that I seriously started working activity into my life. And I've never stopped.

Because—activity is what 'naturally thin' people do. They work activity into their life—every day.

Daily activity is second nature to people who keep their weight under control.

You Have to Walk Before You Can Run

We all know that children learn how to walk by first learning to crawl. Watching "William" pound the track, I didn't think about his journey to fitness, or how he developed the stamina that allowed him to run so long. I needed to restructure my thinking, and accept that he had worked a long time and had learned to challenge himself—to enjoy the effort. No—as so many times before, I compared myself to him as if he were a perfect being—just as I did as a small child, when I had compared myself to everyone and felt lacking.

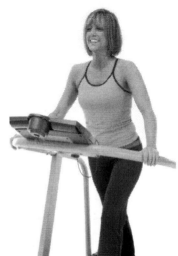

One step at a time is so elementary—and I had succeeded in other areas, right? There was no reason that I couldn't learn to be more active, to make healthy choices. But at the time, I didn't realize that. I thought, *I can't run—so I'm doomed to be fat.* I didn't realize that I could have *walked* around the track. William wasn't running against the clock—he was running for a certain length of time. But, I remember that he was challenging himself---I saw his effort. And that was the point. It wasn't a race, and if I'd have taken just the first step, I could have started on the path toward a better life than the one I was living.

My first steps toward fitness began when I took that walk many years ago on that cool March evening. And

Fitness is My Second Job!

I've developed a "working" attitude toward going to the gym. Just as I wouldn't think of missing work, I show up at the gym at least four days weekly—without fail. It's my second job! Going to the gym is a dedicated part of my life that I have to work other things around, not vice versa. Even on the road, I ensure my travels can accommodate exercise, either in a gym, or outside, or even in a hotel room with videos and equipment (bands, etc.). Again, NOT exercising simply is not an option.

I've taken a similar position with respect to sweets and desserts. On rare occasions I will indulge, but I eat this type of food rarely, so I really don't even have a taste or craving for it. And, when I do indulge, it's often with a "lesser evil" variety of the treat, such as one that's low fat or sugar free.

At home, I avoid temptation by stocking my pantry and refrigerator exclusively with healthy foods—making my choices pre-determined. I don't buy potato chips and then wrestle with whether or not to have one.

Because I've developed these habits, and it's routine for me to make these choices, there is no sense of sacrifice or deprivation, and I don't lament what I might be missing.

I do indulge periodically each week and when the splurge is worthwhile (going to an especially nice restaurant, for example), but these deviations are exceptions to my "normal" way of eating and, as such, usually have little or no affect on my body whatsoever.

My dedication to the "fitness lifestyle" started when I was 18. I had been a small child and adolescent, and then decided to get into bodybuilding. For the first time ever, I had to diet in one way or another (both to gain and then to lose for a show). That changed everything. People who don't know my workout and diet habits make comments such as "you don't need to worry." I tell them that one's weight is relative. I have an ideal for my body (especially after having seen it in "peak" condition) just as an overweight person does. It's this ideal that I continually aspire toward, and which keeps me motivated. I never allow myself to stray too far—if I'm close to it, I can "live a little," if I'm further, I tighten up the reins.

Merilee Kern
Author of "Making Healthy Choices -
A Story to Inspire Fit, Weight-Wise Kids"
San Diego, California

once I began to workout with weights, I found that beneath my fat, I had some muscle. I had a framework to build upon—my own skeleton. I wasn't able to run in the beginning, because my hips hurt when I ran, and I got winded so fast. So I walked. It's amazing what I accomplished by putting one foot in front of the other. I started slowly, and gradually I began to "work it out" and eventually, deliberately striding, and by pumping my arms, I turned my walk into a calorie-burning experience.

Running isn't necessary to lose weight—it's not the 'best' exercise for everyone, and if you're overweight now, it can be uncomfortable and stressful on your joints and tendons—so don't do it. Just as the best diet for you is the one that suits YOU—your lifestyle and food preferences—the best exercise for you is the exercises and activities that you enjoy and will look forward to doing. Purposeful walking will get the job done. You start gradually and keep going forward. Start with a minimum of 20 minutes, which means going out the door and walking for 10 minutes, turning around and coming back. Walk with purpose, dance with abandon, and bike with some effort.

Aerobic means:

- "With air," any exercise that uses a lot of oxygen

- Uses large muscle groups (your legs and arms)

- Can be sustained over time

- Uses continuous effort, as opposed to bowling, tennis, golf, or weight training.

Anaerobic activities will build muscle and tone and use other muscle groups, but aerobic activity is best for burning calories. Regular, deliberate activity develops strength and endurance and reduces stress.

Make your time to do deliberate exercise *your time.* My favorite time for deliberate activity is the morning. During the rest of the day, I use activity strategies to add to my calorie-expenditure diary. Getting out every morning makes me feel wonderful about life. But maybe you're not a morning person—if you want to do it after work, that's fine...as long as you do it. Marking off your activity on a daily diary is going to really pay off because when you write down your goals—and then note your progress—then they become accomplishments. You don't have to write a lot—just note what, when, how long, and if it was easy or still challenging. Do it on the log I've provided, invest in a book that provides a guided program, including logs and fitness guides, or do it online and sign up for a walking program (see Chapter 10—Help Is Here)

A Word about Pets

Your pet's fitness is your responsibility—overweight pets have the same health risks as overweight owners. Schedule time to walk, it's good for both of you and fun, too. I'd be remiss if I didn't mention Cindee, our 15-year-old Doberman Pincher. She was four months old when I adopted her, and it was my lucky day, certainly one of the smartest things I ever have done. She is the sweetest big baby, and from the day I got her, we walked and walked—always an hour in the morning, and at least for 30 minutes in the evening, even more when the weather was warmer. On weekdays we usually walked at 4:30 a.m. so that we'd get at least an hour. Cindee thrived on the activity, and so did I—I slept wonderfully every night, and for years I never had to worry about getting all my "steps" daily. On the weekends, we'd say hello to everyone in the street, and it was a real joy having such a personable doggie. Having a dog is a responsibility, but it is also such a reward, and most dog owners will tell you that they know the names of the neighborhood dogs, even if they don't know the owner's names. Now that Cindee has slowed down and can only walk shorter distances, I've had to use different strategies to get my aerobic activity. I now make deliberate and conscious efforts to take walks, and it seems strange to walk without her. My husband Ken misses walking with Cindee too, and has been very supportive—he says "yes" when I ask him to come along on walks without her.

You—Your Project

I like to think of fitness and diet as a job. How about you? If you are assigned to a new project, the first task is to do some research. Identify the objective—what is your goal? What are you attempting to accomplish? Why is it important to achieve the objective? If you understand the "why" and agree with it, then you will be motivated to get the job done. Next, it's important to identify the resources necessary to achieve your fitness goals just as you would for any project at work.

In this case, your resources will be dependent on the avenues you take to achieve the goal of personal fitness.

So think of yourself as a project. Work *in* your workouts, just as you would schedule your appointments and meetings with a project team. You are your own team leader, and you call the shots. You evaluate your progress, and you modify the goals as needed. Make an executive decision to be the best you can be. Create a schedule that will get the job done.

Fitness is a lifestyle—I don't think of exercise as a chore. Activity is part of my lifestyle, which means I fit it in—every day.

What's More Important: Counting Minutes or Calories Burned?

Most people can begin a simple walking program as long as they have no risk factors such as diabetes, heart disease or other chronic conditions. If you do, please speak with your doctor or healthcare provider, and if you're pregnant, or a new mom, a walking program is great, but speak with your doctor first, and don't let yourself get overheated.

Activities calculators are great for understanding how many calories you can burn doing specific activities, but using them too much is a lot like counting calories in foods. Focus too intently on the trees, and you lose sight of the forest. The idea is to get your daily minutes. Just do it, whatever you do, and do it daily.

The number of calories you're burning during exercise will depend on your personal body type, your bodily ratio of fat to muscle, and how intensively you're exercising and for how long. But as you continue to challenge yourself to do more, bear these two things in mind:

1. You should be able to carry on a conversation while exercising.

2. Your activity should make you feel stronger and energized, not wiped out.

Start with low impact activities like walking. When you're in the *action stage of change*, you may want to jump right into running—don't. Getting fit doesn't happen overnight—but it does happen, one step at a time.

If you have arthritis or you're very overweight now, just take it slow. As the name implies, low impact means one foot is always on the ground so there's less stress on your joints, tendons, and muscles, reducing the risk for injury. Even low impact can improve your cardiovascular function and increase your endurance—and strengthen those same joints, tendons, and muscles.

Getting Started

1. Warm up by just walking (even in place) for five to 10 minutes: Notice, I don't say stretch first, because your muscles, tendons, and joints are "cold" at the beginning—and warm when you are finished exercising. Never stretch "cold".

2. Activity, about 20-30 minutes: Simple walking is genius low-impact aerobic activity. Start slowly, and gradually work up the pace. For the first week, walk normally, and then pick up the pace to about three to four miles per hour.

3. Add Variety: Walking is great, but it's best to alternate with other low-impact activities so you work different muscle groups and don't get bored. Try biking (my favorite!), step machines, elliptical trainers, rowing machines, water aerobics, or dancing.

4. More: Yoga, tai chi, and other meditative exercises are great to strengthen your bones, muscles, and tendons, and they also decrease stress. They perfectly complement the new you—as you're becoming more fit, you're also more in touch with how you feel, breathe, and live.

5. Cool Down: As important to your safety and fitness as your warm up—take five minutes to slowly stretch your muscles, flex your tendons, and breathe deeply.

6. Write it Down: Use your Daily Living Log to record what you did—what time you started, how many minutes you spent, and how you felt afterward.

7. Reward: At the end of the week, take 30 minutes to relax and reflect on how wonderful you feel about your accomplishment. You did it for you, because you're worth it!

Be a Lean, Mean, Fat-Burning Machine!
Male/Female Puzzlement

It's a common complaint. Two people—let's call them "Cathy" and "Carl"—go on a diet at the same time. Both of them go to a nutritionist who determines how many calories they need to maintain their current body weights, and they each get a meal plan that decreases that number by 500 calories per day. Ideally, according to the formula for weight loss used by the experts, this should produce about a pound of weight loss every week.

But after two weeks, Carl loses four pounds, and Cathy only loses two pounds. After a month, Carl has lost almost 10 pounds, and Cathy has only lost five. What is she doing wrong? Most likely nothing—and everything. If Cathy is just dieting and restricting her calories, Carl will most likely lose faster. Carl's body is made up of more muscle, which is metabolically more active than fat, and it's doing some calorie-burning for him. Cathy needs to create a new situation that will help her burn calories at rest, too.

In *She Loses, He Loses*, a book by registered dietitian Karen Miller-Kovach, she describes the physiological and psychological differences between men and women when it comes to weight loss. For example, men wouldn't feel comfortable with being described as "thin" because that implies weakness, but women think that "thin" is complementary. When men decide to go on a diet, they are more confident that they'll succeed. Women more often change their diet first—men exercise more. And because they're made differently—there are differences in hormones, body type, even differences between how they think about food—they lose weight differently, too[1].

Weight loss happens one pound at a time by creating a calorie deficit—either eating fewer calories or burning more calories in increased activity. But most girls don't grow up playing the way boys play. In my generation, girls were less likely to engage in muscle-building activities. And it's natural for girls to have more body fat than boys, for normal hormonal function and menstruation. Consequently, since women have a smaller percentage of their weight from muscle, they're at a weight loss disadvantage since muscle tissue is more metabolically active—that is, a muscular body requires more calories for maintenance than a body with more fat.

Muscle is more calorie-useful than fat. That is, the more muscle mass you have, the more calories you burn at rest. And muscle doesn't disappear from your body—it doesn't turn to fat. When people gain weight, they gain fat stores—they can make more fat storage sites, or fat cells—but their muscle cells don't go away; they just get hidden underneath the fat.

So when a guy goes on a diet, eats fewer burgers, drinks less beer, eats better, goes walking, plays more basketball, and burns more calories—just because he has more muscle underneath to begin with—he loses weight more quickly.

Thus, women need to think *muscle*. Not big muscle, but lean muscle. Think lean! Think muscle. Yes, some bodies are genetically programmed to store fat more easily and efficiently—they wouldn't starve as quickly when the famine came! But, we *can* change our bodies—research shows that women who lift weights at least twice weekly have a huge advantage in slowing down "middle age spread"[2]. Build some lean muscle and look trimmer, feel stronger, and maintain your fitness.

When I was growing up in the 50s and 60s, girls didn't have the opportunity to build muscle. Boys had team sports, had to climb ropes, and do real pushups, but girls could do modified pushups on their knees. As a kid, I never developed upper body strength and remember being mystified that boys could pull themselves up, arm-over-arm. I remember once trying to climb the robes in gym, and I couldn't lift myself an inch from the floor.

Today, I know that the reason I don't have to count calories—the reason I'm able to maintain my weight without going on and off diets—is because, over the years, I've developed muscle mass and decreased my body's fat stores. Recently my body fat measured by a commercial bioelectrical impedance device was about 23%--I've replaced fat stores with lean muscle and burn more calories at rest than when I was overweight.

Gym Transformation

Back in my late 20s, I joined a gym, which helped me change how I thought about my body—and made my dream of weight loss and weight management possible. By using the machines and a few free weights—and doing it regularly—within months, things were definitely looking up for me, and everything started to change.

At my initial visit, they took my measurements, weighed me, and wrote it all in my own log book, which they asked me to use to record my activities every time I worked out. Measurements are a good way to monitor progress, because as you gain muscle and fitness, your weight is less important than how you've been able to transform your body. You don't lose inches overnight, but soon those numbers change, as you increase your fitness, and as your fat stores decrease, you also build muscle. I weigh myself infrequently, but I do use those jeans that I was so excited to fit into to keep a check on my waist and butt!

Back at my gym, the trainer showed me around the weight machine circuit, first demonstrating how to properly use each machine and explaining what I was trying to accomplish by using it. Then she made me show her that I could set the weights as prescribed, and I then finally, I performed each exercise properly. She showed me how she wanted me to complete my workout log, including noting my aerobic activity.

"Don't increase the weight each time you go," she said, adding that the biggest risk for injury is when people start stacking on the weight before they're ready.

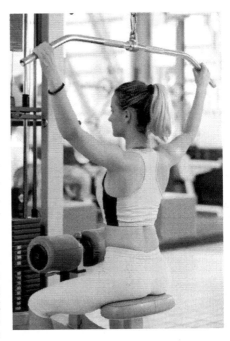

When I was in weight loss mode, I used the step machine and treadmill for aerobic exercise. At first, completing just 10 minutes was so difficult, especially on the step machine. I noticed immediately that most of the people using the step machines were leaning forward—with their hands positioned backwards on the sidebars— and stepping really fast. I thought, *Gee—I'm really out of shape. Look how fast they're going— I'll never get that good.*

But, I soon realized that, while the position allowed them to go faster, they were using less effort than it would take to stand straight, using the side bars just to balance. I kept it up, using recommended form, feeling righteous that I was getting more out of going slowly than those "leaners" were. Experts say not to count on the workout equipment's calorie burn displays because they commonly overestimate by up to 30 percent. A better indicator of effort is whether or not you break a sweat; when you do, you know you're exerting an effort. Isn't that simple!

I gradually gained endurance as I increased my time from 10, to 15, then 20 minutes. Pretty soon I looked forward to getting to the gym by 5:30 a.m. and doing 30 minutes on the step machine, followed by 30 minutes of weight machines.

For the past 25 years, I've kept the gym in my life. Occasionally I ask the floor trainer to show me how to use a machine I've not used or ask for tips on my technique. Each year, I rejoin, weighing the cost per month against my lifestyle. For example, my old gym cost about $40 per month. That's about $1.33 per day. I can afford that. And because I paid in full each year, they added a free month each time I rejoined—what an incentive! When I recently moved from South Florida to North-Central Florida, I had no regrets—except for leaving my gym. I'd found a home away from home there—every morning I could count on seeing my old pals there, even though we never socialized we saw each other at least three times a week. And I found a new gym. My new gym isn't as close to my home as my old gym, but I've turned it into a positive. Like so many years ago, I'm multi-tasking. I ride my bike there, getting in my 40 minutes of aerobic exercise—20 minutes to ride there and 20 minutes back—and then using the machines and free weights for 30 minutes. I'm so happy that I found a new gym—I *love* my new gym. There are people of all ages there very early in the morning, and even though I don't talk at length to anyone—I say hello to everyone—we share the knowledge that we're all there working toward the same goals: Keeping healthy, staying well, and getting our exercise out of the way, first thing in the morning.

On the Machine

Warm up by setting to low speed for five minutes, and either walk or step comfortably, then kick it up gradually. When I break a sweat, I keep going for 15-20 minutes, then back off to a comfortable pace for five more minutes. Never, ever lean on the machine—that's letting the machine do the work, and you will not get results. Avoid looking at the calorie burn estimators—they are not accurate for individuals. Time and effort are individual—so set your own.

Muscle Mass: Burn Calories Without Trying

Just being muscular doesn't always translate into fitness, but building lean muscle helps you age healthfully. The "father of aerobics," Dr. Kenneth H. Cooper, found that—in addition to aerobic activity—including strengthening exercises in your workout routine helps you avoid an inevitable loss in strength and muscle mass.

Resistance training changes your body. After I'd been using the weight training machines and free weights for a few months, I began to notice the difference—my body felt firmer, and as I continued to work out regularly I got excited about the changes.

Now, I'm not saying that I turned my fat into muscle; muscle and fat are different tissues. Both muscle and fat play important roles in regulating body functions, each with their own hormonal secretions and responses. And just as muscle can't turn into fat from lack of use, fat doesn't somehow transform into muscle from exercise. Rather, over time and with effort, stored fat is burned for energy, and fat cells shrink. As you consistently challenge your body by creating resistance, you build new muscles and tone the ones you have.

Your heart is also a muscle that greatly benefits from conditioning, and resistance training and consistent aerobic activity lowers risk for high blood pressure, insulin resistance, heart disease, and diabetes.[3] Depending on your personal goals, start gradually, and stay consistent.

Gyms: Keep it Close, and Choose Your Hour

Gyms don't necessarily mean sweaty, muscle-bound guys lifting huge weights—grunting and screaming and smelling like hell. Well...yes...in some gyms, that's what it's like. I've been there. But all gyms are not the same, and many have family areas, where men and women and teens all work out together. My first gym was great—there was a big room full of Nautilus machines and people of all shapes and sizes, and I never felt intimidated. There was also a free weight area, aerobic rooms, and a locker room. For years, it was my destination before work.

Since then, I've worked out in many different gyms. Over the past few years, I've noticed an increase in the number of older people in their 70s and 80s—not pumping big weights, but they're getting the job done. They are waging the good fight—staying limber, strong, and avoiding muscle loss.

If you join a gym, you most likely will receive an orientation visit that will include a personalized activity schedule and instruction. This is ideal, because your fitness schedule should suit your current level of fitness. Make your motions smooth and strong—if the weight is too heavy and you have to jerk it to lift it, you're risking injury. Don't hesitate to call on a floor trainer to demonstrate proper technique. Don't be shy—it's easy to do it wrong—it's much smarter to ask so you can do it right.

Just like you need a meal plan that suits your eating preferences and budget, your gym needs to be close to your home or office—and the hours need to suit your schedule. If the only time you have for yourself is first thing in the morning, then the gym has to open early, or if your body clock says the best time is later in the afternoon or evening, then your gym needs to be open late.

Today, if I don't work out for a few days, my muscles feel softer, and I don't like it. I prefer the strong feeling I get from a moderate workout. If traveling, I try to stay in hotels with good fitness facilities or in an area that's friendly for walking. Some hotels without fitness facilities will refer guests to a local gym—for free or for a discounted rate. I like to see who else is working out early in the morning. One of my favorite parts of professional conferences is meeting up with colleagues that I only see once a year—I can look forward to seeing the same faces year after year early in the morning—at the hotel's gym. Kindred spirits! I'll get a local map and walk—and pack a resistance band so I can do some simple stretching exercises—it makes me feel great—you can also use a wall to do some shoulder presses and balance for leg lifts. Instead of returning from vacation having to start all over again, I maintain my fitness and strength.

Building muscle can change your life as it did mine. As I began to workout at the gym, my body responded. I noticed that my arms were losing their flab; my legs, my butt, and my abs felt harder. I love feeling strong and continue to build on that feeling of accomplishment.

Other fitness options: Consider the costs; weigh the opportunities

- Group classes: The local YWCA/YMHA associations

- School gymnasiums: Adult education

- Online: Flash technology demonstrates proper fitness protocol; fitness podcasts and online videos

- DVDs or videos: For purchase, by subscription or for free from the library; aerobics, yoga, Pilates

- Equipment instruction: Many fitness tools come with instructional videos

My Bike-Affair

I hadn't ridden a bicycle outdoors since I was a kid. My neighbor Fred was older than my father, but he was so slim and energetic that he seemed much younger.

Every Saturday morning, Fred and a couple of neighborhood boys would set out on their bikes, and one morning, he said, "Come on—we're going for a ride—you can come, too!" I hesitated, but followed, trying to keep up with their 10-speeds, but falling behind on my 3-speed bike. The hills were steep, and I remember the pain and frustration of trying so hard—I was so winded that I turned around and went home. That's why I think it's close to miraculous that some 40 years later, the activity I enjoy the most is biking. I know it's because I have worked hard to develop what I didn't have then—endurance and aerobic capacity. Poor Fred: He never understood why I hid from him. I just wasn't ready—I hadn't developed walking skills, and he and the boys were running.

When I lived in New York City, in my pre-dietitian days, I joined a healthy weight support group. We consistently discussed different ways to keep active. One of the girls loved biking around Central Park, but of course, winter's snow and ice—not to mention rain—made outdoor biking impossible. So she bought one of those contraptions that allowed her to bike indoors. She liked it much better than an exercise bicycle and said it gave her a better feeling about riding in place—she felt like she was really riding. When I first joined the gym back on Long Island, I noticed a guy who arrived on his bike as I drove up in my car. *Hmmm*, I thought, *what a smart guy. He's multi-tasking! I can ride my bike to the gym and get my aerobic exercise at the same time.* What a concept!

Riding to the gym in the morning marked the beginning of my bike-affair. Today, I never drive when I can bike—the time it takes to ride to the post office or grocery store is usually within 10 to 15 minutes of the drive time, and I get the benefit of burning calories, too. My husband supports my bike-habit—in addition to the one he bought for $40 at the garage sale (my errand bike, with a basket) my birthday a few years ago was a bike with fat tires and saddlebags, great for going to the beach, through sand and dirt. My road bike is lighter, with skinnier tires, and it's easy to go longer distances. My bikes always have the tires pumped up and as my husband says, "they're always ready to roll!"

Regain Does Not Have to Mean Relapse

When I started working at eDiets in 2000, I gained about two pounds the first month. I realized it was strictly from my new lifestyle. Working online means sitting all day—if you let it be that way. I had come from working as a clinical nutrition manager at a hospital—where I deliberately climbed the stairs, often three or four times a day. Five flights—18 stairs per flight—up and down and up. Add walking up and down corridors and parking at least three city blocks away—if I even managed to get that close! Urban people are often slimmer than their counterparts in rural areas, who use cars to travel everywhere.

But working online changed my personal calorie-burning equation. Yes, I was still doing my regular deliberate activity—biking every morning, walking my dog at least 30 minutes daily—but I was doing less **everyday** activities.

Get Strong!

The Centers for Disease Control and Prevention advise that strength training is safe and effective for people of all ages—men, women, and especially the elderly—even if they are not in perfect health. Rehabilitation and treatment for conditions such as heart disease and arthritis includes lifting weights a few times weekly. Strength train to avoid these conditions—and if you currently suffer from any of these conditions, consult with your healthcare provider to see if you can get a referral to a strength training program.

- Arthritis: Strengthens bones, muscles, and connective tissue to decrease pain

- Diabetes: Improves insulin sensitivity—helps maintain normal blood glucose

- Osteoporosis (bone loss): Maintain or build bone mineral density; reduce risk for falls

- Sarcopenia (muscle loss): Almost inevitable with sedentary people; strength training to build and challenge muscle avoids this debilitating condition—performed on alternate days and enhanced with good quality dietary protein

- Obesity: Of course, you know already that building muscle helps you lose weight, and it's also helpful to avoid the slowing of the metabolic rate that comes with aging—maintain or increase metabolic rate to maintain weight without dieting

- Sleep: Fall asleep more easily—sleep better and feel better because your sleep is improved

- Depression and Self Esteem: Physiologically shown to reduce depression; I can attest to feeling better because I felt stronger and looked trimmer

What to do? I brought my sneakers to work! Twice a day, I put them on and took a quick 10 minute walk around the parking lot. I was lucky enough to live just a few miles from my office, and I started biking to work a couple of times a week. Within one month, I was back to my usual weight.

Get Addicted to Activity

I'm an activity addict—but it's a positive addiction. I take opportunities to burn calories daily, because I know my body—it just wants to store those excess calories in my fat cells! People who don't know me might say, "Oh, you don't have to exercise—you're naturally thin." But, from years of experience, I have found that my staying thin "naturally" results from my every day habits. Exercise is addictive--it makes you feel really good. Exercise promotes the release of stress-reducing hormones called endorphins, and makes you sleep better, and strengthens your immunity.

Besides the physical benefits, there are social rewards too. When you walk around your neighborhood, you'll get to know your neighbors, maybe make new friends.

Walk regularly, in addition to any other aerobic activities you do, and bring your partner, spouse, and any kids you may have at home along with you. You don't have to make it a long distance walk—just 15 minutes or more is all it takes to find other people to say "hi" to and feel more connected to the community.

Marking the Distance, One Step at a Time

Deliberate activity doesn't have to be complicated or expensive---not at all! For most, walking doesn't take special skills or equipment. Good walking shoes are a must, but you can buy them at the local sports store. Brisk walking, done daily, can keep you fit and help you lose weight—and keep it off.

My idea of fun is getting out on my bike and seeing the sights. I personally dislike aerobic classes, because I don't like being yelled at first thing in the morning. But my sister loves aerobics class. She's not a morning person and wouldn't dream of getting up earlier just to workout. She looks forward to dance aerobics after work—shifting gears and getting pumped up. She's energized by the group's sprit and music and even all the shouting. It's motivating to be accountable to others— when you get to know the instructor and the group you feel motivated to get there and show your face two or three times weekly—it's called a relationship! Unless I get my exercise first thing in the morning, I find it difficult to get motivated later— so, I just get it done, and I don't worry about anyone else's schedule—if I need to get up earlier to accommodate others, I will.

I'm a morning person, and if I get out of bed and right into my sneakers, it doesn't matter what the weather—I do it. If I get it done first thing, it's done for the day...that's so motivating for me. I've hit the street on the coldest winter day, with the temperature at zero, wind howling. I wore two pair of socks, covered my face with a ski mask, and did it—just because my script says "Do It!" Now that I live in Florida, I hear complaints that it's too hot to exercise. Too hot, too cold—hey... there's always an excuse NOT to do it. I get up early, and get my bike out before it gets too hot. I go swimming; I walk at dusk. There are always ways to get it done.

The secret is in the consistency. It has to be done daily—or at least five times weekly. The National Weight Control Registry research found that successful weight loss *maintainers* walk about 28 miles a week. Does that sound hard? Remember, it's not 28 miles all at once, but it accumulates by the end of the week. The goal is to walk about 30-60 minutes daily *or* about 28 miles weekly. Depending on how YOU like to measure the "distance" you can use time, or steps.

Using a pedometer to monitor the distance covered is a great idea. It's one of those techno-tools that make us more active—what a concept! Most technology serves to make us more sedentary—but pedometers make us get up and go. Also, just as a good friend can offer gentle reminds without criticism, a pedometer can be your conscience— in a very good way. Successful step-counters clip on their pedometers every morning, the same way they put on a wristwatch—as part of their wardrobe.

Choose a pedometer based on what you want it to do for you; a simple step counter is great for beginners, and The American College of Sports Medicine has a lot of great information about walking and choosing the right pedometer for you[4]. Log on to the Internet for an integrated program. You can log your steps, and the programs will assess your activity compared to your personal data (height, weight, age, sex) and voila! You can even print reports of the calories you expend, or create online reports that graph your progress.

Your steps per day describe your activity level[5]:

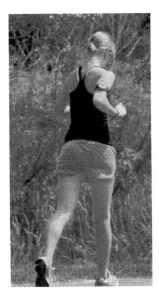

STEPS PER DAY	ACTIVITY LEVEL
Less than 5,000	Inactive
5,000-7,499	Slightly Active
7,500-9,999	Moderately Active
10,000-12,499	Active
12,500 or more	Very Active

Make walking second nature

The average adult takes approximately 2,000 steps per mile, so it takes about 10,000 steps to walk five miles. If you move more, that's great. American adults average fewer than 5,000 steps a day. If that's you, no problem. It's going to get better. Start by making **gradual changes**. Set an easily **attainable**

Pedometers

Make your pedometer part of your wardrobe. It's a friendly monitor and motivator, reminding you to get your steps in.

The Weight Management Dietetic Practice Group, a specialty practice group of the American Dietetic Association, recommends a pedometer that:

- Has a closed case—prevents accidentally resetting
- Has a safety strap—so it can't fall off when you lower your pants
- Has a flip-to-open mechanism and spring-loaded clip versus a molded plastic clip that slides over waist band
- Comes with a warranty
- Accusplit and Digiwalker were recommended by most of the group's online forum members
- Women take note; the Omron HJ can be worn in your pocket or bra, a nice feature
  - Buy online at Amazon.com for competitive prices and variety

goal of increasing your steps by 2,000 more per day, and if weight loss is your goal, reduce your caloric intake by 100 calories. Over time, work your way up to 10,000 steps per day.

Take some time and think about what you are preparing for. You're not dieting, or "going on a diet," you're preparing to succeed by understanding first where you are, and you do that by making your first week a "warm-up week." This week prepares you for increased effort, it prepares your body and your legs, especially if you're not used to walking. If you're currently exercising daily, that's wonderful, and keep it up. But now you're going to be writing everything down, so you can see your progress over the next 12 weeks.

This is *NOT* the week "before the diet", and forget the notion of "going on" a diet at all. Many people think, "Oh, I'm going *on a diet* so I'll eat all my favorite foods this week, in preparation for the deprivation." No—the first week is just the week to *maintain your usual diet and activity*. And to begin to log your progress.

1. Your Calendar: Choose a day to begin---most people like Monday. From that day, count forward **13 Mondays. Circle each day of the first week; that's** your "warm-up week." Then draw a big heart around the second Monday—on the second Monday, you'll start increasing your steps. Finally, draw a big heart around the 13th Monday—to mark 12 weeks of fitness walking.

2. Warm-up Week: As in the stages of change model, this week is to solidify your preparation for the rest of your life. For the next week, wear your pedometer daily and log your steps—plus any deliberate exercises you normally do—and record in your *naturally eating* food diary everything you eat and drink. But don't change a thing from your *usual* diet or activity.

3. Week Two: After your warm-up week, total all your steps for that week, and divide by seven: that's your average daily steps—your baseline to work upward from. *Get Started:* For the first three weeks, add at least 500 more steps daily. Remember, when you wear that pedometer, ALL activities count...dancing, stair climbing, biking, or taking the long way around from the parking lot to the office. It all adds up!

4. Wear your pedometer every day. Use your walking log to write down how many steps you take daily, or go online and track your steps—it's fun!

5. Log where and when you are active. At first, I was intimidated just by thinking about the numbers of steps it takes to walk a mile—about 2,000 for the average adult. But as soon as I put on the pedometer, I realized that every step I took started adding up, and it was easy to get my steps in when I tried.

Warm-up Week: If you determine that you average 3,000 steps daily over seven days, this is your baseline

- Week 1: Aim for at least 3,500 steps daily

- Week 2: Aim for ~4,000 steps

- Week 3: Aim for ~4,500 steps

On your fourth week, step it up and add 600 steps daily.

- Week 4: Aim for ~ 5,100 steps

- Week 5: Aim for ~5,700 steps

On your sixth week, step it up and add 700 steps daily

- Week 6: Aim for ~6,400 steps

- Week 7: Aim for ~7,100 steps

On week eight, step it up and aim for 10,000 steps a day—more, if you're enjoying it.

Weeks 8-20: For the next 12 weeks, keep going and add deliberate exercise to your day, including strength training. If you don't join a gym, that's fine—use an online program, a DVD, or a video to learn and practice strengthening exercises at home.

Naturally Thin Lifestyle Ideas

- Pedometer Ideas: I put on my pedometer when I wake up and take it off to go to sleep. I keep it in the bathroom so I see it first thing in the morning when I'm brushing my teeth. When I first undertook my lifestyle change, we didn't have pedometers, but today—especially when I'm traveling and away from my usual routine—I clip on my step counter to monitor my activity. By the way, weight maintainers often wear theirs daily, long after they've reached their goal. Just think of it as your daily exercise reality check.

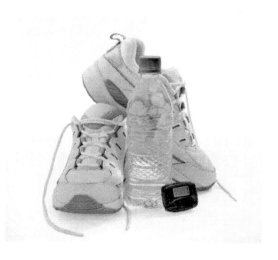

- All Weeks and Onward: The pedometer is your friend—it helps you maintain weight loss because it reminds you of the distance covered toward your goal. How many steps you need to cover depends on you, but experts advise at least 10,000 steps daily. Remember, a 20-minute walk is just 10 minutes one way and 10 minutes back.

- Natural: Monitoring your steps means more than just burning calories—it means maintaining a healthy weight—naturally. What can be more natural then moving more?

- For the first few weeks, pace is less important than distance. After a while, the distance becomes easier, and then it's time to pick up the pace and have some fun challenging yourself. Over time, your fitness level will increase, and you can work toward picking up the pace.

- It Fits: Make exercise fit into your lifestyle. It may mean taking short 10-15 minute power-walks during the day.

- Non-negotiable: My friend, Beth Casey Gold, is a registered dietitian who has spent years guiding people through the process of weight loss and maintenance. As an expert in leading structured programs, she helps individuals identify positive behavioral changes that lead to permanent weight loss. Beth says that since exercise is a non-negotiable aspect of permanent weight loss, walking is the perfect program to get most people moving—most everyone can do it, and it can fit into every lifestyle.

- Guess what? Pedometers measure **all your activity**—that's why they're so much fun. So dance, skip, jump, bike! It will all show up as accumulated activity.

- Added deliberate activity will translate into weight loss and increased strength and agility.

Be Deliberate

- **Deliberate exercise** is also known as *physical activity,* and besides helping you lose weight and maintaining the weight loss, deliberate exercise reduces stress, lowers risk for diabetes and heart diseases, and increases self esteem. Start with a physical and discuss your results with your doctor.

- Once you start walking, make it *deliberate.* Deliberate exercise can be power-walking, aerobics, dancing, or biking at a moderate-intense pace.

- Your walking sessions don't have to be 30 minutes all at once—especially in the beginning. Start with two 15-minute sessions at least three days weekly for the first two weeks. Then bump it up to twice daily for 20 minutes, and so on, until you're walking at least five days a week for at least 45 minutes.

- Just by walking, you will create a calorie deficit of 100-200 calories daily, which means approximately 20 pounds of fat loss in a year. Make it *second nature* and keep the weight off permanently.

Naturally thin thinking: Stay Positive

Are you worried that you won't be able to maintain an exercise schedule? Head off negative thoughts right from the start by acknowledging that it is going to be different, but it's going to be **good**.

Turn negatives into positives by naming your fears—and then name smart solutions:

For example:

FEAR:
I can't exercise because I have to work late and then carpool my daughter to soccer.

SMART SOLUTION:
Instead of standing on the sidelines watching the game, I'll bring my sneakers with me and walk for 30 minutes on the perimeter of the field.

FEAR:
I can't wear a pedometer—it looks stupid!

SMART SOLUTION:
I'll get used to it—it's fashionable to wear electronic stuff clipped to your belt. I like the idea of taking my fitness with me.

Prepare to Succeed

Commit to succeed. Create a plan and identify the resources you need to get started. A pedometer is a smart investment and everyone can afford one (just think—give up one fast food meal and you can afford one) and range from basic and inexpensive (as little as $4-$5) to technologically sophisticated tools that may be used with an online program to graph your progress.

For me, joining a gym made very good sense. I decided to invest in my future and treated my gym membership as the cost of materials needed to make my goals a reality. I looked at my schedule—and at my priorities—to see what could be changed and adjusted so I could fit in my workouts every day.

Of course, joining a gym—a reputable establishment with certified personal trainers, lots of machines for you to build muscle, and aerobics classes to pump your heart—is a wonderful idea, especially when you're starting out. But gyms aren't going to make or break your weight goals—you don't have to pay extra to get fit. Although it's nice, it's just like weight loss diets. You can do it on your own, as long as you have goals for activity, a place to log your activity, and a re-evaluation plan.

Instant Motivation
Online Activities Calculator

If you're like more than 70 percent of Americans, you have access to the Internet. All ages, even seniors, are logging on and learning. Although some may criticize computers for keeping people sedentary, they have become a marvelous way to access fitness and nutrition advice and find tools—lots and lots of tools. Log on and type "fitness program" or "activities calculator" into your web browser—there are dozens of free programs and calculators available. Don't hesitate to keep tracking your activities, so you can see where you're going and stay motivated to continue.

Log on and play with an activities calculator to see how many calories you need to maintain your current weight. To lose weight naturally, cut about 200-300 calories from your usual daily diet. That's a lot easier than you might think! For example, cut out one 8-ounce glass of orange juice and replace with one whole orange (cut 60 calories); eliminate one serving of bread and replace with lettuce and tomato (cut another 60 calories); and change your afternoon snack from a moccachino latte to a skinny latte (cut 100 calories—total deficit about 220 calories). Then add some calorie-burning activity to your usual daily activity, and burn at least 200 calories extra, three times a week. Within one month you can lose a pound just by making very small dietary changes, and by adding deliberate activity, your body responds by shedding more fat.

Activities Calculators:

Find out how many calories you burn by doing your exercise—or tell the program you want to burn 200 calories, and see how many minutes it takes (choose from hundreds of exercises)

www.calorieking.com/tools/exercise_calories.php

www.caloriesperhour.com

www.caloriecontrol.org/exercalc.html

www.bodybuilding.com/fun/calories.htm

www.cancer.org

Log on as see, for example, how many calories a 150-pound person burns doing a bunch of different exercises. For instance, walking briskly burns almost 300 calories per hour. Dancing burns almost 400 calories. Biking vigorously: 440 calories per hour. Experts say that accumulating at least 150 minutes of activity weekly is a good goal

She's Walking Every Day

While getting a manicure, I overheard the woman in the next station saying that she'd just returned from vacation in Ireland. We started chatting about how beautiful Ireland's countryside is and how interesting and wonderful that they have banned smoking—even in the pubs! We agreed that it's fun to explore different cuisines.

She said, "Oh, I gained weight on vacation."

I looked at her more closely; she was obviously thin, and she looked pretty good to me—clear eyes, smooth skin—and I guessed she was in her late fifties or early sixties. *OK, I'll bite*, I said to myself.

I commented that her natural habits must be pretty healthy, and she said, "Oh no...I eat all day long!"

"What do you usually eat for breakfast?" I asked. I usually find that knowing what a person usually eats for breakfast helps me understand her lifestyle.

"Oh, my usual oatmeal, skim milk, and fruit."

"Hmm...that sounds pretty balanced," I said. "What else do you eat?"

"Well, I usually don't eat junk—it's just that on vacation, I didn't do as much activity as usual, and we ate out so much."

"And what kind of activity do you usually do?" I asked.

Casually, she said, "Oh...I swim lengths of the pool for 30 minutes in the summer, and all year round I walk every day for four miles—takes me about an hour."

"Wow, that's great" I said. And I thought to myself, "I rest my case." I think, here's a perfectly illustrative case of someone doing deliberate activity *every day,* which has become second nature to this dear lady—she's adopted second nature living and stays thin, naturally.

for fitness, but don't be intimidated. An hour of exercise may be broken down into two 30-minute sessions or three 20-minute sessions or four 15-minute sessions—over one or two days!

Some websites allow even more personalization—put your unique vitals in—height, weight, age and sex, and the program more accurately predicts calorie expenditure.

I maintain my weight by eating approximately 1800-2000 calories daily—and that is with doing at least one hour of deliberate activity daily. If I eat more than my *usual diet*, I add more *deliberate physical exercise* to make sure my *internal scale* balances in my favor. I don't weigh myself every day, but I make sure my favorite pair of jeans fits just right. When they get a little snug, I change the equation, lower my calorie intake, and step up my deliberate physical exercise.

The American Heart Association and the American College of Sports Medicine Physical Activity Recommendations

Recommendations for physical activity for people ages 18-65 and over: www.americanheart.org; www.acsm.org

Ages 18 to 65: To promote and maintain health, all healthy adults aged 18-65 need moderate-intensity aerobic (endurance) physical activity for a minimum of 30 minutes on five days each week or vigorous-intensity aerobic physical activity for a minimum of 20 minutes on three days each week.

Ages over 65: Similar to the guidelines for younger individuals, these stress the importance of an individualized program based upon each older adult's current fitness level. Activities that maintain or increase flexibility are recommended, plus balance exercises for older adults at risk of falls. In addition, older adults should have an activity plan for achieving recommended physical activity that integrates preventive and therapeutic recommendations. The promotion of physical activity in older adults should emphasize moderate-intensity aerobic activity, muscle-strengthening activity, reducing sedentary behavior, and risk management.

Every Day Fitness	Daily Activity Plus Deliberate Exercise	Monday through Sunday
Start Slowly	Most healthy people can start a walking program.	Consult with your healthcare provider if you have a medical condition, especially heart disease or diabetes. It's a great idea to get a yearly physical: check your blood pressure, blood cholesterol and blood glucose
Stretching and Flexibility: Do this every day—especially on days that you're working out and exercising.	At least 10 minutes—Every Day	Warm up by walking—start slowly to warm the muscles and avoid injury: finish by stretching: hold the stretch—breathe—hold again—and release.
Every Day Daily Activity: Walk the dog, take the stairs, do your housework and yard work, etc.	Every Day, Any Way: Clip on the pedometer	Every Day—use all those smart strategies that burn calories— • Taking the stairs wherever you can • Walking the dog for an extra 15 minutes morning and evening • Walking after lunch for 10 minutes • Walking after dinner for 10 minutes • Walk up the escalator • Walk next to the people-mover in the airport
Pump it Up: Deliberate moderately intense activity	At least 30 minutes—at least 5 days a week	Moderate-intensity physical activity: Means working hard enough to raise your heart rate and break a sweat, yet still being able to carry on a conversation. Fast walking, moderate cycling, jogging, biking 5 miles in 30 minutes, swimming laps, or water aerobics

OR Deliberate vigorously intense activity	At least 20 minutes at least 3 days a week	Aerobic class, racquetball or basketball, biking 6 miles in 20 minutes—anything that keeps you pushing it for at least 20 minutes.
Strength Training	At least 2-3 days weekly, for 20 minutes	Lift, push or pull—to strengthen your muscles, using light weights or exercise bands or gym equipment. If you can, work first with a personal trainer to determine your program, and guidelines recommend 1 set of 8-12 repetitions, 2-3 days weekly. Always warm up and cool down, 5-10 minutes each (warm up is NOT stretching—just walk briskly).

Fitness Programs—Gyms, Trainers, Equipment

You don't have to join a gym to get fit, but if you're able to even go periodically, boy—it helps! The closer to your home or office, the better, and if you think you can't afford it, consider that a gym membership ranges from a dollar to maybe three dollars a day—save that money by not eating out just once a week, or by buying fewer coffees or snacks. Choose a gym that fits your lifestyle; for example, I love a club that is open early because I'm a morning person—I want a gym that's open early on the weekend, that's clean, and whose staff is friendly and knowledgeable. This is what keeps me coming back.

The American Council on Exercise has some common sense information on how to get fit while avoiding injury. Log on to ACE (**www.acefitness.org**) for lots of great fitness info for all levels.

- Stretch After: Don't stretch to start—stretch to finish. Start out by warming up your muscles for 10 minutes—by walking, jogging slowly, or rowing gently on a rowing machine. Then do your aerobics/workout and finish with stretching and cool-down.

- Avoid the all-or-nothing approach. It's not essential to work out for a full hour—that may be discouraging if you try to do that all the time. I multi-task by biking to and from the gym (that works as my cardio), which also warms me up for my 30 minutes of strength training. I aim for two to four times weekly.

- Four gym NO-NOs:
  - Unbalanced strength-training programs
  - Bad form
  - Not progressing wisely (too much weight risks injury!)
  - Not enough variety

For best results, and to keep moving forward without injury, take advantage of the free training session most gyms offer to new members, because it is the best way to understand how each machine works. A personal trainer and will design a program appropriate to your level of fitness, so you don't overdo—especially important when you're getting started.

- Your Machine Size: Take a minute to re-adjust the machine to your size—if you don't, that machine won't give you the results you want and it will increase your injury risk. It's a good idea to use the written schedule given to you in your first training session—there are a lot of different machines, and it's going to take a while for you to get used to your proper settings. Track your workouts and re-visit your certified personal trainer to reassess your program, your progress, and modify your workout as you increase your fitness.

- Focus: Are you concentrating, or talking? I know—it's fun to meet new people at the gym, but stay focused on getting the most for your money, and stay safe—technique is very important for avoiding injury, too.

- Cool down: Take at least 10 minutes at the end of your workout to stretch, breathe, and lower your heart rate—it's a good time to work on your flexibility. Your personal trainer will show you some stretches designed to increase your range of motion and keep your muscles happy and healthy.

- Gym etiquette: Good gym etiquette includes letting others "work in"—you do a set and let the next person do a set. Don't hang out on the equipment and chat; wipe down the machine after you finish, and don't let the weights drop on the floor—put them down gently. Oh, and if you added weight to the machine, return it to the original settings.

- Set realistic goals: As with a weight loss diet, fitness happens one day at a time. Mix up your activities—alternate classes with running with biking, etc. Build up your strength, and I guarantee you will enjoy your firm arms and butt—you won't believe how great you'll feel. Make monitoring your fitness part of the program—work with your gym's or fitness center's trainer to set goals for fitness. Make them specific, realistic, and achievable, and reward yourself with a new fitness jersey or pair of cool gym shoes for each goal you attain.

Home Equipment

How many people do you know whose treadmill or step machine sits in their bedroom, acting as a clothes hanger? I think big, heavy gym equipment is great—in the gym—but everyday fitness is possible without spending a lot of money. Buy an inexpensive jump rope, a couple of exercise bands, and an exercise ball—there are many different sizes, and they come with instructions. They range from about $20-$100. They are quite easy to store and fun to use. I keep an exercise band strapped to the back of my bike—my routine is to bike over the bridge near my house, then when I'm at the beach or on the boardwalk, I do band exercises: I stretch, do leg lifts, then bike home. When I'm working in front of my computer,

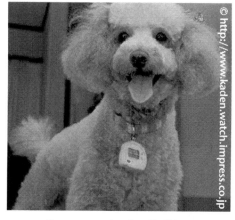

Keep your pet naturally thin too

I sit on a balance ball a few hours every day. I do some curls with hand weights when I'm watching television. I take my jump rope when I walk the dog—and do 20 jumps at the end of the street, 20 more when I get home. Every little bit helps.

Oh…don't forget your sneakers—invest in shoes that are well constructed and fit properly. Don't bother with cheap shoes. If you're a runner, buy running shoes. If you're a walker, good shoes provide different support. If the shoe fits poorly, it can hurt your balance and your back, hips, and knees, so make good sneakers a priority.

- **Exercise Bands:** Easy to use and inexpensive, color-coded resistance bands indicate light, medium, and heavy exertion. These are perfect for traveling: Use them to work deliberate activity into your natural lifestyle—while watching television, for example. For the first four to six weeks, use the light band—then the medium band for the next four to six weeks—then the heavy band. Bands are great for stretching and offer a full range of motion. Buy an instructional video or rent one from the library to see how to use these bands effectively.

- **Jump Rope:** It gets easier the more you do it, and it takes concentration—no wonder it is such good exercise. Today's jump ropes are so much more fun than when I was a kid—if you haven't seen them lately, you'll find them in a variety of colors and styles. Weighted jump ropes act as conditioning equipment. I've attended classes in the gym that utilize jump ropes to increase variety, and it's fun! Start with 10 jumps without stopping—work up from there.

- **Exercise and Balance Balls:** Great for core work—strengthening your abdominals, increasing flexibility. There are videos, books, and instructional podcasts that show you how to use balls—the balls come in all sizes and shapes. I sit on one—not for hours on end, but for about 20 minutes at a time. I remind myself to sit up and bounce—it helps me concentrate.

- **Hand weights:** I have a pair of vinyl-coated, 4-pound hand weights. Good for flexing my muscles when I'm watching television: I boost my workout by power-walking with hand weights. Light hand weights are smart—too heavy, and you risk injury. Don't walk with ankle weights—they increase risk for back injury. Instead, spend six to 10 minutes using exercise bands to strengthen leg muscles.

- **DVDs and television programs:** Some people prefer to exercise in the privacy of their own home—there are dozens and hundreds of opportunities for exercise—from aerobics to yoga to stretching and toning.

You Try It!

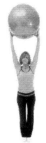
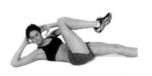
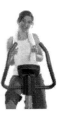
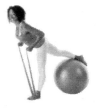

My Second Nature Fitness

Here's a sample log sheet, and I keep it in my night table drawer, either logging last thing in the evening or before getting out of bed the next day.

Susan's Second Nature Fitness Diary

Week of August 25	Monday	Tuesday	Wednesday
My Usual Activities	Walked the dog; sat on the balance ball in front of the computer; stretched for 5 minutes - 3 repetitions	Walked the dog 20 minutes in the morning, only 10 minutes in the afternoon (it was raining!); sat on balance ball; stretched 5 minutes - 4 repetitions	Walked the dog for almost an hour—she was feeling good and made me late to work! Sat on the balance ball; did housework for an hour
My Deliberate Activities	Biked to gym and back about 40 minutes; gym machines for 30 minutes: 5 minutes cool-down stretch	Biked to errands about minutes: used my bands/ stretching/ strengthening (10 minutes)	No time to ride my bike; worked out with exercise bands in front of the television: 30 minutes
My Food Thoughts	Had carrots for snacks— this time I microwaved them for 5 minutes—they taste so much sweeter when I cook them this way	Frozen veggies for a snack: don't forget to pick up some more	Made homemade pizza; a little too much cheese— lots of veggies, though
My Fitness Thoughts	Gym was crowded—it's January! Biked there and back (40 minutes): weight machines 30 minutes	I love when the dog is feeling good—I miss walking her long distances—poor thing	I saw my neighbors walking this morning— the second time this week! Good for them.

Susan's Second Nature Fitness Diary (cont.)

Thursday	Friday	Saturday	Sunday
Walked the dog for only 15 minutes; finished cleaning the floors; sat on the balance ball in front of the computer; stretched only twice today—have to do more.	Walked for about an hour; took a day off from the computer	Short-ish walk this morning. Swept the garage. Walked after dinner.	Walked dog—15 minutes each AM & PM Washed car, did some vacuuming
Biked to the gym and back: about 40 minutes; machines for 30 minutes: 5 minutes cool-down stretch	Took the kayak out for an hour—great arm activity—had a blast.	Husband asked, are you up for a bike ride? He's great—we went south, an hour each way! (120 minutes)	Bike ride to beach—it was really windy; about 30 minutes, but high intensity
Big salad for dinner; bagged greens, canned salmon, tomatoes and onions	Out to dinner with in-laws; Asian buffet; not bad—shrimp, vegetables, soup, and some frozen yogurt—too much salt in restaurant food	Read those labels! Saw another ad on television for a heart healthy cereal—read label-sweetened with high fructose corn syrup!	Husband brought home whole-wheat spaghetti—that's a first. I served with grilled eggplant and fresh tomatoes
Did my workout circuit—there's one lady in the gym who I'm sure is over 80 years old. This neighborhood is amazing.	Shoulders feel sore today—I have to remind myself to keep taking breaks from the computer to stretch.	I want to join a salsa class—I hear it is a great workout and a lot of fun	It was a good week—I put on my jeans today, and they fit the same

YOUR Second Nature Fitness Diary

Month/Date	My Usual Activities	My Deliberate Activities	My Food Notes	My Fitness Notes
Monday				
Tuesday				
Wednesday				
Thursday				
Friday				
Saturday				
Sunday				

Graduated Walking Program

Lace up those walking shoes!

Each day, mark off the distance and frequency of your walking activity in the "Exercise Entries" of your online journal. Estimate:

- 100 calories per mile
- Approximately 20 minutes/mile.
- One mile equals about 2000 steps (for the average person)

*This is a suggested pattern. Accumulate the miles as best suits your schedule.

Week	Mon.	Tue.	Wed.	Thu.	Fri.	Sat.	Sun.	Weekly miles	Weekly calorie burn
1	Baseline	Week							
2	1 mile		1 mile		1 mile			3	300
3	1.5 miles		1.5 miles		1.5 miles	1.5 miles		6	600
4	1.5 miles		1.5 miles		1.5 miles	1.5 miles		6	600
5	2 miles	1 mile	2 miles	1 mile	2 miles	1 mile		9	900
6	2 miles	1 mile	2 miles	1 mile	2 miles	1 mile		9	900
7	2 miles	2 miles	2 miles	2 miles	2 miles	2 miles		12	1200
8	2 miles ST	2 miles	2 miles	2 miles ST	2 miles	2 miles		12	1200
9	2 miles ST	2 miles	3 miles	2 miles ST	3 miles	3 miles		15	1500
10	2 miles ST	2 miles	3 miles	2 miles ST	3 miles	3 miles ST		15	1500
11	3 miles ST	3 miles	3 miles	3 miles ST	3 miles	3 miles ST		18	1800
12	3 miles ST	3 miles	3 miles	3 miles ST	3 miles	3 miles ST		18	1800

*Your goal is accomplished a day at a time, and each day that you walk will make you stronger. If you're not used to walking, do what you can and gradually increase. Rev up your engine, and make your body a lean machine!

ST = Strength train, if desired

Guidelines:

- Logging your miles is a simple way to stay on track. It's easy when you use a pedometer to count your steps

- Most people take approximately 2000 steps per mile.

- Gradually increase your speed to challenge yourself.

- You can walk in smaller mileage increments: Minimum duration 10 minutes.

- Measure a mile (usually easiest by driving it first) to set YOUR baseline distance. Walk the mile at a moderate pace and time yourself. (Most people can walk a mile in about 20 minutes and burn approximately 100 calories.)

- Gradually pick up the pace and try to shave time off your baseline weekly. Pump those arms and move your body!

Bonus: Add the minutes saved to another activity. For example, if it used to take 40 minutes to walk a mile, and now it takes 30 minutes, do 10 more minutes of leg lifts.

If You Love Your Heart, Stay Active

Top 7 Reasons for Staying Active Every Day

Paste this on your bathroom mirror to remind you every morning and evening why activity makes you wonderful!

1. Increase endurance—*Go longer, stronger!*

2. Lose weight and maintain weight loss—*Look trimmer, fitter, younger!*

3. Lower blood pressure—*Decrease your risk for stroke!*

4. Lower "bad" (LDL and total) cholesterol/Increase "good" (HDL) cholesterol—*Lower your risk for heart disease!*

5. Increase insulin sensitivity—*Decrease your risk for diabetes!*

6. Reduce stress—*Increase energy/sleep better!*

7. Set a good example for your family—*Take the lead for fitness!*

Your Second Nature Weight and Waist Worksheet

Use this worksheet to keep track of your progress

Starting Weight		Date	
Your 1st Goal Weight- 10% of Current Weight		Date Achieved	
2nd Goal Weight- 10% of Current **New** Weight		Date Achieved	
3rd Goal Weight- 10% of Current **New** Weight		Date Achieved	

WEEK	Best thing that happened this week	Weight	Measurements Waist/Hip
1 Current weight:	*Log your Usual		Baseline Measurements: Re-measure every 3-4 weeks.
2			
3			
4			
5			
6			
7			
8			
9			
10			
11			
12			

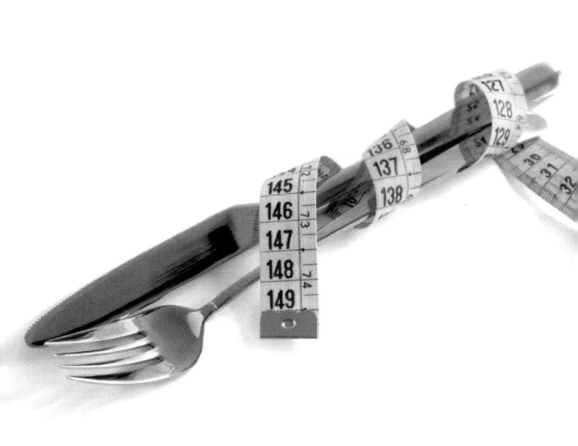

Chapter 9

Dining Out Can Keep You Fat: Dine Out as a Naturally Thin Person

No man is free who is not master of himself.
—Epictetus

I love to eat! I do it every day.

The way I eat every day is what keeps the pounds off. Instead of going on diets, losing weight and then regaining it after returning to my old diet, I choose to have fun enjoying my diet without ever having to deprive myself of fun food.

When people blame their genes for being overweight, I think I understand what they mean. How people are raised—their culture of eating and their family's everyday habits—shapes how they think

An inherited attitude toward overweight may be equally (or even more) important than a genetic predisposition to obesity. When "usual" portion sizes are outsized, it becomes "normal" to overeat. When taking the car to go a half-mile to the store is ""normal," then inactivity becomes the norm.

DEFINITION

Choice

—noun

1. The right, power, or opportunity to choose, "She made her choice and they couldn't change her mind""
2. An alternative action, "My choice is grilled fish instead of fried"

Choose

-verb

1. To select from among possible alternatives after careful consideration
2. To have a preference for

What I consider normal eating can be extremely different from what you consider normal. But I took a look at what was normal for me and made changes. I grew up in a household where overweight behaviors were practiced. I had to overcome my upbringing to discover my second nature.

Changing the Status Quo—At Any Age

My next-door neighbor is a lovely woman who looks far younger than her years. One day, she came over with a question—why, since she hadn't changed her diet and hadn't changed her activity, had she gained weight? Little by little, she said, she'd gained about 10 pounds over the past five years. And she wanted to lose them.

Studies show that our metabolic rate slows gradually beginning at about age 30, and—all things being equal—we accumulate weight naturally. Since she wanted to stay slim and trim, she wanted advice to lose the weight—and to maintain her youthful figure.

We reviewed her usual diet and activity. As long as she wasn't taking any new medications that could contribute to weight gain, I suggested that there were a couple of things she could try for the following 12 weeks.

Eating less wasn't an option, since her usual diet consisted of about 1200 calories daily. At that level, it's important to make smart choices—to make sure her diet provided enough energy, vitamins, minerals, and protein to stay healthy. She could eat differently. For instance, if her usual diet contained higher calorie cheese and meats, she could choose leaner foods and eliminate added fats, such as butter and mayonnaise, to lose weight naturally. Well, she already ate wonderfully and drank lots of water—no alcohol or soda whatsoever. That left activity. At the time, she was walking for about 20 minutes two or three times weekly. But, to tip the scale in her favor, I told her she could add more minutes and intensity, and she could add resistance training, perhaps with bands or light hand weights. To rev up her metabolism and born those calories, I suggested getting a video tape for seniors and checking with her doctor before beginning...just to get the green light.

One evening as we were sitting out on the dock, the sun had set and in that beautiful half-light, we spied our neighbor walking on her second story porch. We could barely see her, but as we walked back into the house, we looked more carefully—trying not to be too nosy—to see what she was doing. She would appear—then disappear—then reappear again. She seemed to be walking—yes, she was exercising! She was power-walking, with hand weights! Back and forth—for 30 minutes, right there, and she got it done. *Wow*, I thought, *she's great*. She got the message, she prepared to succeed—and now, there she was, executing. *She'll lose the weight*, I thought, *and she'll keep it off, too*. I won't give away her age, but boy, this lady can inspire all of us to do it.

Taking My Diet On Vacation

MY *diet* is defined as *what I usually eat,* so I don't take a vacation from my diet. Instead, when I leave my home, I take my *diet* with me, or else, I would miss it! And it travels pretty well—of course, I enjoy some flexibility and include some foods not normally on the menu, but that's what makes vacations fun! If I'm traveling for work, I may be dining out often, but I don't abandon my *diet,* but include it when I'm choosing from menus or dining out at a friend's house.

My husband and I recently met up with our friends, "Rebecca" and "John," for a weekend. I congratulated Rebecca—she'd lost at least 20 pounds and looked wonderful. In a matter-of-fact tone, she related that her success was due to what she'd done in the past—she'd lost the weight before and regained it.

"So," she said, "I know what to do—I just have to do it."

Rebecca said that her main tactic was to banish fast food from her diet—entirely. She stopped her usual daily drive-through for a burger—and said that it was a tough habit to break. She was eating healthier at home, too. She used

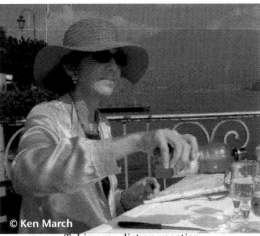
© Ken March

Taking my diet on vacation

to serve her family steak and home fries, buttered bread and creamy salad dressings—now she cooked grilled salmon or chicken breast, replaced sauces with salsa and bought low calorie dressing for salads. She credited her treadmill, which she used in the evening to walk for 30 minutes while watching television, and her resistance band DVD that she used three times a week as making a huge difference in helping her lose weight.

I said, "Wow, girlfriend! You're writing the book on success!"

But over the course of the weekend, I noticed that her ordering didn't reflect what she'd said was her new healthy diet. She ordered a cheeseburger and fries for lunch; she chose an oversized pasta dish, full of cheese and sausage for dinner. We stopped for ice cream in the afternoon—and she ordered dessert after dinner. She had Margaritas at the Mexican restaurant, and beer and wine throughout the weekend.

She didn't walk, run, or jog once during her visit, and at one point she said to me, "I decided that I wanted to take a vacation from my diet."

The question is...can you take a vacation from your diet?

If you take a vacation from your diet, don't go too far or stay away too long. After all, your *second nature* means you should never have to "go on a diet" again.

Are you a chronic dieter? If you have a diet mentality, it's hard to maintain your goal weight indefinitely, because you never completely adopt a healthy diet. A dieter constantly goes on and off a restrictive diet. When you take a vacation from your diet, it may be hard to find your way back. When you consistently make choices without regard to your waistline or health, it shows up on the scale. In order to lose the weight, it takes a concerted effort to reduce daily calories and burn more with exercise.

I'd much rather enjoy my vacation and not return home carrying extra weight. I've heard about folks who bring two sizes of clothes with them when they go on vacation. They are planning on "pigging out" and need larger sized clothes to wear on their way back home. Not me! I'm not going to do it—I'm going to taste a bit of something sweet and have seconds if I want to, but I won't overeat to the point of gaining too much weight—because getting rid of all the excess fat isn't so easy.

Over the weekend when my friend was overindulging, I enjoyed healthier choices and smaller portions, plus I made sure to take a bike ride in the morning and walk every evening. I took a forkful of dessert at one meal, but at others, I took a deep breath, said to myself, *Hmmmmm, I'm too full,* and declined. I never felt deprived and never felt guilty either, although I enjoyed every mouthful of food that I ordered.

My Diet Travels With Me

I may choose one meal to overindulge, but I'm not going to be greedy. If I abandon all my healthy habits, I'd better keep those larger sized clothes...because I'll need them.

- **Breakfast:** I find that I can overeat or choose richer foods for dinner as long as I continue to make breakfast healthy. Hot or cold (low sugar) cereal with nonfat or 1% milk, fruit, and maybe a low fat or nonfat cup of yogurt.

- **Brunch:** A real vacation treat, but I'm not greedy. I stick with egg-white omelets with lots of veggies (a little cheese is what makes it a treat), salad, and fruit, and I just say "No" to pancakes, waffles, and French toast; these foods are just vehicles for fat and sugar.

- **Lunch:** Regardless of what I order, I don't add unhealthy fats to my food. I've worked hard to get in shape, so why blow it by adding mayo, margarine, and butter to my sandwiches and bread? Every scant tablespoon of fat adds another 100 calories. It's not worth it. I like mustard, maybe a little ketchup, and there's nothing bad about nonfat salad dressings, vinegar, and a little olive oil and salsa.

- **Dinner:** On vacation, I may order a pasta or risotto for a main course, and I usually eat the bread on the table—especially if it's an end piece—I love the crust. Yes, on vacation—if the food is great—I'll probably eat too much, but the next day I have my healthy breakfast...after my bike ride.

- **Desserts:** If I'm in the mood for dessert, I may seek out something on the menu when I'm ordering dinner. If I see something that I really want, I'll make it work—and it's always best to share. Maybe I'll choose an appetizer for my entrée and salad as a first course. Sorbet is sweet without fat.

- **Exercise:** I don't take a vacation from my daily activity. I can't remember the last time I came back from a vacation with extra pounds as a souvenir. Vacations to me mean walking...it's one of the best ways to explore a new city, and walking is a very relaxing way to spend an afternoon.

My New Motto

"My new motto is that if it comes through the car window,
it isn't food. If what you eat creates a greasy sack,
eat the sack and throw the food out."

—Mike Huckabee,
twice-elected governor of Arkansas,
who lost 110 pounds and
reversed symptoms of diabetes[1].

Mike Huckabee was the keynote speaker at the 2007 annual American Association for Diabetes Educators symposium, and told us that he was raised poor in rural Arkansas—with a strong family history of obesity and type 2 diabetes. He said that in his world, all food was fried, mainly because poor people learned that frying is the "best" and cheapest way to get as much bang for the buck. But even as he became a successful minister and politician, he kept his eating habits close to home, never giving up his deep-fried favorites, as he says, he was "digging (his) grave with a knife and a fork."

Huckabee knew that he was at risk for diabetes, but nevertheless, the diagnosis hit him hard. He was in his late 40s and weighing nearly 300 pounds when his doctor told him he would be dead within a decade.

On average, a person with type 2 diabetes goes undiagnosed for six years and that's unfortunate, because by the time they are diagnosed and have a chance to start treatment, they've usually incurred irreversible damage to their eyes, peripheral nerves, kidneys, and heart. Since the symptoms are generally silent at the start, chronic high blood glucose causes damage to tiny vessels, arteries and nerves, and that's why type 2 diabetes is the leading cause of blindness, renal failure, and non-traumatic amputation. Heart disease is the primary cause of death for people with type 2 diabetes.

How successful you are at controlling blood glucose means either *living* with diabetes or *getting very sick* from diabetes. But what makes Mr. Huckabee a wonderful example and inspiration is how he handled his diagnosis—very differently from many people diagnosed with type 2 diabetes or any other disease associated with obesity. The day he was diagnosed was the first day of his new life. He made a decision to change. And he's maintaining the 110-pound weight loss by maintaining his commitment to choice. and after losing all that weight in less than a year, he's reversed his symptoms of diabetes, the disease his doctor said was a death sentence.

Obesity and diabetes are unfortunate partners, but there's no denying the relationship and the risk associated with staying together. But Mike Huckabee decided to make his destiny different—he refused to allow his fate to be obesity and premature death. He learned to navigate around his neighborhood, and today makes healthy living second nature.

Planning Equals Success

My challenge with overweight didn't begin until college. Like so many others who gain "the freshman 15," suddenly I wasn't physically active, as I had been in my earlier teens. I also found myself using food to relieve stress.

To lose weight, I 'went on' the popular diet of the time—a very low-fat diet. Some days I ate only 800 calories a day—which produced weight loss, but unfortunately—this led to my eating—then overeating—and I regained, and then gained more weight than before--about 25 pounds more than my current weight.

I knew the only way to end the weight struggle would be to overcome my compulsive overeating. I read books, attended seminars, prayed, and sought therapy. Ultimately I decided that my definition of recovery would be that I could eat anything I wanted—in moderation. About five years later, I was confident that I could say I reached my goal. Without addressing the psychological stress triggers that were at the root of my compulsive eating, I don't think I could have broken the pattern.

Today, maintaining a healthy weight is nothing short of living a lifestyle, not dieting in any way. I schedule time for fitness just as I would an appointment, and that way I'm sure to get it done. I pack my meals, snacks, and water if I am working away from my home or in the office. We keep tempting chips and cookies out of the house, and if I have a craving, I go out and get a single serving of whatever it is that I want. It's important for me to make tempting foods inconvenient; otherwise I might eat them simply because they are there. We limit restaurants to no more than two meals per week. Once a week I can choose my favorite foods, and so I don't feel deprived. Although I treat myself, I do not binge.

I pre-plan what we will eat for dinner once a week and shop from a grocery list. I often prepare three meals at once on Sundays. Though this takes extra time up front, it pays off.

Planning and preparation are two key reasons I'm successful: I can know that no matter how long of a day I've had, or how tired I may feel, I am ahead because I have the right foods available.

Christine Miller, MS, RD, CDE
Advanced Nutrition Concepts, Inc.
Tampa, Florida

Eating for One,
When Everything Ordered Serves Two

"Tell me what you eat, and I will tell you what you are."
French gastronomist Anthelme Brillat-Savarin,
The Physiology of Taste, 1825

Isn't it amazing that by changing a single word in a sentence, the meaning can change significantly? As Huckabee says, we don't have a *health care* crisis in America, we have a *health* crisis. He's so right about that—trying to keep up with treating the diseases plaguing overweight people is a losing battle, no pun intended. We should be funding prevention instead of trying to play catch-up, for example, using a draconian solution like weight loss surgery (gastric bypass or banding). Those considering surgery should weigh the costs because there are always risks, and without permanent lifestyle changes, you're likely to regain weight.

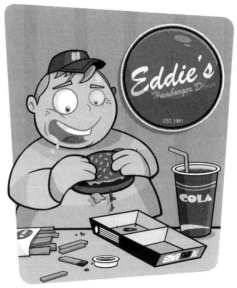

Fast food doesn't *make* you fat. *Eating* fast food too often makes it hard to keep your weight where you want it; no doubt, if you're choosing fried fast food on a consistent basis, it's a recipe for obesity.

Eating too much of just about *any* food will make you fat—so, we can't blame the food for making us fat. All restaurant food has the same obesogenic potential. That said, I won't give fast food a pass because we don't live in a vacuum, and despite our best intentions, there are many factors that influence what we eat, how much we eat, and when we eat. The advertising budgets for some of the major fast food chains run in the *billions of dollars,* vastly outweighing the advertising budget for fresh fruits and vegetables.

Until late in the 20th century, dining out used to be for a special occasion—for birthdays or anniversaries. Not today! According to the National Restaurant Association, Americans are dining out more than ever—more than 945,000 restaurants serve more than 70 billon meal and snack *occasions,* and the numbers are set to grow in 2008 to $558 billion in sales[2].

Are restaurants making us fat? For most Americans, eating out represents almost 50 percent of their total food budget. Surveys show that, in some neighborhoods, it's easier to get a fast food meal than it is to find fresh, wholesome foods—but even in communities with no shortage of grocery stores, people eat out constantly. Some people eat out weekly, some people eat out daily—and I've spoken to people who never eat fresh food prepared at home. They drive through, take out, or sit down in someone else's dining room and give control over their food to strangers.

Now, I know that's harsh. But my point is this: When I took control of what I ate—how much and when—I began to take control of my weight. Once I step outside my door and sit down at someone else's table, I give up control. At a restaurant, it's up to the waiter to translate what I order, and it's up to the chef to prepare it the way I request. And no matter how I try, in some places, I won't get what I ordered, and it will be out of control—it will be overly large, overly sauced, overly salted. Yes, I enjoy dining out. I like feeling pampered. I know that many people are time challenged—I am, too.

Most fast food chains provide nutritional information—either at the point of purchase or on the Web. Some fast casual restaurants do—some don't. Most full-service restaurants do not. That's why it's up to you to know portions, to learn by using measuring cups and scales at the start, so when you're faced with gargantuan restaurant portions, you can modify your intake.

Yes, we are what we eat—and when we dine out, we have no idea what we're eating or how much. Since Americans dine out so frequently—and since portions in restaurants are so over-sized—we wind up eating a lot. Because portions have gotten so large, consumers feel cheated if a restaurant dares to serve what the government considers a normal portion of food.

Americans eat hundreds of calories in hidden fats and sugars daily; the USDA puts the estimate at around 20 added teaspoons of sugar daily—not to mention salt, MSG, colors, and preservatives. When I buy a packaged food, I read the ingredient list and definitely avoid products with long lists of unpronounceable ingredients. But when I dine out, how can I tell what is in my food? I can't.

Food manufacturers try to influence our shopping habits by appealing to our frugal natures. I pay attention when I see *New! Bigger! More!* on the label. Although packaged food labels tell us in black and white what the manufacturer considers a single serving, most people don't eat single servings when the package contains more. Often a container has double or triple what the manufacturer lists as a single serving—think canned soup or bottled soft drinks or ice tea. Similarly, Americans value all-you-can-eat and two-for-one offers, and because food is cheap, people continue to gain weight.

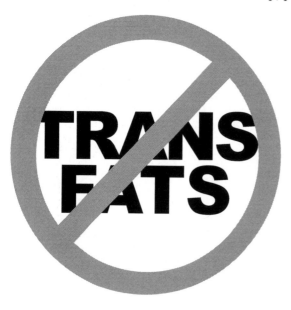

Portion Distortion

The Centers for Disease Control and Prevention have reams of research showing that people who eat out in restaurants eat more when faced with huge portions. And, by the way, people are getting used to eating bigger portions all the time—not only in restaurants, but in movie theaters, at concerts and sporting events, and at home after purchasing prepared foods.

The U.S. Food and Drug Administration (FDA) Nutrition Facts information is printed on most packaged foods. It tells you how many calories and how much fat, carbohydrate, sodium, and other nutrients there are in one serving of food. Most packaged foods contain more than a single serving. The serving sizes that appear on food labels are based on FDA-established lists of foods. (For more information, see www.cfsan.fda.gov)

A "portion" is how much food you choose to eat at one time, whether in a restaurant, from a package, or in your own kitchen. A "serving" size is the amount of food listed on a product's Nutrition Facts. Be a savvy consumer— *serving size* is often different from the portion usually consumed. For instance, when a bottle of sweetened bottled tea contains 2.5 servings, most people will drink the entire bottle—taking in 2.5 times the calories listed per serving. Read the serving size on the Nutrition Facts label to quickly learn the calories and nutrients in a certain amount of food—and then think about what you usually eat—and do the math.

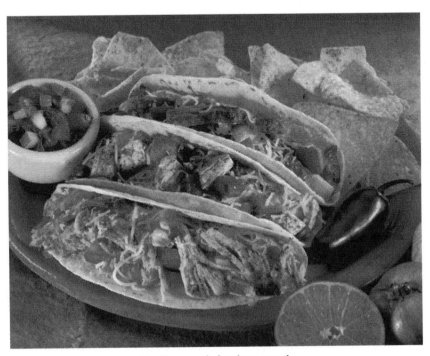

Easily enough for three people

Distorted Portions

The National Heart, Lung and Blood Institute, a division of the National Institutes of Health, has some interesting information about the portion size of common foods—including what we get in restaurants and fast food chains—compared to portion sizes 20 years ago. It's astounding. I've incorporated some of their valuable information here and added some other timely questions, so you can evaluate your own knowledge and see how much you're (over) eating[3]!

1. Twenty years ago, bagels were about 3 inches in diameter, weighed about 1-2 ounces, and had about 120 calories each. Today's bagels contain about how many calories?
  a. 200
  b. 300
  c. 500
	1. Answer: B—300 calories. Bagels are three times the size of the small rolls brought over by Jewish bakers from Poland in the late 1900s. Today's discs weigh closer to 4 ounces or more and contain more than 350 calories—before the 'schmear' of cream cheese and smoked salmon.

2. Twenty years ago, spaghetti and meatball dinners had about 500 calories; today's average pasta dinner contains how many calories?
  a. 600
  b. 800
  c. 1200
	2. Answer: C—1200 calories. Today's pasta dinners are immense, nearly triple that of 20 years ago. At Romano's Macaroni Grill, one dinner serving of spaghetti and meatballs with meat sauce has more than 2400 calories and 57 grams of fat—and that's without a single piece of bread or appetizer.

3. Twenty years ago, an average soda was about eight ounces and about 100 calories. Today, many chains don't even offer a small fountain drink. Today's average size contains:
  a. 12 ounces and 150 calories
  b. 16 ounces and 200 calories
  c. 20 ounces and 250 calories
	3. Answer: C—20 ounces/250 calories. Experts point to soda as a primary contributor to obesity—especially in children and economically disadvantaged people.

4. Today's fast food french fries little resemble the average serving of 20 years ago. Today's medium fries are how big...and contain how many calories?
  a. 3.5 ounces and 490 calories
  b. 4.5 ounces and 500 calories
  c. 6.9 ounces and 610 calories
	4. Answer: B—4.5 ounces and 500 calories. Fries are not only high in fat, but sodium, too. One medium serving is high in total fat and, unless stated, trans fat, too.

5. Twenty years ago, the average cheeseburger contained about 333 calories. Today's burger contains how many calories?
  a. 425
  b. 500
  c. 590
	5. Answer: C—590 calories. Today's fast food cheeseburger averages 257 more calories than a portion 20 years ago.

6. In the 1950s, fast food restaurants offered only one size of french fries. Today's small size is how large compared to the original?
   a. One quarter of the original
   b. one-half of the original
   c. two-thirds of the original
	6. Answer: C—Today's small sized fries are two-thirds of the original size, which means today's medium is yesterday's large, and today's large is gargantuan.

7. True or False: If you drink a soft drink, it fills you up as well as a glass of milk.	7. Answer: False. Studies show that soft drinks don't put a dent in your appetite, so the excess calories are junk nutrition. However, milk (nonfat or low fat) satisfies, adding protein and important nutrients.

8. An American croissant contains how many more calories on average than a French croissant?
   a. 20
   b. 50
   c. 100-plus
	8. Answer: C—A plain croissant has about 150 calories, but one Starbuck's Butter Croissant with Almond Glaze has 320 calories.

9. If you eat an additional 100 calories a day beyond your needs, how much weight could you gain in one year?
   a. one pound
   b. three pounds
   c. six pounds
   d. ten pounds
	9. Answer: D—It's possible to gain ten pounds in one year, just from eating an extra 100 calories per day.

10. True or False: The larger the portion served, the more you will eat.	10. Answer: True. The larger the portion offered, the more we eat.

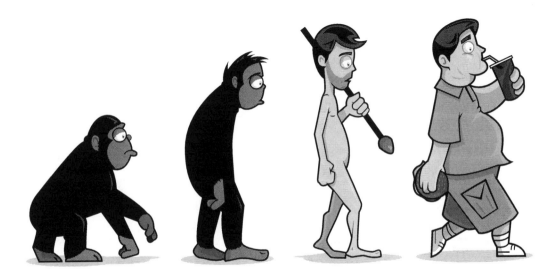

Take a Break from Dining Out

In the beginning I found that having fewer choices worked effectively. For the first three months of my committing to a weight loss program, I stayed close to home and worked it. Every evening, I reviewed my menu for the next day, and made sure I knew in advance what I was going to eat. A printed plan worked very well for me; I found it reassuring, because it provided me with structure and took away a lot of the anxiety that I was used to experiencing over food. I knew in advance what I was going to eat, and when I tracked it every evening, I felt as if I had done something good for myself—I felt like I had accomplished something important for myself, and I had.

By removing my trigger foods and eliminating temptation, I took the pressure off—if it wasn't there, it wasn't an option. My usual bagels with cream cheese, oily bran muffins, and greasy burgers were no more. I put myself into diet boot camp, for sure. But boy, that changed my taste buds—and my tolerance for fatty, greasy, and over-sauced foods. As I worked at my fitness and fed myself simple foods, I lost my taste for greasy, oily, sugary, stale foods—I used to eat them without tasting, because taste wasn't the point of eating. I discovered I could enjoy food without worrying about eating it.

While I was in weight loss mode and sticking close to my program, I decided that eating out was too tempting. I was serious about losing weight, and by staying in control of my portions at home, I was eating according to my stomach—not my eyes—for the first time. From late March—when I went through my pantry and refrigerator and identified and eliminated all my trigger foods—through mid-June, I made healthy eating my first priority and stayed out of restaurants completely. I knew that the less choice I had, the better off I'd be, and it worked.

My resolve was being formed, and I gave myself a chance to succeed by staying prepared—eating smaller meals more frequently, so I never felt ravenous. I also felt secure because if I needed to eat something (and I often felt this even if I wasn't hungry), a snack was just around the corner.

Of course, you cannot always avoid dining out—it's a cultural necessity, especially if you're in a line of work that requires you to dine out. But avoid "all you can eat" for at least the first six months of a new naturally thin lifestyle. That's because it's not natural to eat all you can or even all you want. We are modern humans; we are not cave men and women who need to stock up on calories in case of a drought or famine. We don't have to worry that there won't be enough to eat tomorrow, but when I go to a buffet restaurant, I'm often amazed at how people are eating as if there is no tomorrow. People eat with their eyes, not their stomachs.

No matter how disciplined you are, being faced with a huge expanse and variety of foods isn't easy. It is natural to eat more when faced with your favorite foods. Although I am familiar with my usual diet portions and my daily dietary needs, when I get in that buffet line, I'm likely to eat more.

Thus, eating simpler, fresher foods changed my taste buds. Suddenly the restaurant foods I used to enjoy tasted greasy or salty—and why? Because they are. Even the finest establishments commonly add butter to everything—and over-salting is a tradition. I've had expensive meals ruined because the chef coated fresh vegetables with butter. I don't want to eat butter—I want to eat fresh vegetables, prepared tastefully but healthfully, but when I dine out, that isn't guaranteed. That said, some restaurants make it their mission to prepare fresh food healthfully—those restaurants get my vote.

Here's the way I stay naturally thin: I make healthy choices second nature, even when someone else is cooking for me. Remember what I said about the choices we have in life? Food is one of the few choices we have control over—no one can make you eat it. You are the arbiter when it comes to food—no one can tell you what to eat, when to eat it, or how much to eat.

When young adults are suddenly given *carte blanche* to eat all they want of a variety of foods, the result is the Freshman five or 10 or 15 (or more) pounds of weight gain. When they lived at home and were limited to the meals served, weight control was easier. The same is true for everyone: The more variety and choice we are given, the more we tend to overeat. When I took control, I learned what I needed to lose weight. Those first three months became my foundation for the future. The more I followed my menu, the more I became fit, the more I wanted to continue to feel great. I gradually began to go out again, but I have not returned to my old restaurant habits.

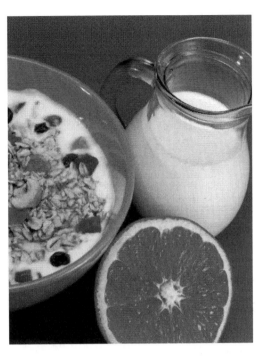

My *second nature diet* means I don't eat *differently* because I'm dining out—I don't change my diet just because it's on the menu. I've been there, done that.

When You Love Them Enough to Say "No"

When I'm traveling, I always throw a baggie full of mixed dry cereals (my favorites are Kashi GoLean and Bran Buds) into my luggage, because often the only choices at a breakfast buffet are sweetened breakfast cereals, whole milk, sweet rolls, or danish. I can deal with the 2% milk, and if I'm lucky there is a non-sugary cereal like Cheerios or Total, but since I make a point of being prepared, I make sure to pack my own. If I find fresh fruit, nonfat milk, and whole grain breads and cereals, I'm happy as a clam.

And although healthier choices are available, most of the time I see people go right for the sweet stuff. Instead of whole fruit, they pour a big glass of juice. Instead of oatmeal or less sugary cereals, they grab frosted flakes, and sugary sweet rolls, donuts and muffins. Even though the better choices are right there, most people don't choose wisely.

On a recent trip, we stayed at a motel that featured a hot breakfast. There was the usual sweet stuff; a Plexiglas display case full of danish, donuts, sliced white bread, and bagels. There was a juice dispenser with apple and orange juice; there was a cold cereal display with single-serving packages of Froot Loops, Frosted Flakes, Sugar Snaps, and Cheerios. There was a bowl of bananas and oranges. They also had a "hot" breakfast: a waffle maker flanked by cups of pre-measured batter; pre-cooked sausage patties, egg discs, and hash brown potatoes. For five mornings, I watched as kids *and* adults made a beeline for the sugary cereals and juice. One or two adults had Cheerios and whole fruit. Some had pastries and hot stuff, too.

The worst day was on Sunday. A little girl, about six years old and obviously overweight, came in with her overweight grandfather. He guided her to a table right next to mine and proceeded to the breakfast buffet. First, he returned with two cups of juice. Then he fetched a full-sized plate of waffles, drenched with syrup and butter, for her. He returned with eggs, sausage, and hash browns for himself, and they both polished off their plates.

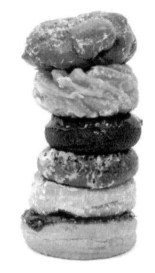

He then went back and returned with bagels with cream cheese. As they polished off the food, and I thought, *poor kid, he's feeding her just like he feeds himself.*

Suddenly, two little girls ran in, followed by their father. The girls appeared to be close in age to the little girl with her grandfather, but were normal weight. They rushed toward the donuts and sweet rolls, but their dad said quickly, "Girls! First get the Cheerios, and then you can share something else." As the little girls opened their boxes of Cheerios their dad sliced a banana over their cereal, and I felt so sorry for that other little girl who was off to such a poor start. I thought about the uphill battle she would have to control her weight, starting off as she was with such an overwhelming handicap.

Navigating the Neighborhood

I have created my *second nature*, and if I can't find healthy options, it doesn't mean I give in and eat whatever is there. If I'm dining out with friends, I don't feel obligated to eat what everyone else is eating—and if I'm traveling, I go prepared. It took me a while to understand that whatever I eat today will show up on me tomorrow. I'm exaggerating, but my body is awfully efficient—if I overeat and get fewer minutes of exercise than I need, I'll feel the added weight on my torso in no time at all.

There's no magic to staying slim—just consistency. If that's magic, then I am a wizard.

For example, I distinctly remember the first time I went to the movies and deliberately didn't stop first at the concession stand for a bucket of popcorn. That took some doing! I habitually anticipated popcorn when I went to the movies, and bought it even if I wasn't hungry. And I always finished every kernel, even though by the time I was halfway through the bucket, it tasted awful and my fingers were greasy. I reasoned that if I didn't put butter on it, I was fine. I finally faced up to the fact that movie popcorn is just not worth it—and I was eating it out of habit.

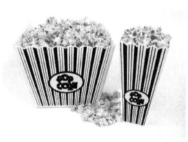

Movie popcorn--usually popped in trans fat-laden oil---often "pre-popped" and not worth the calories.

Did you know that a medium-sized plain popcorn has 900 calories and 60 grams of fat? What's worse, most movie popcorn is popped in unhealthy hydrogenated oil, and often, movie popcorn is pre-popped—just sitting in the display, slightly stale. Brian Wansink, who has done a lot of research about how big portions influence people to eat more, famously gave movie goers buckets of stale popcorn. Even though the stuff was old, people didn't seem to mind and just kept munching[4].

No more will I lose my mind in the darkness of the theater. Just as restaurants earn their biggest profits from beverages, so do movie theaters. Today's movie theaters resemble amusement parks, selling everything—from popcorn, candy, chips, dips, and tacos, to hamburgers, hot dogs, ice cream, and of course, big, big cups of soda. Theater owners have learned from fast food chains and bundle the offer, making it seem like such a deal to spend a few pennies more and upgrade to king- or giant-sized portions.

When you go to the movies—or to any entertainment venue—here are some smart *second nature* strategies:

- Eat first: If you're not hungry when you arrive at the theater, it's easier to stroll on by the refreshment stand.

- Popcorn: I dare you to find movie popcorn not popped in hydrogenated fat—trans fat. Bring your own air-popped popcorn or some peanuts in the shell—use the bag for the shells.

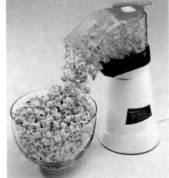

- Plan for a sweet: If you arrive with a sweet tooth, share a small box of licorice, gummy bears, or Jujubes (1.5 ounces has about 120 calories and no fat).

- Skip the soda: One 20-ounce serving has about 200 calories. Save your money or buy bottled water.

- Cut up fruit, baby carrots, and celery: Fresh, crunchy snacks that are good for you, too.

This Presto® PopLite® hot air corn popper uses hot air, not oil, making popcorn a healthy, low-calorie treat.

Dining Out: Stadium Events

Navigating the neighborhood means taking stock wherever you go. When you go to a stadium for a hockey game, to the circus, or to an outdoor fair, you'll usually find the same concession stands, and most don't offer much in the way of healthy choices. Fire up your motivation and practice some winning tactics for staying slim.

Instead of Overweight Stadium Selections	Try a Naturally Thin Stadium Selection
Chili Cheese Dog: 340 calories, 17g fat	Plain Hot Dog with Sauerkraut: 260 calories, 12g fat
Nachos: 700 calories, 35g fat	Pretzel with mustard: 340 calories, 2g fat
French fries: 570 calories, 30g fat, 5g trans fat	Bag of peanuts: 340 calories, 26g fat, 0g trans fat
Large soda (32-ounce cup): 400 calories, 0g fat	Water or diet soda: 0 calories/0g fat
Total calories Old: 2010 Total fat Old: 82g (5g trans fat)	Total calories New: 940 Total fat New: 40g (0g trans fat)

Take me out to the ball game!

- If possible, dine al fresco at the stadium.

- Sandwiches: Scoop out the doughy part of a hard roll and layer in turkey, chicken breast, or lean roast beef; top with thin-sliced cucumber, leafy romaine lettuce, and sliced tomato.

- Fruit: Easy to transport apples, pears, and plums travel well.

- Whole grain: Crackers, pretzels, or rice cakes—1 ounce has about 100 calories.

- Container of yogurt or cottage cheese: Bring a plastic spoon and enjoy a healthy snack.

- Bag it: Raw veggies, such as baby carrots, celery, bell pepper, cucumber, and broccoli florets. Bring a cup of homemade nonfat yogurt dip (mix with 2 Tbsp of low sodium onion dip).

From Theory to Practice: Second Nature Dining

There are almost a million dining establishments in America with countless ways to enjoy a variety of cuisines—American, Italian, Chinese, and Greek. In my own city, I can dine around the world. I'm not going to talk about each and every ethnicity, because that would be an entire book, but I will review the basic principles of dining out by focusing on a few of the restaurants that I frequent most often. The most important point to remember is that I *do* enjoy dining out in restaurants—but, I *don't* change my *diet*.

Remember, my definition of diet is *what I usually eat*. I don't change my basic diet principles—or portion size—just because I'm not eating at home. Of course, on special occasions, I will try a dish prepared with a rich sauce—but I'll ask for it on the side. On occasion, I'll enjoy a dessert—but I'll share it. If I indulged too often, the pounds would creep back on, and pretty soon I'd gain weight just like anyone else.

So when I'm dining out, I take my diet with me. I go in fully informed—and warned—and enjoy the experience without undoing the hard work I did to get where I want to be, size-wise.

Second Nature Dining Out

1. Arrive informed: Communicate—that's a valuable tool in my arsenal. I am not shy about asking—or researching—the restaurant menu in advance. I've phoned ahead or gone to the website to see if there's a menu to review before I dine. Most quick-casual chains—and just about all fast food chains—have online menus. Some have nutritional information right there—just click. Hope Warshaw, a registered dietitian and diabetes educator, offers pocket-sized dining out guides—keep one in your car so you are always prepared. Get a *Healthy Dining* book, with nutritional information on a wide variety of restaurants. Be an educated consumer[5]!

2. A quick study: Learn to read. A naturally thin diner will quickly scan the menu to ascertain the dishes that are heavily sauced or fried or breaded. When you know the lingo, it is easy to differentiate between well-prepared foods and food that are high in fat and calories.

Dining Out: Plan in Advance

Restaurant portions are double, or triple, what experts consider appropriate for most people. Knowing approximately how my calories translate into the portions of food I need for the day lets me stay on track. Knowing how much food I *usually* eat per meal allows me to plan in advance and allows for some leeway when dining out. For example, I'm on vacation, and I know that at home, my usual lunch meal totals about 400-500 calories. But, I'm going to need to eat more at lunch and dinner, so I'll need to transfer calories from other meals to stay on track. So, I'll plan for it. I'll cut back on breakfast—and limit to maybe a cup of cereal, a cup of berries, and a cup of milk (about 300 calories); I'll have just a piece of fruit for a mid-morning snack or just a cup of tea instead of my usual raisins and nut mixture, and save about 200 calories there. That means I've already earned about 300-400 calories that I can add to lunch or dinner. I'm not counting calories per se, but I translate calories into portions, and stay on track.

Usual Breakfast	Usual Snack	Usual Lunch	Usual Snack	Usual Dinner
500	200	400	200	500

3. Don't be shy: I always speak up for myself. I'm always polite, but I never hesitate to ask—and I politely make my requests. I always quickly scan the menu to zero in on descriptions that fit my natural way of eating—grilled, baked, broiled, or steamed, for instance. If the menu doesn't specify the prep, I merely ask. Asking is always better than being unpleasantly surprised with a dish covered with cheese or floating in fat. Here's how I do it: "I hope you can accommodate my order—and thank you for your assistance. I'd like my fish prepared grilled (or broiled or baked) —no sauce, gravy, or butter, please." It works most of the time.

4. Out of sight: When you sit down at many full service restaurants, there's usually a basket of bread or crackers—even dips—on the table. And of course, we know all about the basket of chips in Mexican restaurants. It's too easy to polish off an entire basket before ordering a single thing. Take a deep breath—and repeat: "Been there, done that!" That's my favorite saying—have I had that chip or bread before? Yes! Is it especially tasty or wonderful? Nah! I'll skip it and save my appetite for the main course.

    •   Bread and Butter: I don't add fat and extra calories to my food, especially not to bread. If the bread isn't good enough to eat without butter, leave it alone.

    •   Chips: If you can't eat just one, consider that just a dozen restaurant tortilla chips may have more than 200 calories.

    •   Dips: Avocado dip, or guacamole, is rich in healthy monounsaturated fat, but it's still fat and adds up quickly—about 200 calories per half-cup. And don't forget to count the calories in the chips!

5. On the Side: Make this part of your restaurant vocabulary, and never hesitate to say it. Most servers understand this request, but it can never be said too often, because salads, vegetables, entrees may all have a fatty sheen of butter or sauce slathered on top. Yes, fat tastes good—but doesn't look so good when you're wearing it.

6. Portion Control: Remember, the entrée will usually suffice for two or more, so order one entrée to share, and start with an appetizer salad or soup. Or order two appetizers—and enjoy one as your entrée.

7. New Take on Taste: If fatty, fried foods are the only thing you're used to eating, then changing your taste buds is going to take some work. But it will happen.

8. Log On: Go to www.HealthyDiningFinder.com and punch in the zip code for your dining destination. This company partners with restaurants around the country and shows the establishments that feature dining options for consumers who want to take their naturally thin dining habits with them. It's a great tool for when you're traveling, too, so you won't get stuck at a place that won't honor your healthy requests—no matter where you go.

9. About twice a year, I find myself in a full-service restaurant (not fast food or fast casual) that offers something very special—such as fried calamari, fresh-made french fries, or hand-cut potato chips. I consider it a special occasion and share an order.

I Don't Add Fat to my Food:
A special note about fat on the table

I have a motto: *If the bread isn't good enough to eat without butter, I don't eat it.* Here is where the rubber meets the road, calorie-wise. Freeing your food from fat is a small change that pays off in extra-big savings—saving calories, that is. Of course, like most people, I *like* butter. Fresh, creamy butter is great. I like olive oil; if you've never tasted high quality extra virgin olive oil, you must—good quality oil is fruity and delicious. My tongue sings for butter—my taste buds revel when coated with succulent and fragrant oil. That's natural. Fat brings flavor to food—but at nine calories per gram, adding extra fat to food is the quickest way to add pounds to my hips.

And that's the point! I changed my attitude about adding fat to my food when I lost 40 pounds. I do not use bread or vegetables as vehicles for bringing extra fat to my daily diet. I dine out, I cook, I enjoy food—but I have not put butter on my bread in more than 25 years. I don't dip my bread into little dishes of oil.

I've adopted the *been there, done that* philosophy about fat. I've tasted the best butter—I gained weight from unceasingly "tasting" butter. And it tastes great. And yes, it makes food taste good, but at a big cost.

Fat doesn't discriminate. From butter to oil, margarine, or mayonnaise, all forms of fat contain about 100 calories per scant tablespoon, and that's a *level* tablespoon. When you're sitting at a restaurant, you're not measuring what you're adding to your bread. Each "dip" into that cunning pool of olive oil and—poof—you've just added perhaps another 100 calories. Each time you butter your bread or dip your bread into olive oil you're adding calories—sometimes hundreds of calories—fat calories, easily stored in your fat cells.

Consider what it takes to **burn** off extra calories, and maybe you'll think again before dipping. I wanted to see how long I'd have to walk to burn off a couple of pieces of bread dipped in olive oil—I'll estimate 200 calories. I logged on to the Calorie Control Council Calorie Calculator (www.caloriecontrol.org) and first entered two slices of sourdough bread (136 calories) plus two tablespoons of olive oil (240 calories); in total, 376 calories and 30 grams of fat. Then I logged into their Exercise Calculator to find out that I'd have to walk *very briskly* for more than one hour just to burn off the excess calories. What I've found is that it's hard to stop dipping, so I don't start. It's too easy to make just one little dip, then another, and yet another. Two, three, four hundred calories, and I haven't even eaten a bite of salad yet, let alone any other food.

No, get rid of that oil please, and "thanks, but no thanks" to the butter. It's not worth it to me. I will save my calories for my entrée and maybe a glass of wine, and I'll leave the table feeling great about what I just consumed...not guilty for overeating.

Don't get me wrong. If I'm dining out and the chef uses some butter to finish a wonderful piece of fish, I'll enjoy the flavor, but I don't make a habit of ordering sauces and fatty foods. By not overloading my taste buds and constantly coating them with fat, I'm primed for flavor and can more easily discriminate between overly greasy foods and tastefully prepared cuisine. Dipping my bread into fat add hundreds of calories to my diet, which means pounds of fat to my waistline, butt, or thighs.

Choosing to be Naturally Thin

A lot of people don't like to make special requests. Well—how else are you going to get what you want unless you ask for it? There aren't many things in the world you can control—but food is one of them.

I read menus the way I read food labels, with a skeptical and practiced eye. Restaurant menus don't commonly display nutrition facts, so find common clues to the type of preparation—buzzwords, if you will. Once you know the lingo, you can't be fooled again. When the dish is labeled "fried" or "creamy," that's a no-brainer. But menus can deceive—the dish you thought was healthy may be topped with high-calories sauces, cooked with too much cream and butter, or topped with cheese. It pays to be knowledgeable about some common preparations.

Some dishes are named for the creator, such as *Alfredo*; or a famous personality, such as *Caesar, Rockefeller, Wellington,* or *Benedict*; or a place, such as *Monte Cristo* or *Bolognese*. Did you know that all these preparations mean lots of butter, sauce, and calories? I didn't. I had to learn. Dishes described as "Primavera" or "Mediterranean" often mean a lighter preparation with vegetables and tomatoes, but it pays to ask before you order, because each establishment has their unique way of serving and preparing different favorites.

Learn more about food by logging on to the Internet. Many popular restaurant chains feature ingredients; many have nutrition facts, and others allow you to personalize your order—see what happens when you change the ingredient list and remove some fat-laden sauces and cheese—voila! A better burger! All of the sudden that "special sauce" isn't so appealing. Be a wise consumer, and make smart choices second nature.

Please, take it back!

It's perfectly fine to ask your server to modify your order. Recently, my husband and I realized that we had over-ordered, but it didn't end there.

We were on the road for a month, working all day and staying in local motels. We had our usual breakfast of cereal, fruit, and nonfat milk, but we didn't have a kitchen, so we were dining out every night. One evening, Ken chose a Mexican restaurant. Mexican-American can be hard on a healthy diet because of the chips—you know, that basket of chips appears on the table, and it's hard to eat just one or two, and before you know it, you're halfway through the basket, and you haven't even ordered your meal. A mere 10 or 12 chips have more than 200 calories, and that's a recipe for weight gain. But Ken was right about this restaurant; yes, there were the usual tacos, burritos and other cheese-laden casserole-type dishes, but they also had great grilled meats, poultry, and fish, prepared with interesting sauces like pico de gallo or tomato-based salsa.

We ordered two ceviche appetizers—citrus-marinated fish—a very delicious and low-fat preparation. Since we anticipated small appetizer-sized servings, Ken went ahead and ordered an entrée of fish tacos, and I ordered the Mexicali Salad—described as lettuce, tomatoes, hearts of palm, avocado, and onions.

The appetizers were enormous. Two platter-sized portions of gorgeous chunks of white fish, shrimp, scallops, red onions, and celery; easily two full cups of seafood for each of us. We looked at each other.

Ken said, "Gee, I don't need the tacos!" I said, "Wow—there's plenty of food without!"

We quickly looked around for the waiter. "Could we please change the order if it's not too late? Could you cancel the fish tacos? There's plenty of fish here for both of us."

With just a little smile, he said, "Of course."

We left the table satisfied, but not overstuffed.

	Do You Know the Lingo? How menu savvy are you? Take this quiz, and see if you can match the Number (preparation) with the Letter (description)	
1.	Alfredo	
2.	Benedict	
3.	Bolognese	
4.	Caesar	
5.	Monte Cristo	
6.	Rockefeller	
7.	Primavera	
8.	Mediterranean	

A	This oyster dish's original recipe is kept secret in Antoine's restaurant in New Orleans, but other restaurants have adopted and adapted the recipe; it contains butter, oyster liquor, spinach, and the distinctive anise liquor, *Pernod*, and is topped with bread crumbs and sometimes Parmesan cheese.
B	Based on traditional cuisine from countries including Greece, Italy, Portugal, Spain, and France, ingredients are likely to be fresh; preparation is grilled or broiled, and dressed with olive oil, capers, and garlic.
C.	This is a sandwich of ham, turkey, and Swiss cheese that's batter-dipped and grilled or deep-fried.
D.	This means *spring* in Italian and usually applies to a pasta dish made with vegetables.
E	This is the name of a creamy white sauce made with butter and Parmesan cheese, usually paired with fettuccini pasta.
F	This describes a rich dish of poached eggs on buttered and pan-fried English muffins, topped with ham or Canadian bacon and Hollandaise sauce.
G.	This describes a wine-based, creamy meat sauce.
H.	This romaine lettuce salad is dressed with a thick, creamy dressing made from oil, egg (raw or coddled—briefly cooked), and anchovies, and is often topped with Parmesan cheese and croutons.

Answers:

1. Alfredo	E	This is the name of a creamy, white sauce made with butter and Parmesan cheese, usually paired with fettuccini pasta.
2. Benedict	F	This describes a rich dish of poached eggs on buttered and pan-fried English muffins, topped with ham or Canadian bacon and Hollandaise sauce.
3. Bolognese	G	This describes a wine-based, creamy meat sauce.
4. Caesar	H	This romaine lettuce salad is dressed with a thick, creamy dressing made from oil, egg (raw or coddled—briefly cooked), and anchovies, and is often topped with Parmesan cheese and croutons.
5. Monte Cristo	C	This is a sandwich of ham, turkey, and Swiss cheese that's batter-dipped and grilled or deep-fried.
6. Rockefeller	A	This oyster dish's original recipe is kept secret in Antoine's restaurant in New Orleans, but other restaurants have adopted and adapted the recipe; it contains butter, oyster liquor, spinach, and the distinctive anise liquor, *Pernod*, and is topped with bread crumbs and sometimes Parmesan cheese.
7. Primavera	D	This means *spring* in Italian and usually applies to a pasta dish made with vegetables.
8. Mediterranean	B	Based on traditional cuisine from countries including Greece, Italy, Portugal, Spain, and France, ingredients are likely to be fresh; preparation is grilled or broiled, and dressed with olive oil, capers, and garlic.

Taking My Naturally Thin Diet Out to Eat

The fastest growing segment in the restaurant market is *fast casual*, a blend of quick service fast food and restaurants with table service. Although fast casual may be perceived as a better and fresher alternative to fast food, consumers still need to consider portion size and added ingredients. Generally, with the exception of restaurants that offer just a few menu items, wherever there's a menu, there's a choice. My Old Overweight Choices kept me from attaining my weight and lifestyle goals. I use the second nature eating principles to guide my new *second nature* choices wherever I go.

Ordering Naturally Thin

I try to relax and deliberately drink a glass of water before I order, to take the edge off my appetite. Try to take a little time with the menu and don't rush to order.

Restaurant dining is a matter of choice. If the menu doesn't detail the way the food is prepared, I'll ask—and if necessary, I'll clearly and politely make my request.

"Salmon? Great. I'd like it grilled, please—no added butter, please...and medium-rare." Most restaurants add butter or oil to vegetables automatically—so you may want to request steamed veggies with or no added fat.

I may opt for the vegetable and a salad with my entrée. Since most restaurant portions can easily top eight ounces, I plan in advance—either I'll share the entrée, or take half home. A general guideline is that three to four ounces of meat, fish, or chicken looks like the palm of your hand.

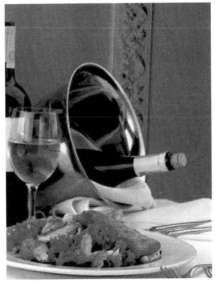

Savor your restaurant meal; take some time to enjoy it.

"Living Thin Naturally" Cooking

A heavy sauce may undo even the healthiest cooking techniques. Remember those four little words—"On the side, please!"

Roasted: Food cooked uncovered in the oven. A good choice is roasted fish or chicken—leave the skin to avoid hundreds of fat calories. Of course, I know you like the skin, and why not? Fat tastes good, but it sure looks bad on the hips and thighs.

Broiled: Cooked directly under the heat source. A restaurant that's worth its salt will always deliver this option. Serious eaters will order their food broiled or grilled—they know they're getting the most unadulterated food, and the kitchen can't hide poor quality under heavy sauces.

Baked: Cooked slowly with gentle heat. Baked fish or chicken may be a good choice, but restaurants tend to heavily sauce baked foods. Ask the server if the fish is baked in papillote, or if it's a casserole.

Grilled: Cooked directly over the heat source, with coals or a gas grill. I love that so many restaurants have become grilling experts. One of my favorites is a grilled salmon steak—medium rare.

Pan-broiled/Pan-seared: Cooked in a heavy skillet (without adding fat), draining off fat as it accumulates. Request sauce on the side, as this preparation often comes dressed and sauced.

In Parchment paper/En papillote: Cooked in a bag, using special heat-resistant paper. Traditionally, this dish is made with fish or chicken breast, spices, and sometimes fruit—the result is tender and healthy—using little or no fat. Look for this one, and ask request that the chef not add butter to the bag.

Poached: Cooked in simmering broth, water, or wine: traditionally fish or chicken, and the result is tender, with little or no added fat. Poached salmon is a treat—the fish comes out moist and delectable.

Sautéed: Cooked quickly over direct heat, with just a little added fat or broth. Depending on the amount of added fat, sautéed foods can be high in calories.

Steamed: Cooked over boiling water in a covered pan. Steamed foods are usually lightly cooked, remain crunchy, and retain their nutrients. Look for steamed vegetables, fish, shellfish, or chicken, especially in Asian food restaurants.

Stir-fried: Foods cooked quickly in a wok (a high-sided pan). A superior option to deep fried or fried food—the Chinese use a wok to sauté meats and vegetables, and by quick-cooking with high heat and little fat, the dish comes out flavorful yet low calorie. Request cooked without added fat, ask for broth instead.

Dining Deliciously "Around the World"

As you dine around the neighborhood, or travel around the world, there are a number of different ethnic cuisines to enjoy—different flavors, different preparations. A common comment from those dining globally is that in America, everything is bigger—and so are we. But countries that were once known for their healthy cuisines, such as Greece and Turkey, are now facing an epidemic of obesity. Even the French, who historically were thought to be able to eat whatever they wanted, are wrestling with a childhood obesity problem that's on pace with the United States.

Paring Back the Menu

OK, it's easy when the menu says "fried" or "deep fried." But here are code words that mean excess calories, and knowing the lingo helps make your choice easier. These terms mean that the food has been either fried or battered or both. Or it's been topped with high-calorie sauces, cheese, or other fried bits, such as won tons or other cracker-type additions.

- Creamy

- Crisp or Crispy: For example, a description of an appetizer called Crispy Green Bean Fries describes "snappy green beans, breaded and deep-fried to a golden brown crust." Or a salad "topped with crisp tortilla strips."

- Breaded: Usually indicates excess calories, both from the batter and the cooking method—usually fried or deep fried.

- Crunchy: Usually indicates fried, or with an added fried topping.

- Fritters: Foods battered, then deep-fried.

- Loaded: As in "loaded with sour cream and cheese."

- Smothered: As in "smothered in bread crumbs and cheese."

- Stuffed: As in an entrée called Stuffed Chicken Florentine; *stuffed* means stuffed with high-calorie cheese and/or creamy sauce. "Stuffed potato" means added cheese and fat.

Menu Terms: Describing characteristic ingredients

- Alfredo: As in Fettuccini Alfredo, describes a white, creamy sauce with Parmesan cheese—high in fat and calories. Instead, choose a marinara sauce, a "red" sauce with vegetables. May be called "primavera," but ask the waiter if it's a red or creamy sauce.

- Cordon bleu: Pounded veal or chicken, topped with ham and cheese, then battered and fried.

- Gorgonzola: As with Alfredo, indicates a sauce laden with cheese.

- Au Gratin: Foods covered with a sauce, sprinkled with cheese or breadcrumbs (or both) and baked to a golden brown. Very rich and high in calories.

- Parmigiana: Generally means double trouble—breaded, then fried chicken or eggplant; topped with marinara sauce and melted cheese.

- Foods topped with

  o Melted Cheese! Especially in Mexican and Italian restaurants. Most all the platters in Mexican-American restaurant foods are loaded with cheese, sour cream, or both.

  o Crispy wontons: Many otherwise healthy salads are topped with fried bits of crackers, otherwise known as won tons, or tortilla strips, but both mean extra calories.

  o Nuts—glazed nuts! A garnish of nuts makes a salad crunchy and interesting, but if they're coated with sugar and called "glazed," then we're talking candy.

Appetizers: I avoid certain appetizers entirely

- Dips: As in "Hot Artichoke Dip—a blend of artichokes, cheese, and cream cheese." Stick with a tossed salad or appetizer-sized portion of pasta with red sauce.

- Ranch dressing or any other creamy dressing: As in "Buffalo wings with ranch dressing"—and while we're on the subject...

- Wings: Fried wings don't compute. It takes too long to burn off 1000 calories for just nine wings with buffalo wings sauce.

- With Dipping Sauce: As in "breadsticks with dipping sauce."

- Stuffed stuff: As in "Stuffed mushrooms"—prepared with butter and breading and not worth the 100+ calories per piece.

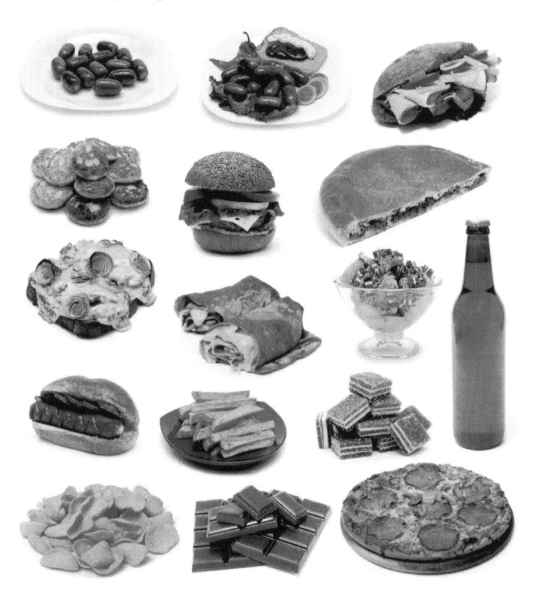

Dining Out—Restaurants and Fast Food

Order Smart

Dining Out means that sometimes, regardless of how I try, I have NO control over what I'm served. The establishment can write the nutrition facts, publish a beautiful menu, describe the food as low fat, and say "no added salt," but the chef may—or may not—be telling the truth. So, it's safer just to avoid some foods and situations, and choose smart substitutes.

Old Overweight Order	New "Living Thin Naturally" Order
Sandwich Salads: Thinking that tuna salad was better than roast beef, I forgot that regular mayonnaise has 100 calories per tablespoon. I could tell how much added fat I was eating by how white my salad was. The creamier the tuna or shrimp salad, the more mayo and/or sour cream added.	Colorful Foods: I've given up white foods, foods made with mayonnaise or sour cream. Specifically, commercially prepared shrimp, tuna, and potato or macaroni salad—packed with extra calories from pure fat. White foods aren't worth it to me. I'll stay naturally thin by making smarter choices.
Heavy cream or half-and-half in coffee: Oh, I used to dump at least two tablespoons of half-and-half into coffee—at least two in the morning, one mid-morning, and at least one mid-afternoon. That added up to eight tablespoons of cream—about 40 calories per two-tablespoon serving. 160 calories per day, 80% fat.	Dairy Defined: Italians don't put cream in their coffee. In fact, espresso is the brew of choice—a small, demitasse cup of strong, brewed coffee with one or two sugars—never artificial sugar. The first time my husband and I visited Italy, I asked him to take a stand against adding half-and-half to his coffee. Although he was quite used to creamy coffee, he decided that it was a good time to do as the locals—and never looked back. Black coffee, brewed and fresh, has no calories.
All You Can Eat: When all you can eat becomes eat all you can, it's a recipe for weight gain. It's so easy to lose track of calories when helping yourself from a huge platter. Family style dining means eating for you—and for your family, too.	A la Carte: Even when dining out, I can approximate my usual diet—the diet I use to stay naturally thin—by ignoring dinner entrees and sticking to appetizer portions for my entrée, sometimes adding a salad or soup to start.
Fat On the Table: Dipping bread into olive oil adds hundreds of calories; each pat of butter adds another 100 calories.	Better Bread: I enjoy the end pieces of crusty bread—if it's really good, I'll substitute the bread for rice or potato.
Creamy Dressings: A salad's calories can double or triple depending on the type of salad dressing and how much is put on.	On the Side: The most important words in dining out—save hundreds of calories by asking for oil and vinegar, and dress your salad yourself.

Dining Out: Bagels

OK, I admit it. I love bagels...and giving them up ranks next to that huge bran muffin as my "Rosebud" foods, the foods that kept me fat, that I fixated on when I was feeling stressed and needed comfort food.

During my early 20s, my overweight years in Florida, I went out to breakfast every morning with my best friend, Barbara. She had one scrambled egg, a toasted buttered bagel, and coffee. I had

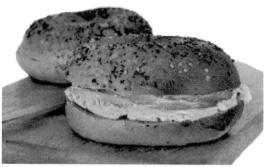

One regular bagel is equivalent to 5-6 slices of bread—plus a couple of tablespoons of cream cheese—total almost 1,000 calories!]

a bagel and cream cheese, plus a scoop of shrimp or tuna salad. That was my nemesis. The bagels were huge, the shrimp salad was made with mayonnaise, and I put cream in my coffee.

Today's huge bagels have little resemblance to those of my youth...they're huge! Unlike the old two- to three-inch bagels, today's giants represent at least three or four servings (slices) of bread, up to 400 calories—maybe more.

And beware the little plastic cups of cream cheese—each adds another couple of hundred calories. Bagel stores offer a range of quick casual breakfast and lunch meals, but wherever you go, remember that before you add anything to that bagel, you're starting out by eating a lot of calories from refined white flour (unless you can find a real whole wheat bagel.) Scoop it out, stuff it with salad, and stick with low fat cheese—maybe a 'schmear' of hummus.

Old Overweight Bagel Order	New "Living Thin Naturally" Bagel Order
Toasted everything bagel: 390 calories, 6g fat Serving of cream cheese: 200 calories, 19g fat Small scoop of shrimp salad: 50 calories, 3.5g fat Orange juice, 6 oz: 77 calories, 0.3g fat 2 cups coffee with cream: 140 calories, 12g fat	Scooped out, toasted whole wheat bagel: 195 calories, 3g fat Light cream cheese: 60 calories, 4.5g fat Lettuce and tomato: 15 calories, 0g fat Coffee, black: 0 calories, 0g fat
Total calories Old: 856 Total fat Old: 41g	Total calories New: 264 Total fat New: 7.5g

Scoop it Out! I remember the first time I heard someone order a "SOB." What? That's shorthand for Scoop Out the Bagel. You'll never miss the doughy insides if you stuff your sandwich with lettuce, tomato, and cucumbers.

Regular cream cheese has about 50 calories per level tablespoon, reduced fat cream cheese has 25% fewer calories than the original (about 25 calories). Additional lower calorie options include "light", "lite", and "fat-free" (about 15 calories). Scoop out that bagel and save 100 calories, too.

Dining Out: Breakfast Restaurant

Breakfast can be the easiest meal to eat out safely—as long as you choose right. Almost every restaurant has a la carte options, such as hot or cold cereal, fruit cups, fresh melon, grapefruit, and of course, eggs done your way. Oatmeal is high in fiber and protein and, with skim milk and fruit, keeps me satisfied until lunch. A higher protein choice is eggs—again, I've adopted *second nature* ordering habits and make my requests specific to the way I want to eat. For example, here's a "before" and "after" menu. You try it—log on to a breakfast restaurant like Denny's, www.dennys. com, to see how easily different choices dramatically affect calorie and fat count.

If I go out to breakfast, I order a la carte and save HUNDREDS of calories, while still enjoying breakfast out with my friends.

Old Overweight Breakfast Out with Friends	New "Living Thin Naturally" Breakfast Out with Friends
Scrambled eggs and ham: 1080 calories, 53g fat Toasted bagel: 310 calories, 1g fat Whipped margarine: 87 calories, 10g fat Orange juice, 10 oz: 126 calories, 0g fat Coffee with cream: 50 calories, 5g fat	Scrambled Eggbeaters: 120 calories, 0g fat English muffin, toasted, dry: 150 calories, 2g fat Grapefruit half: 60 calories, 0g fat Lettuce and tomato on the side: approximately 25 calories Coffee, black (*if you don't like Eggbeaters, order 2 scrambled eggs—request cooked dry: 240 calories, 20g fat*)
Total calories Old: 1653 Total fat Old: 70g	Total calories New: 355 Total fat New: 2g

My old overweight breakfast was a diet-disaster, with almost an entire day's worth of calories and fat, not to mention sodium and cholesterol. Other good choices at restaurants include:
- A "short stack" of pancakes or silver-dollar pancakes. Skip the butter and syrup: Add fresh fruit and request sugar-free syrup.
- Hot cereal with nonfat or 1% milk.
- Melon, berries, or grapefruit.
- Lean Canadian bacon is a better choice than bacon or sausage, which is loaded with saturated fat, sodium, and nitrates.
- Egg white omelets: Ask for the whites with vegetables—tomatoes, peppers, onions, mushrooms, and broccoli are usually available—cooked dry with whole wheat toast. I put mustard on my omelet!

Dining Out: Hotel Breakfast

Breakfast is the place to get some of those nutrients that could be lacking in the rest of the day's meals—fiber and fruit—especially when you're on the road.

Old Overweight Breakfast	New "Living Thin Naturally" Breakfast
Cheese Danish: 370 calories, 18g fat Orange juice, 8 oz: 102 calories, 0.5g fat Coffee with cream: 140 calories, 12g fat	1.5 cups Cheerios: 150 calories, 3g fat 1.5 cups nonfat milk: 136 calories, 0.9g fat 1 cup blueberries: 83 calories, 0.5g fat
Total calories Old: 612 Total fat Old: 30.5g	Total calories New: 369 Total fat New: 4.4g **Plus 9.5g fiber**

When I'm traveling, I take cereal. Otherwise, I try to locate Cheerios, usually offered in hotels and motels, because it's very low in added sugar and has a few grams of fiber. When I'm flying in the morning, I portion 1-2 cups of Kashi GoLean and ⅓ cup Bran Buds into a covered plastic container, and add ½ cup dry nonfat milk and a couple tablespoons of raisins. After I've passed through the security line, I get a cup of coffee, add water to my cereal, mix and voila! Breakfast.

Dining Out: Brunch

Here's just an example of how I used to order brunch at my favorite diner—and how I order brunch now. I think my new way is so much better—certainly it tastes great, but look at the calorie differential—it's naturally brilliant, if I may say so myself!

Old Overweight Brunch	New "Living Thin Naturally" Brunch
Scrambled eggs (in butter) with bacon, home fries, buttered bagel, orange juice, and coffee with cream	Omelet, made with 2 egg-whites and 1 whole egg, tomatoes, and mushrooms (cooked without butter in a nonstick pan); whole-wheat toast; lettuce and tomato; a small wedge of melon; and black coffee
Total calories Old: A whopping 1200 calories Total fat Old: 70g (only 4g fiber!)	Total calories New: Only 300 calories Total fat New: 9g Total fiber: 7g

My new habits are now second nature—I don't even think about it anymore. I just ask nicely---*I'd like an omelet, prepared dry please—no added butter—and please tell the chef to add onions, tomatoes, peppers, mushrooms—I love vegetables, as long as they are not buttered or oiled. I'd like whole wheat toast—dry, please—no added butter, thank you! And if you have a half-grapefruit or piece of melon that's ripe, I'll have that too. Thanks again!*

Wherever they prepare breakfast to order, you can have it your way. I've had a perfect egg white omelet at the Cheesecake Factory—it came with the reddest, freshest sliced tomatoes, a big orange slice, and crisp dark green lettuce.

Dining Out: French

Ah, the cliché that "French women don't get fat" is untrue. More and more French women, men, and especially French kids are getting fat. The lifestyle that formerly meant small portions of deliciously prepared food eaten slowly with family and friends is a thing of the past. However, it is possible to enjoy many French preparations—especially the Mediterranean French dishes, traditionally with lots of seafood. Small portions of really tasty food are smarter than huge portions of mediocre, over-sauced, and fatty food.

Old Overweight French:	New "Living Thin Naturally" French: Nouvelle Cuisine
French Fat Terminology • Béarnaise: Sauce made from egg yolks and butter. • Fromage: Au fromage means "with cheese" • Beurre: Butter	• "Entrée" means appetizer. Start with consommé (clear, broth-based soup), bouillabaisse (tomato-based shellfish soup), or a small salad with oil and vinegar. Speak with the waiter and ask him to recommend a dish that is baked, broiled, or grilled, such as seafood, chicken, lean veal, or filet mignon—and steer clear of heavy sauces and butter.
• Buttery croissants were my undoing in Switzerland. I noticed the athletic German girls had muesli instead. • Fondue appears to facilitate a fatty diet--dipping white bread into hot cheese. • Crepes may be filled with calories from cheese and topped with white sauce	• For a light lunch or dinner, a Salad Nicoise (lettuce, hard-boiled egg, potatoes, string beans, and anchovies) or a salad with grilled chicken or fish are always smart selections. Request dressing on the side.

Dining Out: Mediterranean

Greek, Turkish, Moroccan, Israeli, Spanish, Southern Italian, and Southern French

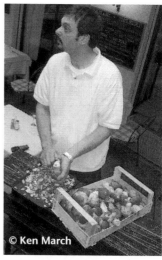

© Ken March

The Mediterranean way includes fatty fish, olives and olive oil, nuts and seeds, and avocado—all heart-healthy, but my portions suit my calorie needs. All these foods are heart-healthy, but high in fat.

The Mediterranean, or Cretan diet (Crete is an island off the coast of Greece in the Mediterranean) may be (or used to be) the most heart healthy on earth, because it traditionally contained a predominance of foods known for their antioxidant qualities, including whole grains, and all different legumes and beans. This way of eating includes an abundance of fresh vegetables, including eggplant, tomatoes, and potatoes; and all kinds of fruit. Fatty fish and shellfish are commonly on the menu, but meat and poultry are eaten occasionally.

Getting morels ready for dinner; Bellagio, Italy

Beware of popular Greek "taverna" style restaurants—portions are American-sized and huge—many formerly healthy dishes are transformed and are covered with cheese.

Mediterranean Dining

Dining out the Mediterranean way means that if I'm in the mood for fish, my first choice is a roasted fish—such as red snapper—and maybe a salad of fava beans and tomatoes as a first course.

- Think **Grilled**—and avoid dishes in phyllo dough (thin sheets of dough layered with fat), loaded with sauce and cheese. Yes, it's delicious, but hey—been there, done that. All these recipes are better prepared at home, because you can modify the ingredients.

- Souvlaki, kebabs: Skewered meats, chicken, and fish—grilled or roasted with vegetables. (Choose chicken for fewer calories and fat, compared to beef, lamb, or pork.)

- Greek salad: The "Greek" means feta cheese and olives, high in calories, but also in taste and good fats. Request dressing on the side to control calories.

- Pita: Whole-grain is best.

- Gyros: Sandwiches made from pita wrapped around ground beef or lamb; can have more than 700 calories and 40 grams of fat. In general, Greek dishes made with ground meats are high in fat—opt for grilled meats and chicken dishes instead.

- Tabouli: A salad made with cracked wheat, chopped herbs, and vegetables. It is a light, healthy option.

- Tzatziki, or "yogurt sauce," may sound diet-friendly, but—even though the other ingredients are mere herbs and garlic—it's typically made with full-fat yogurt.

- Hummus: Chickpea dip, made from mashed chickpeas, olive oil, garlic, lemon juice, and a little tahini (sesame paste). Hummus is high in protein and healthy fat—portion size counts (two tablespoons have about 50-100 calories, depending upon the amount of oil in the preparation).

- Baba ganoush: Eggplant dip, made from roasted eggplant, olive oil, garlic, lemon juice, and a little tahini for taste. Can make this with roasted red peppers, too.

Dining Out: Indian

My first job as a nutritionist was in a senior healthcare clinic in Queens, New York home to one of the most diverse populations of immigrants in America—many from Southeast Asia, namely India and Bangladesh. My usual clients were overweight or obese seniors—mostly women—with type 2 diabetes, heart disease, and/or hypertension. In their countries, they'd shopped daily in the market and walked everywhere—portion size was smaller compared to now, in New York, where most of them lived in walk-up apartments, and they rarely left their homes. The inactivity and larger portions of food meant significant weight gain in just a few years after immigrating. Most had "syndrome X," now known as metabolic syndrome, with symptoms of insulin resistance, high triglycerides, high blood pressure, low HDL, and high LDL cholesterol.

Old Overweight Indian Food	New "Living Thin Naturally" Indian Food
Many dishes are deep fried, served with "ghee" (clarified butter) and are high in calories. Served with white rice, portion size can be double or triple—or more—than what you need	When dining out in Indian restaurants, I request foods to be prepared without ghee, and choose: • Dal: Made from lentils, tomatoes, onions, and spices. • Tandoori: Fish, meat, or chicken baked in a clay oven, or tandoor, often without added oils or sauces. • Pullao: Basmati, or long-grain rice, which usually accompanies the main entrée and is a good option for a low-fat side. • Raita: A yogurt-based side dish with shredded onions, cucumbers, and occasionally additional vegetables. • Naan or Chapatti: Breads prepared without butter. Avoid deep-fried breads or those made with butter, such as poori or paratha.

Dining Out: Italian

Italy is a country of different climates—and food preparation. Many think that all Italian food is made with red sauce and gargantuan bowls of spaghetti and meatballs. Not so. My husband and I have traveled in Italy, and the first time we dined out in southern Sicily, we took note of the manageable first course of pasta with olive oil and garlic. At first we thought, gee—that's not very much. But the flavor! Traditionally, Italians enjoy dining in a relaxed and unhurried way, and the food is served with gracious attention to detail. Eating slowly is so much more satisfying. In America, I seek out a restaurant that duplicates the type of service found in Italy, where meals often begin with a cup of soup, followed by a small first course of pasta with olive oil and garlic or maybe fresh pomodoro sauce—fresh red tomatoes. An entrée is simple grilled fish or meat, and most Italians enjoy a small salad to finish. Unfortunately, there's a trend in the U.S. for Italian-American restaurants to serve in bowl-sized dishes, enough to feed three or even four people—with more than 1000 calories per serving.

Old Overweight Italian Restaurant Meal	New "Living Thin Naturally" Italian Restaurant Meal
• Fried mozzarella sticks, half order: 440 calories, 31g fat • Eggplant parmesan: 1240 calories, 64g fat • Tiramisu: 1000 calories, 64g fat	• Mozzarella a la Caprese (with tomato and basil), half order: 260 calories, 21g fat • Pollo (chicken) grilled with zucchini: 330 calories, 5g fat) • Italian sorbet with a small biscotti cookie, half order: 160 calories , 2g fat
Total calories Old: 2680 Total fat Old: 159g	Total calories: 750 Total fat: 28g

---

Naturally Thin Italian Appetizers

• A cup of broth-based soup, such as minestrone or lentil.

• A half-portion of bruschetta (toasted bread with chopped tomatoes, garlic, and olive oil).

• A small tossed salad with a tablespoon of balsamic vinaigrette, or dress your own with a little olive oil and vinegar.

• Order from the side dishes, especially vegetables such as broccoli rabe or the vegetable of the day, drizzled with a touch of olive oil.

• Steamed mussels or clams in red sauce.

• Calamari, not fritti or fried, but sautéed, grilled, or marinated.

• Shrimp cocktail is always a good choice.

Naturally Thin Italian Entrees:

Meats, fish, poultry, and shellfish, prepared simply—grilled; Cacciatore-style recipes mean red (tomato) sauce. Marsala means cooked with wine.

Pasta: Most American-Italian restaurants serve huge pasta and casserole dishes—an appetizer is typically entrée-sized. Marinara or pomodoro mean red (tomato) sauce. White clam sauce means wine and garlic; primavera means tossed with vegetables, but some chefs may use cream to finish, so ask.

Dessert?

Traditionally, Italians finish with a salad or piece of fruit. A fresh ending with an espresso coffee, and perhaps a double-baked cookie (biscotti), is ideal. Otherwise, for a special occasion, tiramisu is my favorite, but watch out for the calories! Made with espresso-soaked ladyfingers and creamy mascarpone cheese, at Macaroni Grill, one serving has 1000 calories! Share it with at least four people—there's no rule that says you have to eat the whole portion.

Dining Out: Buffet

When did all you can eat become eat all you can? For many, buffets seem to be offering endless opportunities to overstuff. Gee, I don't leave my mind behind just because I'm faced with too much choice. I just zero in on the good stuff.

Buffets are easy to navigate when they have boiled shrimp; steamed or poached fish; and lots of salad offerings. I find that Chinese buffets can be a challenge—some appear to put oil on everything, including vegetables. But I persevere and get out my compass. When I see foods glistening with oil—or white with mayonnaise—I keep on searching. When I see fatty meat drowning in gravy, I keep on going. When I see fish smothered in creamy sauce or breaded and fried, I skip it. But when I see steamed shrimp, or baked turkey breast and cranberry sauce, and undressed salad, I know I've arrived at my *second nature* diet destination.

Old Overweight Buffet: Chinese	New "Living Thin Naturally" Buffet: Chinese
Sweet and Sour Chicken, ¾ cup: 465 calories, 27g fat Pork Fried Rice, ½ cup: 500 calories, 16g fat Egg roll: 190 calories, 8g fat Ice Cream, 1 cup plus 2 tablespoons chocolate syrup: 255 calories, 8g fat	Steamed shrimp and vegetables, 2 cups: 250 calories, 12g fat Fresh pineapple and watermelon, 1 cup and a small slice: 120 calories, 0g fat 1 Fortune cookie: 30 calories, 0g fat
Total calories Old: 1410 Total fat New: 59g	Total calories New: 400 Total fat New: 12g

Old Overweight Buffet: American	New "Living Thin Naturally" Buffet: American
1 cup broccoli cheese soup: 280 calories, 18g fat 1 serving (leg quarter) barbeque chicken: 480 calories, 22g fat 1 serving (3.5 oz) mashed potatoes: 120 calories, 6g fat ½ cup creamed spinach: 180 calories, 13g fat 1 yeast roll (no butter): 195 calories, 2g fat ½ cup vanilla soft serve ice cream: 100 calories, 2g fat	1 cup chicken gumbo soup: 140 calories, 3g fat 4.5 oz marinated chicken breast: 120 calories, 1.5g fat ½ cup steamed vegetables: 66 calories, 5g fat 1 small sweet potato: 137 calories, 0g fat 2 Tbsp 'lite' vinaigrette: 60 calories, 6g fat ½ cup sugar-free gelatin: 10 calories, 0g fat 1 cup fresh fruit: 60 calories, 0g fat
Total calories Old: 1355 Total fat New: 63g	Total calories New: 593 Total fat New: 15.5g

On the Buffet Line:
Log on to a buffet or salad franchise to learn the nutrition facts before you drive over. All the info is there—from the soups and salads to the bakery, breads, and beverages. Pay close attention to serving size when you're perusing the nutrition information because calories listed depend on serving size, and they may differ among restaurants.

More Buffet Basics:

- Fill Up, not Out: Start with fresh salad, but avoid pre-prepared salads with a oily sheen (lots of added calories). Nonfat salad dressing is a better choice than full fat. For example, 2 tablespoons of regular blue cheese salad dressing has ~190 calories, versus only 35 calories for 2 tablespoons of fat-free ranch dressing. Calories add up, so make visible cuts first.

- Start with a cup of clear soup or steamed vegetables to take the edge off your appetite.

- Rethink these Additions—every little bite adds up:
  - All add about 100-200 extra calories per scant 2 tablespoon serving
    - Full-fat salad dressings
    - Croutons
    - Olives
    - Nuts, seeds, and bacon bits

- Avoid "White" Foods: Mayonnaise-dressed salads, such as egg salad, chicken salad, and tuna salad have hundreds of extra fat calories; white usually means high-calorie sour cream, too.

- Think Salad: Carrots, celery, radishes, cucumbers, broccoli, cauliflower, etc.

- Skip breaded and battered fish and chicken and foods loaded with cheese or glistening from butter.

- Go for some lean protein: baked ham, turkey, chicken, and fish.

- Steamed shrimp or steamed crab is tasty, extremely low in fat and saturated fat, and satisfying.

- Cocktail sauce counts: each tablespoon has about 35 calories.

Dining Out: In the Deli

I grew up with fresh, Jewish rye, corned beef, and pastrami, but I've left them far behind because these salty meats are so high in fat and calories. I put them in the "been there, done that" column. I usually skip the soup—also too salty and fatty. Nevertheless, dining in delis can be delicious—just take a fresh look at the menu board, because there are naturally thin choices to be made.

Old Overweight Deli Dining	New "Living Thin Naturally" Deli Dining
Matzo ball soup: 400 calories, 14g fat Pastrami sandwich on rye bread with mustard: 1843 calories, 78g fat Cream soda, 12 oz: 188 calories, 0g fat	Lite turkey club: Smoked turkey breast, low fat ham, lettuce, tomato, low fat Swiss, and fat-free dressing on toasted whole grain wheat. 533 calories, 15g fat Seltzer with lemon: 0 calories, 0g fat
Total Calories Old: 2431 calories Total fat Old (oy vey!): 92g	Total New calories: 533 Total fat New: 15g

Go online before you go. Type "deli restaurant" into your Web browser and review menus—there are number of healthy dining options. Delis often offer half-sandwiches—a smart selection for most everyone who needs to stick to 2000 calories a day or less. If your deli doesn't offer nutrition info, use your Nutrition Tracker from MyPyramid.gov. Keep it simple and avoid casseroles—more likely to have high-calorie ingredients. And share—portions tend to be oversized and overstuffed.

Deli Defined:

- Order a half-sandwich: Avoid fatty meats, and opt for lean turkey or chicken.

- Add lettuce and tomato to sandwiches for more fiber.

- Hot dogs are high in fat, sodium, and nitrates; share a turkey sandwich instead.

- Pickles are "free" food because they're so low in calories. However, they are high in sodium, so if you're sodium sensitive, avoid pickled food.

- Avoid white salads made with full-fat mayo, such as potato or macaroni salad.

- Opt for vinegar-based cucumber or garden salad with low fat, low calorie dressings.

- Try a cup of vegetable or bean soup.

Dining Out: Japanese

Traditional Japanese food is low in fat and saturated fats and features fish and all types of vegetables, including sea vegetables.

Appetizers	Entrée	Sushi and Sashimi
• Miso soup (clear soup made with fermented soy, scallions, and tofu) • Edemame (steamed soy bean pods) • Mixed greens with miso or carrot-ginger dressing on the side • Ohitashi (boiled spinach) • Seaweed salad • Oshinko (pickled cabbage) • Shumai (steamed dumplings) • Yakitori (chicken and onions broiled in teriyaki sauce on a skewer) • Yaki-udon (stir-fried udon noodles) • Yutofu (hot, soft tofu in soy sauce) • Ebi-su (shrimp)	• Steamed or broiled fish • Shabu-shabu: Thin slices of beef, quickly cooked with mushrooms, cabbage, and other vegetables. • Soba (whole wheat), Udon and Ramen noodles with chicken, meat, fish, or vegetables in broth • Teriyaki chicken (can be high in sodium): Grilled or broiled in sweet soy sauce • Yakitori: Grilled chicken skewers • Yosenabe: Fish, vegetables, and noodles in broth	High-quality raw fish, served plain or with rice. Health experts advise people with weakened immunity or pregnant women to avoid raw fish. • Sashimi: Sliced raw fish with wasabi (Japanese horseradish), soy sauce, and pickled ginger. • Sushi: Sliced raw fish served atop vinegar-seasoned rice. Ask for all sauces on the side. • Maguro: Tuna • Tako: Octopus • Saba: Mackerel • Ika: Squid • Ebi: Prawn • Sake: Salmon • California roll: Avocado, cucumber, and cooked crabmeat wrapped in a thin sheet of seaweed and packed against rice • Futomaki: Fat sushi roll

I ignore battered and fried tempura, and focus on fresh, simply-prepared food—my naturally thin diet choices. Sushi generally comes with white, sticky rice—½ cup of rice per serving—or 100-200 calories, depending upon the size of the roll. If you can find it, brown rice sushi is the best choice. Sashimi is sushi-grade fish without the rice. My favorite meal is seaweed salad or miso soup to start, followed with broiled fish—maybe in teriyaki sauce. Miso, or fermented soy paste, is quite delicious—and high in sodium, so make it an occasional menu choice. Go online to www.sushifaq.com and learn more about different types of fish and nutritional values for different sushi rolls. Finally, green tea is antioxidant-rich, a perfect accompaniment to your Japanese meal.

Dining Out: Steakhouses

In order to understand American's girth, stop into a steakhouse—where they appear to champion distorted portions of food, where a "regular" sized steak means 8-12 ounces, double or triple a "normal" portion of beef. It's quite easy to dine naturally thin at a steakhouse—as long as you order smart. Realistically, I already know what I'm going to order, and it's fish, salad, and asparagus. I don't avoid steak houses, but don't eat beef, and the appetizers with rich cheeses and sauces never tempt me —I ignore them. Thin dining means sharing entrees, or choose restaurants that offer smaller or half-sized portions.

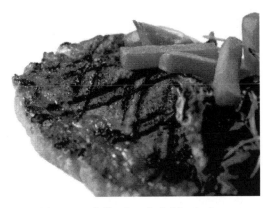

Eat with your waistline in mind—big steak means big calories, saturated fat and cholesterol

The January/February 1997, Nutrition Action Newsletter, published by the Center for Science in the Public Interest, featured a story on American steakhouses. They analyzed 15 of the most popular entrees, appetizers, and sides, and found that "Steak can be a decent meal or a disaster. But the worst food you can buy at a steakhouse isn't steak. It's the appetizers" (Center for Science in the Public Interest 1997).

Twelve years later, nothing has changed. There are more steakhouses to choose from— some expensive fine-dining establishments and some casual chains. They have in common big cuts of steak and prime rib; lots of deep-fried appetizers, such as onion rings and creamy soups; big sides; and big desserts, too. But you can choose! If the restaurant doesn't provide nutrition information online, do a little menu sleuthing and log on to your favorite nutrition tracker, such as MyPyramid.gov, or any weight management website. That's what I do! If they don't list the nutrition, you can "guesstimate" the calories served per menu item. Skip all the appetizers—all the wings and dips and fries and other deep-fried foods weigh you down. There are healthy options, such as fish, and chicken, too.

Dining Out: Steak Houses

Appetizers and Starters		Entrees	
Old Overweight Steakhouse	New "Living Thin Naturally" Steakhouse	Old Overweight Steakhouse	New "Living Thin Naturally" Steakhouse
Shrimp and Lobster Dip with Tortilla chips	Tossed salad: I request olive oil and vinegar	A 20-ounce steak: Estimate the yield of a 20-ounce steak is about 14 ounces	Grilled salmon: Be smart and opt for a smaller 7-ounce portion size (instead of the 10-ounce) Recall that my naturally thin diet means my regular portion of fish is about 4 ounces—so 7 ounces is almost double. I can share or take some home for the next day. Request extra lemon and hold the sauce.
Total calories Old: 800 Total fat Old: 50g	Total calories New: 60 Total fat New: 6g	Total calories Old: 1300 Total fat Old: 64g (including 32g saturated fat)	Total calories New: 350 Total fat New: 15g

Entrée:

•   Bigger is never better—it's just bigger. Opt for the smaller size when they offer it—it'll still be too big.

•   Cut counts: The loin cut is the leanest.

•   Go for grilled or poached fish, broiled chops or sirloin, grilled chicken, or steamed shrimp. If ordering steak, opt for lean loin cuts; share an entrée—it's usually enough for three or four people (normal serving size is four ounces)

•   Request your food prepared without added butter, sauce, or gravy

•   Some entrees come with sides and starch: Ask to hold the starch and double up on steamed or grilled vegetables.

Appetizer:

•   Skip the deep-fried onions for appetizers—just one has more calories than an entire meal of grilled salmon and baked potato with salsa

•   Forget the french fries smothered in cheese and/or ranch sauce

•   Order a tossed salad with dressing on the side

•   Select some sliced tomatoes with onions

•   Order shrimp or crab meat cocktails with cocktail sauce on the side

•   Try tomato-based Manhattan clam chowder; skip creamy New England or bisque made with heavy cream

Sides:

•   Baked potato—skip the butter; request tomato salsa or chopped tomatoes

•   Steamed asparagus: Hold the Hollandaise and butter

Dining Out: Mexican

There's a major difference between authentic Mexican—which I'll call "South of the Border" food—and fast Mexican-American food. The latter is usually covered with cheese, sour cream, and fat-laden refried beans. Even traditional South American restaurants have often modified their menus to cater to typical American tastes—so keep the chips off the table. Just one ounce can mean more than 200 added calories. See Mexican-American Fast Food for more naturally thin tips.

Appetizers and Sides		Entrees	
Old Overweight Mexican	New Naturally Thin South of the Border	Old Overweight Mexican	New Naturally Thin South of the Border
Nachos: fried tortilla chips covered with cheese and sour cream	*Ceviche:* Citrus marinade cooks fresh fish and seafood	*Quesadillas* with cheese and beans	Mesquite grilled *camerones*, shrimp, or skinless *pollo*, chicken
Quesadillas: fried and stuffed, covered with cheese and sour cream	Black bean soup; *gazpacho* (chilled vegetable soup)	Read the menu to discern preparation and added ingredients. Watch for descriptive terms, such as crispy (deep-fried) and *queso* (added cheese)	*Arroz con Pollo:* stewed chicken with rice
Refried beans	Black beans (*frijoles negros*) and rice	*Enchiladas, empanadas*—usually cheesy and high calorie	Fish or chicken *Veracruz*, in a spicy red tomato sauce
Guacamole and chips: Avocado contains healthy, monounsaturated fat, but chips are generally fried and fatty and very salty; a couple won't hurt.	*Pico de gallo* and salsa made with fresh chopped vegetables—usually tomatoes and other raw vegetables, with lime juice, fresh cilantro, and mild, medium, or spicy chili peppers	Combination plate: usually a sample platter, including a *burrito, taco,* and *enchilada*—and cheese, refried beans, and more cheese	*Fajitas:* Grilled fish, meat, or poultry—or sometimes shellfish, even tofu, with fresh vegetables; request no cheese or sour cream, and extra salsa; skip the tortilla—there's usually enough food for two or more

Dining Out: Vegetarian

If you are a strict vegan, it's best to inquire when you're dining out. You can make your wishes known, but what comes out of the kitchen is out of your hands. Some vegetarian soups or other menu items may include ingredients such as chicken stock.

Don't be shy about telling your server specifically what you want—if you do, you're more likely to get what you need.

If you avoid all animal products, unless you're visiting a restaurant that states that its policy is vegetarian, it's best to speak with your waiter before ordering:

- Soups: Beef and chicken broth are common ingredients in soups, as well as gravies and sauces.

- Salads: Ask your waiter to be sure there are no hidden items, such as bacon bits, eggs, or luncheon meats in salads.

- "Vegetarian": If an entree is labeled vegetarian in a non-vegetarian restaurant, it may be prepared using animal-based fats and/or meat products. Ask your waiter to be sure.

- Gelatin: Made from animal bones; avoid aspic and other gelatin-containing foods.

- Complications: Dishes made with many ingredients are harder to discern— casseroles, in particular, may contain cream, cheeses, and other meat or dairy ingredients.

Best Vegetarian

Ethnic restaurants with plant-based cuisines are easy picks for vegetarians. My favorite Mediterranean and Middle-Eastern cuisines feature grilled vegetables with different marinated salads and mushrooms, hummus (chickpea dip), and baba ganoush (eggplant dip). Japanese offers miso soup and vegetarian sushi; Chinese favorites include steamed vegetables with tofu; in a Greek restaurant, I love salads with feta cheese and olives; if you eat fish, any restaurant will be easily accommodating.

Appetizers, Starters, and Sides	Entrée
Soups: Gazpacho, lentil, bean, and minestrone. If they don't specify, ask if the broth is vegetarian or meat-based, to assure it's not made from chicken or beef stock	Grain and pasta: Try a pilaf or pasta entree with marinara sauce
Salads: Start with the house salad or order a dinner salad with dressing on the side, of course. Salads with grains, such as couscous, are delicious.	Rice and beans: Ask your waiter to assure it's not made with lard or animal fat
Appetizers: Order hummus and a salad with pita bread	Soy: Vegetarian casseroles with soy protein

Sides: Make a meal of grilled vegetables and baked potato	Salad Bar: Vegetarian options include all greens, crunchy vegetables, tomatoes, peppers, cucumber, baby corn, garbanzo/red kidney beans, artichoke hearts, hearts of palm, tofu chunks, optional cottage cheese, low fat or fat-free dressing, olive oil, and balsamic vinegar
	Fast Food: Burgers: Some chains offer vegetarian burgers. Avoid the full-fat dressings and cheese. Pizza: Vegetarian pizza often means loaded with cheese—request all the veggies and just a sprinkle (or no) cheese. Sandwich and subs: Roasted vegetables Mexican and Southwestern: Beans and rice; vegetarian burritos—make sure that no animal fat or butter is used, and hold the cheese.
Dessert: Fresh fruit plate, fruit sorbet (dairy-free), or sherbet (with dairy).	

Fast Food: An Infrequent Proposition

> *"If It Comes Through A Car Window, It Isn't Food"*
> —*Mike Huckabee*

In an article in *USA Today* (April 3, 2002), writer Bruce Horovitz reported that drive-thru represents *half* of the $129 billion spent yearly at fast food restaurants. Recently, I've seen higher estimates—up to *70 percent* of some privately owned and franchise fast food store's revenue comes from drive-thru customers. Some people just live in their cars—they get in line first thing in the morning for coffee or breakfast; lunch comes through the car window; and they stop for take-out on their way home. Lunch is the most popular meal served at fast food restaurants, but breakfast is the new proving ground. With coffee increasing in popularity, the big franchises like McDonald's and Burger King are beefing up their breakfast menus, with McDonald's making a special push to promote better-brewed coffee. From Starbucks to Dunkin' Donuts, from Arby's to Subway, fast food is going *hot* breakfast. Hot equates to hot sausage, eggs, and hash browns—usually with cheese—which means lots of sodium, fat and calories. Order any of the big breakfast meals, and usually, they'll contain a combination of eggs, sausage, hot cakes and hash brown potatoes—in excess of 2000 milligrams of sodium and enough calories to supply an average person with enough calories for breakfast and lunch. Depending on your weight goals, eat one breakfast, and you're almost past your total calories for the day. Drive-thru guarantees a private dining experience—but dining while driving is one of the major causes of automobile accidents, in more ways than one.

DEFINITION

Occasional
--*adjective*

1. Occurring or appearing at irregular or infrequent intervals; occurring now and then

---

Fast food is a way of life for many people who insist that they need (and are used to) the convenience. In 2001, I was working as nutrition director for eDiets.com and noted increasing numbers of fast food franchises putting nutrition facts on their websites. Although some franchises offered nutrition information at the point of sale, on menus or on placemats in the restaurants, the Internet meant that consumers could simply click for a comprehensive menu, including all sizes offered and the corresponding calories, fat, protein, fiber, sodium, and even cholesterol per serving! All the nutrition facts were as close as a click of the computer mouse.

Members were asking our nutrition support staff for information about dining out—what to choose instead of the meal listed on their menu. They wanted their menus to change if they were going to eat out—they wanted their shopping lists to change, too. *Here's an idea*, I thought, *let's create the fast food option*. Why couldn't we use the information published on the Web to create hypothetical meals for members—we could show them how to eat fast food and still stay within their calories suggested for their meal plan. We used the published data from a variety of restaurants to create meals at different calorie levels, so that breakfasts, lunches, snacks, and dinners would be similar in calories to the meals in the member's program.

Online franchises help teach you about nutrition. From burgers, chicken, pizza, and subs to donuts, bagels, and coffee, quick serve restaurants' nutritional information is increasingly available and allows the user the ultimate in flexibility. Log on to the "build a meal" or "personalize your meal" page and start modifying your order the way a naturally thin person does. For example, click on a big burger sandwich and unclick the processed American cheese. That saves 50 calories. Then unclick any special sauces, and save another 80-100 calories. Click again to recalculate—and you've eliminated up to 150 calories. Now, if you do visit fast food, just tell the order taker exactly how you want your meal assembled and served.

If you *do* frequent any fast food establishments, log on and take a spin. Most every fast food franchise has nutrition facts and armed with serving size and calories per serving, you are prepared to make better choices.

That said, although most quick service (fast food) restaurants feature website technology and nutrition information, fast casual establishments are slower to follow, and you won't find most fine dining establishments' menus online. There's no national consensus or regulation that requires restaurants to publish nutrition facts.

> Studies confirm that poorer neighborhoods have fewer grocery stores and more fast food franchises, and the unavailability of fresh food is linked to higher risk for obesity. Other studies link consuming fast food frequently to increased risk for obesity—a condition that significantly raises the risk for type 2 diabetes.
>
> **Many years ago, I visited New Orleans and noticed that fast food franchises littered just about every corner. There were also a few convenience stores every few blocks, but I couldn't find one grocery store. Studies have confirmed the association between poorer, urban neighborhoods, the availability of fast food, the lack of grocery stores selling fresh food, and the rate of obesity in the people frequenting fast food restaurants. So, in principle only—since I can afford not to—I don't eat fast food[7,8,9].**

Is driving through faster than parking and walking in?   Not always, and in some neighborhoods, vehicles stack up in lines that wrap around fast food franchises, spilling out onto the street. I think, *Gee...I wonder if these kind people realize the amount of pollution they're causing by idling in line—and wouldn't it be smarter for them to pack a breakfast or lunch? Not to mention all the dollars—and calories—they'd save by skipping the drive-thru.*

Fast food can be a cultural addiction—after all, people are time-challenged, and yes, it's easier to just drive through, have food handed to you through the window, and eat in your car. No one sees you, and in some cities, you don't even have to reach for your wallet—there's actually a speed pass function at some franchises. Fat tastes good—and studies show that salt is an acquired taste. If you're used to all your food tasting salty, naturally unsalted food will taste bland. So what happens when you consume more than a day's worth of sodium in one breakfast sandwich? You're going to be taking in way more than you need over the course of the day—and the next, and the next.

Fast food appeals to people who are traveling—they're in a strange place, traveling from point A to point B, and the last meal was breakfast—five hours ago. But I don't think the solution is to drive-thru—eating with one hand on the wheel. If fast food is the choice, choose to take the time to get out of the car—stretch and breathe. If I'm going on a road trip, I travel with a cooler and a bag of baby carrots, a couple of small cups of yogurt, some fruit and some water.

Personally, I don't think that fast food is a good fit for weight loss and maintenance menus. Healthy eating has become *second nature* for me. I've developed my own convenience menus so that even if I'm busy, I have healthy meal strategies. Fast food's negative environmental impact is something I don't want to contribute to—people eat too much beef and chicken, and both industries tax the environment by producing an inordinate amount of waste. Although some local communities have recycling laws that govern fast food restaurants' container disposal, there are no federal laws or regulations in the U.S. specifically aimed at getting fast food chains to reduce, reuse, or recycle their waste. Even though some chains have gone away from Styrofoam boxes, there's evidence that the replacement containers are little better, in terms of their breakdown in landfills.

Finally, I'd rather beef up my savings by packing my own lunch when I'm working or traveling, and you can do it, too. Leftovers, turkey sandwiches, fruit and yogurt save me dollars I apply toward fitness. Lunch can certainly be quick, but it's almost never fast food.

How Expensive is a Value Meal?

When restaurants bundle menu items and promote them with a discounted price, what's the savings? If you order a small burger, fries, and a coke as a bundled value meal, there's a price to pay—in terms of calories, fat, and health. The food company's strategy is to promote brand loyalty, because consumers think that more is better. For just a couple of cents more, you get a large- or king-sized portion, but where's the value in that? Researchers have determined that "value marketing," or providing more food for less money, is profitable for food companies, but expands waistlines, too[10]. Although the regular size is plenty big enough in calories, fat, and sugar, who can turn down a bargain?

Go online to investigate the price of one of those huge convenience store drinks. They're offering 40 ounces for the price of a 32-ounce drink. Who needs 32 ounces of high fructose corn syrup? Forty ounces has about 600 calories, which represents a third of my entire day's needs. Plus, soda doesn't put a dent in our appetites—but it does add inches to our girth. The more we're offered, the more we eat—no matter if we're hungry or full. As portion size increases, so does our girth[11,12]. A kid's meal at a burger franchise—hamburger, french fries, and chocolate milk—contains more calories than an adult requires. In some communities, the only opportunity for kids to play in a playground is at the fast food franchise.

Studies show that diets high in saturated and trans fat are linked to high "bad" LDL cholesterol, and eating too much trans fat may also lead to lower "healthy" HDL cholesterol. All packaged foods in the U.S. must include ingredient lists--hydrogenated or partially hydrogenated oil means trans fat. Unfortunately, food label rules say that even if the label reads "0 grams" of trans fat, a serving may contain up to 0.5 grams of trans fat, so always read the ingredient list for nutrition information. To improve your diet, avoid deep-fried foods, especially in fast food chains. Some chains have announced that they no longer cook with trans fat or shortening, but have possibly substituted other cooking oils such as palm oil or palm kernel oil, highly saturated fats. The same chains may still include trans fat in other food items. Choose fresh and simple, save fast food for an occasional treat, and read labels.

Here are a few options for fast food dining—this list isn't all-inclusive, but it's a representation of what I do when faced with fast food. I went online to find menus that would give an approximation of calories per meal.

Instead of frequenting fast food, I try to stay prepared by pre-making salads, sandwiches, and healthy trail mix. I stock up on single servings of yogurt and cottage cheese—in a pinch, I will usually stop in a grocery store for single-serve items and fruit.

That said, there are a number of chains that encourage healthy dining—modified orders to eliminate added fat (cheese, mayonnaise) and options for grilled poultry, lean meat, or fish (hold the tartar sauce!).

Fast Food Franchises: Take Charge Get to know the lingo			
Best	**Avoid**	**Instead of**	**Try this**
Grilled, baked, or broiled	Fried, deep-fried, battered, dipped, breaded, crispy, melt, ranch	French fries, onion rings	Baked potato with salsa or small chili; side salad with fat-free dressing
Whole grain roll, wrap, or tortilla	Added cheese, cheese sauce, gravy, sour cream, guacamole, special sauces, mayonnaise	Regular soda, lemonade, sweetened tea	Water, low or nonfat milk, iced tea (unsweetened), diet soda
Small size—even a medium is more like a large; for example, a medium soda at McDonald's or Burger King is 20 ounces	Supersized, large, big, thick, grande, deluxe, ultimate, whopper, monster, loaded, stacked, generous	Double or triple hamburgers, cheeseburger, value meals, double decker	Personalize—make your meal fit your needs—bigger isn't better; broiled burgers; grilled chicken breast or fish; baked potato
Light or Lite, fat-free dressings	Sandwiches on croissants; breakfasts on biscuits	Salads with mayonnaise or topped with *crispy* tortilla strips or croutons; full fat salad dressing; fried fish sandwich; fried chicken	Salads with grilled meat, chicken; fat-free salad dressing

Coffee 'N Donuts

When did coffee become dessert? Today's "chino" drinks are full of sugar and topped with cream, and the flavors are foreign to those who treasure the slightly bitter and decidedly un-sweet flavor of coffee. Coffee is internationally loved but, historically, was consumed as a food, not a drink. In the 11th century, we started to consume the hot brew, and coffee's popularity has increased with each decade. America is the world's largest consumer of coffee, importing 16 to 20 million bags annually (2.5 million pounds), representing more than a third of all coffee exported. More than half of the United States population consumes coffee and typically drinks at least three to four cups of coffee a day. Coffee is the most popular drink worldwide with over 400 billion cups consumed each year[13].

Healthy or Candy?

Coffee can be good for you, as part of a healthy diet. Moderate coffee consumption (two to three brewed cups daily) is fine for the average healthy adult. You can even count moderate coffee servings as part of your daily fluid intake. Studies point toward some health benefits from regular coffee consumption, including a lower rate of Parkinson's disease, colon cancer, and asthma, and there's evidence that coffee's antioxidants are akin to those in red wine. I'll be the first to admit that a morning without coffee is like an engine running without all its spark plugs. It might start up, but it's going to be a very rough go.

Coffee morphed into candy because of the American penchant for sugar and all things sweet. I see too many overweight people with their hands attached to "chino" drinks—*frappuccino, mochaccino, and chocolate-chino.* They're sweetened with flavored high fructose corn syrup and topped with whipped cream. And they sell. Coffee drinks pack on the pounds, no doubt about it.

The good news is that you can choose—choose to gain, or choose to lose. There's no excuse for ignorance, because nutritional info is just a click away for most franchises. If you can't get the nutritional information either online or at the point of sale, use your common sense—any creamy drink topped with whipped cream —coffee, tea or other—is dessert.

Fast Food: Donut Shop

I mistakenly thought I was improving my diet by switching from a donut to a fat-free bran muffin—I was wrong! No wonder I got so jittery after eating—that muffin was more like dessert than breakfast, with 33 grams of sugar (I went online to find the nutrition facts). Reading the ingredient list, I found that the "fat-free" muffin's first ingredient is white flour, and the second ingredient (and therefore, second most by volume) is sugar—so, my muffin was just as bad as a donut—even worse in some cases. What you drink counts too. Instead of a creamy/sugary coffee drink, stick to nonfat milk and a little sugar (16 calories per teaspoon). Log on to a foods database such as www.caloriescount.org and compare menu items. Hot or cold, any coffee drink that says creamy or whipped will be topped with whipped cream, and contain a similar nutrition profile to cookies, cake, and candy.

Old Overweight Fast Food Donut Shop	New Naturally Fast Food Donut Shop
• Raisin-honey bran muffin: 480 calories, 15g fat • Latte, mocha-almond: 290 calories, 10g of fat	• Toasted English muffin: 160 calories, 1.5g fat • Lite vegetable cream cheese, 2 oz: 100 calories, 8g fat Or • Egg and Cheese English Muffin Sandwich • Coffee black
Total Calories Old: 770 calories Total fat Old: 25g	Total Calories New, English muffin with lite cream cheese: 260 calories Total fat New: 9.5g Or Total Calories New, Egg and Cheese English Muffin Sandwich: 280 calories Total fat New: 9g

I've faced down many a donut—especially at the office or at a breakfast meeting. That's why I always come to meetings prepared to deal with the menu—and think about how great my jeans will look, and continue to look great, as long as I don't give in to the donuts. Fried donuts are double-trouble for me. A huge dose of empty refined carbohydrate causes a correspondingly large release of insulin to cover the sugar surge and sets my body up for a reactive low that leaves me feeling jittery—then, I have to eat again! And soon!

No problem: I bring a small yogurt and a cup of cereal, and mix them together when I get to the office. That sets me up for a nice, slow energy release, and I feel great instead of guilty.

Fast Food: Coffee Companies

Besides donut shops, coffee franchises are responsible for making coffee the most popular beverage after water. The good news is that you can go online and click on menu items to see how changing the serving size affects the calories, grams of sugar, and other nutritional facts. If you think tea is a better choice than coffee, make sure it's not a tea blended with cream and topped again with whipped cream—a mistake often made by consumers who think that tea has more health benefits than coffee and don't consider the hundreds of added calories.

If you're in the mood for something sweet and creamy, order a "skinny" cappuccino drink. Skip the whole-milk varieties and opt for nonfat milk. A "skinny" version still features steamed, foamy milk, but for a mere 100 calories—it's a good way to get one of your daily servings of nonfat dairy. If you like, add a packet of sugar (about 20 calories) or the artificial sweetener of your choice.

Old Overweight Coffee (or Tea!) Breakfast	New "Living Thin Naturally" Coffee Breakfast
Large or grande-size coffee with mocha syrup: 600 calories, 15g fat Low fat blueberry muffin: 400 calories, 5g fat	Reduced-fat breakfast sandwich, with low-fat cheese and turkey bacon: 350 calories, 11g fat Skinny (nonfat milk) Latte, tall: 100 calories, 0g fat
Total calories Old: 1000 calories Total fat Old: 20g	Total calories New: 450 calories Total fat New: 11g
A typical work year is 250 days (5 days a week/50 weeks a year). Suppose you spend about $3.50 per day buying coffee—not including any food items you may occasionally order or the $1 tip you may occasionally leave. That's $850 per year. Brew your own coffee for a mere quarter per cup, and put that money into a gym membership or new fitness equipment. Breaking for coffee is an American way of life, but consider your bank account—and how fat it would be if you skipped the stop.	

Fast Food: Burgers and Fries

Descriptive terms like *Jumbo, Whopper, Big, Hearty, Loaded, Stuffed,* or *Deluxe* mean more calories, more fat grams, and more sodium. Before driving-thru, go online—decide before you drive. All the nutrition facts are there—if you dare. I logged on to a variety of fast food websites, and here are some representative meals. As you can see, depending on the franchise, the nutrition facts for similar items change—for example, a medium soda in one restaurant has 200 calories, another has 210. It's similar for fries—one's medium has 380, but another has 420. Do some online sleuthing before driving in. I don't have to worry, because I never order regular soda or french fries—but if you do—!

Craving a burger? Make it a single—plenty of calories for any single person. Think outside the box and order a grilled chicken sandwich (no sauce) and feel the difference—feel *so much* better. I'll go for a baked potato—pass on the cheese, but take added vegetables, salsa, or even chili. Make it second nature to order better:

- Grilled, baked, broiled; not fried

- No mayo—leave off the sauce

- When in doubt, assume that they add mayonnaise or sauce to all sandwiches—so have it your way and be polite, but firm and say "no mayo or sauce, please"

Old Overweight Burgers and Fries	New "Living Thin Naturally" Burgers and Fries
Big burger: 520 calories, 29g fat Medium french fries: 380 calories, 20g fat Medium soda, 21 oz: 210 calories, 0g fat	Grilled chicken wrap sandwich, no cheese: 220 calories, 6g fat Small yogurt and fruit *parfait* (no granola): 130 calories, 2g fat Water
Total calories Old: 1110 Total fat Old: 49g fat	Total calories New: 450 Total fat New: 8g
Old Overweight Burgers and Fries	**New "Living Thin Naturally" Burgers and Fries**
Bigger *burger sandwich*: 670 calories, 39g fat Medium french fries: 360 calories, 20g fat Medium soda: 200 calories, 0g fat	Grilled chicken salad, with fat-free ranch dressing: 240 calories, 9g fat Low fat (1%) milk: 110 calories, 2.5g fat
Total calories Old: 1230 Total fat Old: 59g	Total Calories New: 350 Total fat New: 11.5g

Old Overweight Burgers and Fries	New "Living Thin Naturally" Burgers and Fries
Quarter-pound double cheeseburger with all the fixin's (with mayonnaise, lettuce, tomato, and cheese): 430 calories, 23g fat Medium french fries: 420 calories, 20g fat Small chocolate shake: 330 calories, 8g fat	Grilled chicken sandwich (with lettuce, tomato, mustard, and dill pickles): 280 calories, 4g fat Small yogurt *parfait* (no granola): 140 calories, 1.5g fat Water
Total Calories Old: 1170 Total fat Old: 52g	Total calories New: 430 Total fat New: 5g

Other Options:

- Baked potato: Make a meal of a baked potato and personalize it by adding broccoli and a 3-oz chili: 370 calories, 3g fat

- Salads: Not always the best choice—when they're made with fried chicken or topped with fatty croutons or fried tortilla strips. For example, a salad with croutons and honey mustard dressing has 690 calories and 47.5 grams of fat; some franchises' Asian-style chicken salads have nuts, fried tortilla strips, and full-fat dressings. Trim them down by eliminating nuts and fried tortilla strips, and opt for the fat-free or low fat dressing.

- Kid's Meals: Often have enough calories for adults—no wonder kids are growing so heavy. A few chicken nugget meals allow substitutes; for instance, apple slices with caramel instead of french fries—apple juice instead of chocolate milk. Yes, there are fewer calories in sugar than fat, but why put candy on apples? Apple juice is fructose in water. Milk is a better choice, even 1% chocolate milk.

- Carb Conscious? Some restaurants advertise "low carb" burgers—they just eliminate the bun. No doubt.

Fast Food: Chicken

A close second to burgers and fries, chicken comprises about 20 percent of fast food purchases. Don't spoil a grilled chicken sandwich by adding excess fat calories from mayo and special sauce. Instead, request extra lettuce and tomato and add flavor (without fat) with mustard and ketchup.

Log on to your franchise and check out the nutrition facts for accurate calorie counts on your sandwich.

Old Overweight Fast Food Chicken	New "Living Thin Naturally" Chicken
A regular order of boneless wings with teriyaki sauce, 10 pieces: 1000 calories, 40g fat Small order of coleslaw: 200 calories, 10g fat Medium soda: 180 calories, 0g fat	Grilled chicken salad with fat-free ranch dressing: 250 calories, 8g fat A small piece of steamed corn on the cob: 70 calories, 1.5g fat Water
Total calories Old: 1360 Total fat Old: 50g	Total calories New: 320 Total fat New: 10g

Chicken Choices:

- Skip breaded or fried chicken: Choose grilled, roasted or rotisserie-style chicken.

- Skin the bird: All the fat and cholesterol lies in the skin.

- Skip the sauce and mayonnaise: Order ketchup, mustard, or salsa.

- Portion size counts: Instead of a half- or quarter-bird, order a grilled chicken breast with a side salad and plain baked potato (if available) or unbuttered corn on the cob. (I love salsa on my potato.)

- Skip the high-calorie gravy.

- White breast contains less fat than dark thigh chicken, but as long as the skin is removed, the difference isn't that important.

- Char-grilled and flame-grilled marinated chicken.

- Steamed vegetables and side salads with salsa.

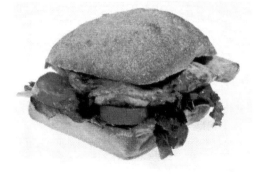

Fast Food: Pizza

All pizza is not created equal! For instance, a fast food chain pizza stuffed with cheese and meat is a recipe for weight gain, but a thin-crusted pizza made with vegetables, some goat cheese or a "light" coating of mozzarella satisfies me without damaging my natural diet.

Log on and, with a click, you can *see* the difference an order makes.

Old Overweight Pizza Order	New "Living Thin Naturally" Pizza Order
6" individual pizza with pepperoni and extra cheese: 700 calories, 34g fat Medium soda: 190 calories	2 slices thin-crust pizza, with extra green pepper, red onion, and diced tomato: 600 calories, 8g fat Water
Total calories Old: 900 Total fat Old: 34g	Total calories New: 600 Total fat New: 8g

In Italy, pizza is often made without any cheese at all, but most American pizza more resembles cheese platforms and are covered with a thick layer of white cheese—did you know that a mere ounce of whole milk mozzarella cheese has about 85 calories and almost 7 grams of fat? To cut down on fat, don't be shy and tell the waiter how you want it. And avoid high-fat, high-calorie meats, such as pepperoni, sausage, and meatballs—they're full of fat and sodium.

My order:

- Share a salad and a personal-size pizza (oil and vinegar or vinaigrette on the side; request "go lightly" on the cheese, please!)

- Opt for thin-crust pizza instead of deep-dish or stuffed crust, which indicates more cheese—more calories.

- Top with all the vegetarian options available: I like onions, mushrooms, peppers, broccoli, tomatoes, and artichokes.

- Vegetarian doesn't necessarily mean low calorie—when loaded with cheese, the pie may have more calories per slice than a meat-topped pizza.

- Three-cheese pizza means three times the calories—goat or feta cheese has fewer calories per ounce than whole-milk mozzarella.

Fast Food: Sandwiches and Subs

I like Subway's ad campaign. It's great to see a real life guy like Jared take control, lose weight, and keep it off. Made-to-order means that you dictate how you want that sub or sandwich assembled, so request extra added lettuce and tomato to beef up your grilled chicken sandwich with extra vegetables and fiber. A new option is "smaller sized" subs. Take advantage of online nutritional information and see what happens when you *don't* add cheese and regular dressing.

Old Overweight sub sandwich	New "Living Thin Naturally" sub sandwich
6" tuna salad sub: 500 calories, 30g fat Bag of baked chips: 130 calories, 1.5g fat Regular soda: 200 calories, 0g fat	6" turkey breast sub (hold the mayo): 280 calories, 4.5g fat Cup of vegetable soup: 80 calories, 1g fat
Total calories Old: 830 Total fat Old: 31.5g	Total calories New: 360 Total fat New: 5.5g
Old Overweight roast beef sandwich	**New "Living Thin Naturally" grilled chicken**
Large roast beef sandwich: 550 calories, 30g fat Medium fries: 400 calories, 25g fat Container of dipping sauce: 200 calories, 20g fat Sweet tea: 120 calories, 0g fat	Grilled chicken sandwich (hold the mayo): 309 calories, 5g fat Water
Total calories Old: 1270 Total fat Old: 75g	Total calories New: 309 calories Total fat New: 5g
Old Overweight hot sub sandwich	**New "Living Thin Naturally" hot sub sandwich**
Turkey and cheddar sub (with cheese and dressing): 500 calories, 13g fat Plus dressing: 400 calories, 45g fat Medium soda: 180 calories, 0g fat	Small turkey and cheddar sub with cheese (no dressing): 310 calories, 8g fat Water: 0 calories
Total calories Old: 1080 Total fat Old: 58g	Total calories New: 310 Total fat New: 8g

Log on to Subway, www.Subway.com for healthy menu options with about 300 calories and 6 grams of fat or less.

At Arby's, www.arbys.com, they've got turkey and roasted chicken besides roast beef—just remove the skin, and hold the gravy and mayonnaise. Improve any sandwich and make it better—choose lean meats and lots of vegetables, and ask the server to scoop out the doughy inside of sub rolls and stuff with lettuce, tomatoes, peppers, onions, and pickles. Quiznos.com has a special page listing options with 500 calories or less. They now offer smaller-sized sandwiches for about 180 calories—when you hold the full-fat cheese and regular dressing. Can you believe that just by removing the dressing on the chicken Caesar salad, you eliminate 440 calories? Stay online!

Fast Food: Chinese-American

Like most ethnic-American cuisines (Mexican- and Italian-American come to mind), traditionally plant-based Chinese cuisine has become almost unrecognizable in American fast food franchises. Either quick-serve or fast casual, most Chinese-American menus feature deep-fried egg rolls and oily combination plates. Often, healthy shrimp, chicken, and tofu lie beneath the coating of batter and fat. Unfortunately, consumers are wooed by the discounted combo plates, but to order smart, order *a la carte*.

Old Overweight Chinese	New "Living Thin Naturally" Chinese
Egg roll: 130 calories, 8g fat Orange Chicken: 500 calories, 27g fat Fried rice, 1 cup: 450 calories, 14g fat Regular soda, 20 oz: 200 calories, 0g fat	Hot and Sour Soup, 12 oz: 110 calories, 3.5g fat Shrimp and vegetables: 150 calories, 5g fat Steamed rice, ½ cup: 160 calories, 1g fat
Total calories Old: 1280 Total fat Old: 49g	Total calories New: 420 Total fat New: 6.5g

- If you are sensitive to MSG, ask the waiter to eliminate it. But you're more likely to gain control by ordering *a la carte* instead of from the combo menu.

- Best options: Steamed chicken, fish, tofu, and vegetables.

- Descriptors such as *crispy* and *sweet and sour* means fried and sugar—more calories.

- Fatty appetizers include egg rolls and spare ribs.

- Seek out Asian restaurants with tofu, bean sprouts, bok choy, broccoli, cabbage, string beans, eggplant, and spinach: All provide fiber, vitamins and minerals.

- For dessert, opt for pineapple or other fresh fruit. And munch on your fortune cookie for about 50 calories and no fat.

- Opt for steamed rice over fried rice: Some restaurants offer brown rice, but make sure the waiter doesn't confuse "brown" with "fried" rice.

- Watch out for sodium, notoriously high in restaurant soups—maybe even more so in Chinese. Wonton, egg drop, and hot and sour soups are your best bets.

- When ordering stir-fried items, stress "light on the oil" or ask the chef to stir-fry your meal in broth.

Fast Food: Mexican-American

OK—you KNOW that the cheesy stuff in fast food restaurants is not real Mexican food—any more than the huge white flour discs covered with white cheese are anything like the thin-crusted pizza of Naples, Italy. The obesity rate in Mexico is soaring—and it's not from eating traditional Mexican fare. Health experts say that Mexicans are eating too much *American* fast food burgers and chicken—and drinking too much soda.

Traditional Mexican food—grilled meats, fish, and shellfish, black beans, rice, and veduras (green vegetables)—is poorly represented by American facsimiles, but it's still possible to get a decent meal—it's your choice.

Old Overweight Mexican	New "Living Thin Naturally" Mexican
Single beef burrito: 500 calories, 18g fat Small guacamole: 70 calories, 5g fat Regular soda: 200 calories, 0g fat	2 grilled chicken soft tacos (hold the cheese and sour cream) with extra lettuce, tomato, and tomato salsa: 200 calories, 8g fat Small guacamole: 70 calories, 5g fat Water
Total calories Old: 770 Total fat Old: 23g	Total calories New: 470 Total fat New: 13g

Living Thin Naturally—

- Choose soft tortillas over hard taco shells.
- Skip the Nachos: Tortilla chips smothered with fatty cheese, sometimes meat and sour cream, too.
- Quesadillas: Usually stuffed tortillas, covered with cheese.
- Refried beans: Usually prepared with lard or other fat—instead, opt for black beans or pinto beans.
- Request "no cheese": An otherwise healthy dish becomes high in calories when smothered with cheese.
- On the Side: Ask for sour cream and guacamole on the side—or not at all.
- Request extra salsa.

Some Mexican-American Developments:

- Chipotle Grill, www.chipotle.com, focuses on fresh and natural ingredients—they've been trans fat-free since 2004. Log on for a PDF with nutritional facts and portion size; put together a meal to suit a naturally thin diet.
- Taco Bell has technology! Point and click to see the difference smart selections can make. Order anything "Fresco Style," and the dish is improved by holding the cheese and sauce. I do that naturally at any fast food restaurant, but Taco Bell has put a cute and catchy name to the order and made it a no-brainer.
- Moe's Southwest Grill features "Southwest flavors with a healthy twist." Online, Moe's has fun technology so diners can see how much healthier the burrito is when you cut the cheese and sour cream. Here's a chain that offers tofu instead of chicken or meat—in just about all their menu items. Fajitas with grilled tofu—I do love it. Order a salad with grilled tofu, lots of veggies, and salsa—with a click, remove the fried tortilla shell, and save 200 calories. Another click—nix the cheese (minus 110 calories)—and then click to add guacamole.

Fast Food: Fish and Seafood

Fish is a smart and healthy food, because it is low in saturated fat and contains heart-healthy omega-3 fatty acids. Healthy, that is, until they bread and batter the fish and toss it into the deep-fryer, then slather it with white sauce—usually mayonnaise-based dressing. Keep fish lean by sticking with grilled, broiled, or baked, but watch out for bread crumbs and butter. Keep an eye on the sides in fast-food chains—best options are steamed or grilled vegetables or a side salad. Request no butter or oil.

Old Overweight Fast Fish Order	New "Living Thin Naturally" Fast Fish Order
Fish sandwich with the works; fried fish with tartar sauce: 550 calories, 28g fat Medium french fries: 300 calories, 20g fat Medium soda: 200 calories, 0g fat	Grilled fish sandwich with extra lettuce, hold the tartar sauce: 420 calories, 19g fat Corn on the cob: 90 calories, 3g fat Water
Total calories Old: 1000 Total fat Old: 48g	Total calories New: 510 Total fat New: 21g

- Nix fried fish: Most of the major chains offer fish sandwiches, but when breaded and fried, they have more calories than a grilled hamburger (without the mayo).

- Hold the Butter! Dipping it into melted butter can ruin any seafood choice. Just a quarter-cup contains more calories (400+) than an entire order of shrimp.

- Hush! Avoid deep-fried hushpuppies—they sound cute, but they're just fried cornmeal batter.

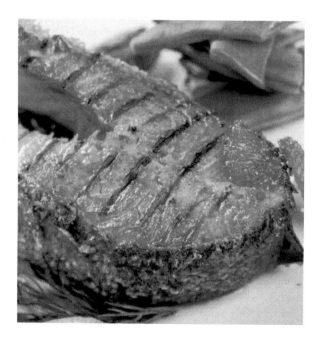

Dining Out: Dessert

Order Dessert First! OK, I got your attention—but hey, most people would think I was kidding if I gave such advice. Well, the point is, are you going out for a meal—or for dessert? I think differently about dining out, and when I dine out, I enjoy my dinner and stay mindful of portion size and calories. Restaurant dining means I'll probably eat more calories than if I'd eaten at home—so, I'd better rethink dessert.

Usually, I'm thinking, *Been there, done that*, and I'll likely be full at the end of the meal. That's better than being stuffed.

That said, dessert is definitely on the menu for a celebratory occasion—or, if I know in advance that they have something I'd love. Of course, it's second nature to not eat dessert daily when you want to stay slim.

Old Overweight Dessert	New "Living Thin Naturally" Dessert
Chocolate cheesecake	A cup of sorbet, or a dessert shared between four
Total calories Old: 700 Total fat Old: 46g	Total calories New: 100-200 for a cup of sorbet or two bites of cake or pie Total fat New: 3-5g

My old overweight eating habit was to eat dessert, but I wasn't paying attention to my stomach. Regardless of how full I was, I'd think about dessert—even as I was eating my appetizer. But now I pay attention to how I feel when I'm eating, and when the waiter offers dessert, I usually decline—I'm plenty full, and think, *is it worth it?* Most of the time, I put restaurant desserts in the "been there, done that" column.

Most restaurant desserts are not worth the calories. I order dinner and eat slowly. Then I stop. I ask myself, how many calories did I consume in the dinner I just ate? Am I full? Is dessert worth it?

Just recently, I ordered dessert—I don't usually. But this time, I had a half-sized salad for an appetizer and an appetizer for my entrée, and when everyone was finished and the waiter came around with the dessert menu, our dining companions said, "Let's share one piece of pie for dessert—it's very special." So that was smart. We ordered tea and coffee, one piece of pie, and four forks. We all had one bite, and my husband had the last, leftover bite.

My favorite treat: Ice Cream!

- There's no need to give all frozen treats the cold shoulder. There's a wide variety of frozen options that fit into a naturally thin lifestyle.

- Soft-serve frozen yogurt is generally available in low fat, fat-free, and sugar-free varieties. Even McDonald's now has a reduced-fat ice cream with just 150 calories and 4.5 grams of fat. A 4-ounce portion is generally 100 to 150 calories.

- Sorbets are a lower calorie, usually fat-free choice. They're also dairy-free—good news for anyone with lactose intolerance.

- Watch out for added toppings—nuts, sprinkles, and chocolate chips add calories: A teaspoon of chocolate syrup has about 100 calories; 2 tablespoons of chopped walnuts, another 100 calories; that means added toppings can easily total more calories than my ice cream.

Healthier Choices

Natural and organic foods' restaurants are a growing segment of the quick casual and take-away market. For instance, New York City is home to *Pret a Manger* restaurants, which feature sandwiches made with naturally grown ingredients—such as avocado and hummus—and freshly-made soups and breads. *Organic to Go* is a new chain of cafes, currently located in California and Washington, that offers certified organic and natural foods. Some grocery stores offer healthfully-prepared foods; many have salad bars—great options for take-away when you're too busy to cook or on the road. Skip the white foods; choose undressed salads, vegetable and bean soups (if sodium is an issue, skip it), small portions of whole grain salads, couscous, and fruit salad.

My Food Made Fast

If you're in the mood for a breakfast sandwich, make your own food—fast. In a quick half-hour each week, create breakfast sandwiches, freeze, and enjoy. Save money! Of course, the nutrition will be better and more reliable when you do it yourself. Modify my recipe by trying different breads and fillings. When you're ready, just microwave on low for a minute or two and go.

Grab 'N Go Egg Muffins

- Package of 6 whole wheat English muffins, split in half. Place each bottom on a square of plastic wrap.

- 1 15-ounce carton of Egg Beaters

- ½ cup *each* chopped onion and fresh green and/or red pepper

- One bottled jalapeno pepper, diced—if like me, you like it hot

- ½ cup low fat cheddar cheese

Assemble Sandwiches

- Cook vegetables over medium heat in a nonstick pan sprayed lightly with cooking spray; add eggbeaters and cook until done (approximately 2 minutes); season with freshly ground black pepper and a dash of salt (optional).

- On each muffin bottom, portion 1/6 of the egg mixture.

- Top with 1/6 of the shredded cheese.

- Top with muffin top, wrap in plastic wrap, and freeze.

- When ready to eat, just heat in the microwave and top with salsa or mustard.

Nutrition per each Egg Sandwich

251 calories, 15 g protein, 10g fat, 2g saturated fat, 783mg sodium, 5g cholesterol

Log On Before Dining Out

Here is a list of websites for some of the popular restaurants I've logged on to. There are many more! And always, if in doubt, log on and check it out.

Additionally, I obtained nutritional information for some individual menu items by logging on to the USDA's food database:

http://www.ars.usda.gov/Services/docs.htm?docid=8964.

U.S. Department of Agriculture, Agricultural Research Service. 2007. USDA National Nutrient Database for Standard Reference, Release 20. Nutrient Data Laboratory Home Page, http://www.ars.usda.gov/ba/bhnrc/ndl

- Applebee's (www.applebees.com): *Quick casual dining with varied menu—click on "Weight Watchers" and you'll see the menu items suggested—with calories and Weight Watchers Points.*

- Arby's (www.arbys.com): *Roast beef and more—has complete nutrition information on all menu items. Has interactive program to personalize menu and modify items by deleting fatty ingredients. Also has printable nutrition facts and ingredient list.*

- Boston Market (www.bostonmarket.com): *Quick serve chicken—has complete nutrition information on all menu items and printable nutrition guide. Provides list of meal combinations; "Entire meal 550 calories or less."*

- Burger King (www.burgerking.com): *Has complete nutrition information on all menu items. Interactive website technology lets user personalize their menu by eliminating high calorie ingredients, such as mayonnaise and special sauce. Click on suggested "Eating Strategies" for detailed nutrition facts for lower-calorie meal options.*

- Chick-fil-A (www.chick-fil-a.com): *Quick serve chicken—has complete nutrition information on all menu items.*

- Carrabba's Italian Grill (www.carrabbas.com): *Italian-American casual dining—suggests diabetic exchanges for specific menu items.*

- Chili's (www.chilis.com): *Quick-casual dining—everything from deep-fried foods to smart salads. Website features printable nutrition guide for all menu items. Huge portions—share an entrée and a salad.*

- Chipotle Grill (www.chipotle.com): *Quick-casual Mexican—has downloadable PDF file with all ingredients; choose your menu to your own tastes.*

- Denny's (www.dennys.com): *Quick casual with varied menu—has printable nutrition guide lists nutrition facts for all menu items.*

- Dunkin' Donuts (www.dunkindonuts.com): *Quick serve donuts, and now breakfast and lunch too—has printable nutrition guide lists nutrition facts for all menu items. Click on each menu item for ingredient list.*

- Einstein Brothers Bagels (www.einsteinbros.com): *Has printable nutrition guide that lists facts for all menu items, and lists all ingredients contained in all menu items.*

- El Pollo Loco (www.elpolloloco.com): *Has complete nutrition information on all menu items; can build a healthy meal by clicking on Healthy Dining link for smart meal recommendations.*

- Jack in the Box (www.jackinthebox.com): *Quick serve hamburgers—has complete nutritional information on all menu items. Build your meal and click to modify ingredients in menu, for healthier meals.*

- Golden Corral (www.goldencorral.com): *American buffet restaurant chain— click for nutrition facts on all menu items. Pay attention to portion size, because it's all too easy to overeat when you serve yourself from huge platters—research shows that the more you're offered, the more you eat.*

- LongHorn Steakhouse (www.longhorn.com): *Steakhouse menu, with description of menu item preparation and occasional portion size description.*

- McDonald's (www.mcdonalds.com): *Complete nutrition information on all menu items. Choose/customize a menu item and modify ingredients: "Meal Suggestions" lists nutritional details for lower calorie menus.*

- Moe's Southwest Grill (www.moes.com): *Quick casual Tex-Mex with complete nutritional information on website—click to add or take away any ingredient(s). No need to recalculate—it's done for you automatically. Makes it fun to modify the order—and informative, too.*

- Olive Garden (www.olivegarden.com): *Italian-American, casual dining—defines a limited number of lower fat options with calories and fat grams per serving.*

- Organic to Go (www.organictogo.com): *West Coast locations—certified organic restaurant features both organic and natural ingredients. All food is 100% natural, without antibiotics, growth hormones, or chemicals.*

- Outback Steakhouse (www.outback.com): *Provides "Healthy Dining" suggestions and "Diabetic Diet" suggestions. Large-sized portions of grilled meat, poultry, and fish—can opt for steamed vegetables and baked potato (or sweet potato) without sauce or added fat.*

- Panda Express (www.pandaexpress.com): *Quick serve Chinese-American—has complete nutritional information for all menu items.*

- Pret a Manger (www.pret.com/us/): *Quick casual and take-away—natural foods; whole grains and some organically grown produce and meat; nutritional info available by clicking on each menu item, and you can also see the price of the item.*

- Romano's Macaroni Grill (**www.macaronigrill.com**): *Quick casual Italian-American fare—huge portions, so take care to share. Kudos to Romano's for providing the nutritional information for all their menu items in printable form. Also offers "Sensible Fare" icon, indicating menu items lower in fat and calories.*

- Quiznos (www.quiznos.com): *Quick serve hot and cold sandwiches—truly inspired online technology shows the consumer all the nutritional options; with a click, you design a naturally thin sub sandwich: See how the calories add up when you add cheese and regular dressing. Think small at Quiznos.*

- Souplantation/Sweet Tomatoes (www.souplantation.com): *Salad buffet—offers lots of healthy options, but portion size counts—remember that when filling your plate. Log on for all the nutritional information for all menu items*

- Starbuck's Coffee (www.starbucks.com): *Quick serve coffee company—enter your zip code, because menus depend on location (and local providers). Printable nutrition and ingredient information for all menu items, including drinks: Can review differences in portion size—click for suggested healthier options; click "make a drink that fits" and learn the lingo that lowers calories/fat/sugar—such as "hold the whip," which will save 130 calories per serving. Twenty drinks under 200 calories.*

- Subway (www.subway.com): *Quick serve subs, soups—has printable nutrition information and ingredients for all menu items; can click on "6 grams of fat or less" tab for list of healthy menu items.*

- SushiFAQ.com (www.sushifaq.com): *Information—Want to know how many calories in an average sushi roll? I did too! This website is chock full of info about Japanese sushi—from preparation to nutritional information to Japanese etiquette—all you need to know with a click of your mouse.*

- Taco Bell (www.tacobell.com): *Quick serve Mexican—has complete nutrition information on all menu items. Kudos to Taco Bell for their sophisticated online nutritional guidance. Point and click, and everything you need to know about healthy dining is at your fingertips. Have fun playing with their nutrition calculator: Build your meal, or just click on Fresco and see what happens when the cheese and sauce are replaced by salsa.*

- Wendy's (www.wendys.com): *Quick serve burgers—great website; personalize each menu item and recalculate total. Easy to read ingredient list leaves nothing to chance.*

- Yum! Brands: *All operate under the Yum! Brand group of quick serve and quick casual dining (a division of PepsiCo). All Yum! Brands websites have complete nutrition information on all menu items. Log on for useful computer technology, and personalize your menus. Practice smart modifications by clicking on the "Nutrition Calculator" and see the calories and fat grams get lower as the cheese, sauce, and mayonnaise are deleted. Click again for an Ingredient Statement that lists all for each menu option; click for an Exchange List planning guide, grouping foods by nutrients and naming amounts.*

  - KFC (Kentucky Fried Chicken): www.kentuckyfriedchicken.com; www.kfc.com

  - Long John Silver's: www.longjohnsilver.com

  - Pizza Hut: www.pizzahut.com

  - Taco Bell: www.tacobell.com

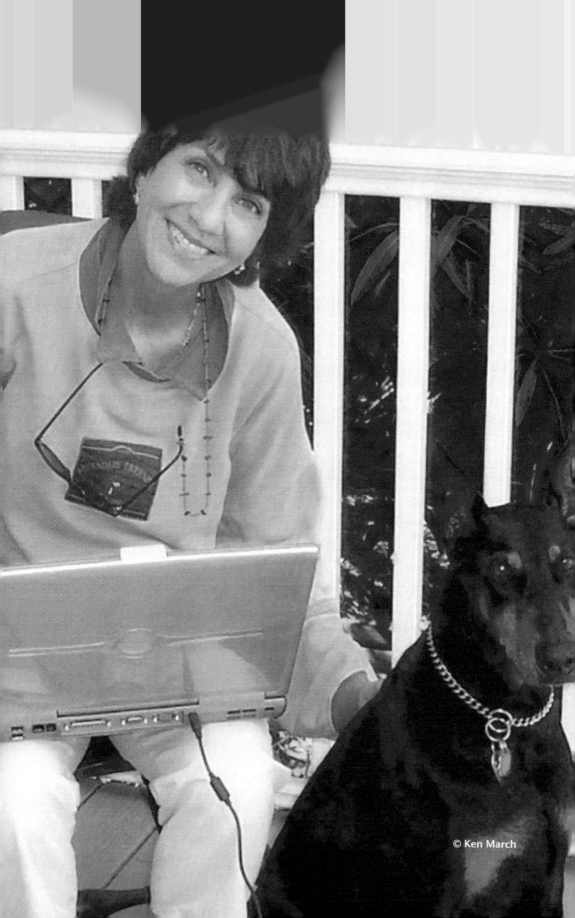

© Ken March

Chapter 10

Help is Here:
Programs and Resources
to Help You Get Started
and Stay Focused

We can do anything we want to do if we stick to it long enough.
—Helen Keller

I must admit it—I'm a news hound. A dietitian I worked with in New York dubbed me "Ms. Informed"; she thought it amusing that she could count on me to know what was going on in the news. I read my New York Times with breakfast. I decided long ago that the "no reading while eating" rule interfered with my natural lifestyle. It's important for dietitians to stay current with scientific news, nutrition knowledge and food safety, and the latest *diet news—a new* program or supplement, for example. We need to comment intelligently when a client says, *does this diet work?*

Nutrition news is often confusing—new science and discoveries constantly lead to new recommendations—and sometimes the news contradicts what's been accepted for a long time. For example, just a few years ago, all fat was grouped together in the narrow top of the USDA Food Guide Pyramid; all carbohydrates formed the base, or largest part of the pyramid. Recommendations for weight loss meant a low fat diet. But today, we know about the health benefits of certain fats, including monounsaturated and omega-3 fatty acids, and recommendations for weight control may skew toward a higher percentage of calories from lean proteins and healthy fats. No longer is a strictly low fat diet the best strategy, especially if your diet is top-heavy with simple, refined carbohydrates. No longer should a healthy diet absolutely require a minimum of 50 percent of calories from carbohydrates. Today's watchword is *customized diet*—for example, some people do better with a higher percentage of calories from protein and healthy fat, and they can adapt their *natural diet* to keep the weight off.

As I learned more about food, I became a better cook; I learned to use technique and ingredients to make food taste good. I learned more about different cooking techniques, cuts of meat, fish, and poultry from *The Joy of Cooking*. I don't use many of the recipes from the book but I think it is a good all-around reference guide. I often read recipes and think, *gee—why did they have to use a whole stick of butter—wouldn't it be better with half?* So, I experiment and reduce fat and sugar, and maybe add more flavors or ingredients, and make them better—just because the fat is there, you don't have to include all of it. Fat makes food taste better, so the challenge is to make it taste better naturally—by using different herbs and spices and cutting back on some ingredients that cooks seem to think is necessary to make it good.

It's not just dietitians who need to stay current—consumers who care should beware. Learn all you can about the food you are eating. The aim of food manufacturers and restaurateurs is to get you to buy—so be a smart consumer and go out to eat armed with as much information as it takes to make healthy choices. Go online to a foods database website, such as the USDA National Nutrient Database http://www.nal.usda.gov/fnic/foodcomp/search/, or go directly to the product or company website. I've called many consumer hotlines when I can't find ingredients or to learn about ingredients listed and can attest to how difficult it is find out the truth behind the labels for some food items.

Weight Loss and Maintenance Programs

As discussed in Chapter 7, what you need to eat to lose weight will certainly be different than what I need to eat—we're not identical. Your body type will be different, and you may be more active—or less active than I am. That's why weight loss isn't usually a straight line to the number on the scale, because as you change your calorie needs change too. As you continue, if you increase your activity you may need *more* calories to fuel your fitness and eating too few calories may stall your weight loss—certainly being hungry will derail a weight loss program quicker than anything I know. Your menu is going to be flexible, customized to your unique likes and dislikes (although please give "old" foods a new try)—and then modified when needed. And remember, a diet is only part of the equation that creates a naturally thin lifestyle. If you think diet means changing your eating style only temporarily, and once you lose weight you can return back to your old style of overeating, then think again. If you return to the way you used to eat—return to the overeating habits that made you overweight—you will return to your old weight, too.

When I talk about fitness, I mean activity. It's not necessary to run miles or do daily aerobics to be active. All weight loss programs should, at the very least, include activity guidelines. Just as a meal plan can reflect your food preferences and your lifestyle, a fitness program may be customized to your current fitness levels and equipment. What works permanently is making smart choices 99% of the time and including activity 100% of the time. Does that sound daunting? Here's a suggestion: wear your pedometer for motivation. I'm not asking for perfection—but weight loss and maintaining your new weight does require consistency. Weight maintenance doesn't happen *naturally*, without effort. Make effort *second nature*—you can do it!

Finally—monitor your progress. If you use a structured workbook program, then paste that calendar on your refrigerator. Write out your goals and graph your progress. If you use an online program, log in and track your goals—track your medical indicators if you need to—it's important. Now that I've maintained my lifestyle for years, I track my weight by wearing my favorite jeans at least once a week. If they get a little snug, the first thing I do is add more activity. A pedometer could be a very important investment in creating a naturally thin lifestyle, and the return on your investment, if you choose to use it consistently, you'll see—it will help you stay on track. If I regain, I'll walk for an additional two thousand steps daily, or about one mile, and will eat an apple as a snack (instead of peanuts and raisins) to create a calorie deficit.

Choose a Weight Management Program

Best Diet for Me (bestdietforme.com): Provides detailed descriptions, expert evaluations, and links to expert-recommended commercial and free weight loss programs, including commercial chains, medically supervised programs, online programs, celebrity and diet bestseller books, health clubs, residential facilities, and more. "The U.S. Weight Loss & Diet Control Market": the ninth edition of this study was published in April, 2007. Take their Diet Quiz for an assessment of what prompts you to overeat—and the best program to address your needs. The website also offers articles and reviews of new trends, diet books, new fads, diet drugs, and more.

Books & Workbooks

1. **"Overcoming Overeating"** and **"When Women Stop Hating Their Bodies"** by Jane R. Hirschmann and Carol H. Munter; Ballentine Books. I think this book helps readers address the emotional aspect of compulsive overeating and eating disorders, such as binge-eating. Go to www.overcomingovereating.com for more information and to buy the books. From the website you can find a local support group, a therapist trained in eating disorders, or join an online support group. Joining a support group helped me give up the preoccupation with dieting.

2. **The Way to Eat,** by David L. Katz and Maura Gonzalez. Naperville, IL: Sourcebooks, 2002. When I saw Dr. Katz recite his soliloquy about polar bears in the Sahara at the Florida Dietetic Association annual meeting in 2002, I became a Katz convert. This book provides a guide to weight management by helping readers identify barriers to healthy eating, and helps readers find ways to eat healthfully in our obesogenic environment.

3. **Active Living Every Day: 20 Weeks to Lifelong Vitality,** by Steven N. Blair, Andrea L. Dunn, Bess H. Marcus, Ruth Ann Carpenter, and Peter E. Jaret. Human Kinetics Publishers, 2001. Experts in diet, fitness, and behavioral change guide you through a 20-week program designed to incorporate healthy behaviors into your life—permanently.

4. **The LEARN Program,** by Kelly Brownell. **The Lifestyle Company (American Health Publishing).** LEARN stands for Lifestyle, Exercise, Attitudes, Relationships, and Nutrition. Start at page one, and with each chapter, you gain a new awareness of unhealthy behaviors—then set goals for better behaviors, learn new skills and strategies for choosing better foods and increasing activity.

5. **The Step Diet Book: Count Steps, Not Calories to Lose Weight and Keep It off Forever,** by James O. Hill, John C. Peters, Bonnie T. Jortberg, and Pamela M. Peeke. Workman Publishing Company, Inc., 2004. This paperback edition comes with your own pedometer. An expert-written lifestyle program to incorporate daily walking and healthy eating into an active lifestyle.

6. **Trim Kids(TM): The Proven 12-Week Plan That Has Helped Thousands of Children Achieve a Healthier Weight**, by Melinda S. Sothern, T. Kristian Von Almen, and Heidi Schumacher. New York: HarperCollins, 2001. Based on a clinically-proven program, this book is written for parents to accurately assess their child's weight, and parents and kids work together through a 12-week program, exploring new ways of eating, plus kid-friendly fitness exercises and behavioral modification strategies.

7. **The Volumetrics Weight-Control Plan: Feel Full on Fewer Calories** By Barbara J. Rolls, PhD, Robert A. Barnett, Harper Paperbacks, 2000. This book provides valuable visuals to show readers that just making different choices from "lower energy-density" food (lower calories), helps you stay satisfied and motivated while you lose weight.

Online Information, Weight Management, and Fitness–Personalized Programs

Log on and join in to lose weight, get fit, and get involved. Online programs help simplify the tracking process—the more you know about your usual lifestyle, the easier it is to pinpoint when you can make changes to improve your choices. Track your food, your activities, your blood pressure, and blood glucose—with just a click of your computer mouse, you can create reports to see how many calories you've burned just doing your everyday activities. You can estimate how many minutes of deliberate activity you need to do to burn that donut; you can create a report that shows you if you're getting enough calcium in your usual diet, and then if you add a cup of nonfat yogurt, see your diet improve! Some programs are free, some are a few dollars a week, and some—with structured lessons and personalized feedback—cost more. Many offer great support systems, ideal for those who don't have a lot of free time and may not have the time or financial ability to meet face-to-face with a coach or trainer.

In the first months after joining eDiets.com, I realized that purchasing an online weight loss plan seemed to be an *impulse buy* for many consumers. With best intentions, they'd sign on for the three-month program, but weren't prepared to do anything differently. Some would log on for a couple of weeks, but many never returned to the website, to get their meal plans and to set up their fitness program. And it's just as if you bought a diet book or joined a gym---you need to work the program, and commit to staying with it.

Are you ready for a "self-help" program? Are you motivated to log on or to follow the written program in the workbook?   But, studies show that participants in programs with *scheduled participation* obtain the best results, and even better results come from personalized, expert feedback and consistent self-monitoring of diet and activities.

The best programs collect your personal information, including your current weight, your current activity, and your goals (lose weight, increase fitness, improve health, for example) and then (if appropriate) should allow you to set a personal first weight goal of about 10 percent of your current weight. A meal plan should consider your current weight and your goal weight, and then display menus or allow you to create your meal plans approximating your calories for gradual weight loss—about one to two pounds per week. Initially, for the first couple of weeks, you may lose more, but the goal is consistency, and changing your current way of eating to one you will maintain permanently.

How to choose an online program depends on a number of factors. Consider if you're ready to change—are you in the *action stage* and looking for resources, such as tracking tools, new recipes, or fitness ideas? Then a self-help program—one that you use to suit your schedule without pre-determined meeting times—may be ideal. Consider your personal needs—will you benefit from structure—regular and personalized email or even phone feedback? Then invest in a program that offers more. Some online programs offer real-time phone support and some offer group meetings, weekly lessons, and personalized feedback. Some websites have very lively and interesting communities—including Web blogs, message boards, online meetings, and podcasts demonstrating how to cook—for beginners or more complicated recipes. Some fitness programs are quite sophisticated and provide animated demonstrations and/or videos demonstrating proper technique. I think you should log on and take a tour---many websites offer a promotional period, or a virtual program tour.

Online Weight Management Programs

- **Calorie Control Council** (www.caloriecontrol.org): A free website with nutrition and exercise tracking tools.

- **Calorie Count Plus** (www.caloriecount.about.com): Good recipe analysis feature—add your own recipe to their database of thousands—just click for instant analysis and to add a single serving to your food log.

- **CalorieKing.com** (www.calorieking.com): The CalorieKing University is a structured, 12-week online lesson program covering nutrition, improving activity, lifestyle, and positive behavioral change. (approximately $55 per year: offers a trial period with a money back guarantee).

- **Diet.com** (www.diet.com): Take a Personality Profile created by obesity expert Dr. Robert Kushner of Northwestern University. The program "pinpoints your styles of eating, coping, and your activity preferences: get your personalized lifestyle modification plan, including meals and activities, and content. From $2.29 wk + $19.95 initiation fee.

- **eDiets.com** (www.eDiets.com): Choose from different diets or meal delivery service: offers real-time phone and email support from registered dietitians and diet techs, diabetes, and fitness experts. Minimum offer: $53.88 for three months. Early termination fee $25.

- **FitDay** (www.fitday.com): A free, easy-to-use and comprehensive foods database and activities calculator.

- **MyPyramid Personal Plan** (www.MyPyramid.gov): A free comprehensive guide to healthy eating—workbooks, trackers, calorie and physical activities calculators, and fun graphics show you how to eat. Use MyPyramidTracker to log your diet and your activities, and graph your progress toward your weight goal.

- **Nutrihand.com** (www.nutrihand.com): Created to help people with diabetes gain blood glucose control by improving diet and activity. Basic service is free, and includes meal and activities trackers and glucose monitoring. Your dietitian or diabetes educator can work with you securely and privately online with this program.

Online Weight Management Programs (cont.)

- **SparkPeople.com** (www.sparkpeople.com): Access free diet and fitness plans, a comprehensive array of e-tools, reminder emails, recipes database—enter your own recipes and instantly see how modifying them improves nutrition. Has a vibrant online support peer community

- **Slim·Fast.com** (www.slim-fast.com): A good example of a commercial plan with menu flexibility: include Slim-Fast products in your meal plan or switch out products—free tools, support and information.

- **Jenny Craig** (www.jennycraig.com): Jenny Craig online or off-line includes a plan for diet, fitness, and behavioral modification. Online e-Tools and recipes are free: face-to-face service costs $20 plus the cost of food.

- **VTrim—University of Vermont Weight Management Program** (www.uvm.edu/~vtrim) Designed to recreate the "look and feel" of a face-to-face group meeting: each week receive personalized feedback and meet weekly online with your expert team facilitator; complete weekly lessons and build healthy behaviors for permanent weight loss. Costs $595 for six months (offers maintenance program).

- **WebMD Weight Loss Clinic** (www.diet.webmd.com): Complete comprehensive eating analysis, and see your personal evaluation and 21 key recommendations for change. Menus reflect your usual eating patterns and foods, with modifications for weight loss. Fitness and community included. Costs $21.62 per month.

- **Weight Watchers Online** (www.WeightWatchers.com): Weight Watchers online offers same diet program options plus comprehensive web tools. Online costs $65 for the first three months and then $16.95 per month.

- **Pharmaceutical-sponsored programs** to help people with diabetes manage weight with healthy menus and activities: Free guidance for people with diabetes:

    - **ChangingDiabetes-us.com (from NovoNordisk)**: www.changingdiabetes-us.com

    - **Diabetes Control for Life from Abbot Labs (Glucerna.com)**: www.diabetescontrolforlife.com.

Exercise & Activity

Personal Trainers—go online to find a credentialed personal trainer:

- American College of Sports Medicine: **www.acsm.org**
- American Council on Exercise: **www.acefitness.org**
- National Strength and Conditioning Association: **www.nsca-lift.org**

Walking Online: When you're walking, you're getting fit and burning calories. Experts say to take 6,000 to 10,000 steps daily for weight loss and maintenance, depending on your current weight and goals.

- **America On the Move** (www.americaonthemove.org): Join as an individual or as a group with your office friends or family. Log on for a personalized plan, plus log your daily steps on a route of your choice. My route is The Colorado Trail, but yours could be the China Silk Road or the Iditarod! A lot of fun, and it keeps you coming back. You can also learn a lot about food, nutrition, exercise, etc.

- **America's Walking** (www.pbs.org/americaswalking/index.html): Connecticut Public Television produces this television series. Log on, view the motivational series on the Web, and then read all the info and recommendations; get a walking plan.

- **About.com** (www.About.com/walking): In addition to expert information on almost every topic imaginable, About.com has a free, personal walking program. Log in your current fitness level, and you receive a walking program detailing how to step daily, plus a free, online log to post your progress. Lots of great calculators and assessment tools.

Nutrition News—Stay In the Know

Vitamins and Minerals: How do you know if that vitamin you just bought really contains 100 milligrams of vitamin C? You don't—unless the manufacturer performs valid laboratory testing and analysis of their finished product. Since 1994, the U.S. government has exerted little oversight over the manufacturing and merchandising of vitamins, minerals, amino acids, herbal preparations, or other such combinations of products. Historically, the Food and Drug Administration (FDA) has only taken action to remove a dietary supplement if a problem arises—for example, if people are getting sick. The FDA's newly expanded Good Manufacturing Practices (GMPs) take full effect on June 25, 2009. The new ruling requires manufacturers of all dietary supplements to perform at least one scientifically valid test on final products to ensure they conform to packaging claims.

The average consumer actually knows fairly little about dietary supplements. Because there is no official agency which currently confirms the purity or potency of dietary supplements, consumers should use products with independent testing until tighter regulations are in place. Examples of such agencies include:

- ConsumerLab.com (www.consumerlab.com) Brands that pass Product Reviews or the Voluntary Certification Program are posted on CL's Web site as having "passed" the specific test performed. If the product passes, the manufacturer may then purchase a license to use the CL Seal of Approval.

- United States Pharmacopeia (USP) (www.usp.org): An independent testing agency. If product passes ingredient and product integrity, purity and potency tests, then the manufacturer may display USP Verified Dietary Supplement mark on their product labels.

- NSF Dietary Supplement Certification program (www.nsf.org): The NSF mark means the product has undergone third-party testing for identity, purity, quality, and consistency.

My Regular References

I subscribe to a certain number of print and online publications. Knowing what's behind the label—and what's coming down the pike, in terms of research on unique foods—makes the difference between just living and living smart.

Print

Just about everything I read is available online, but sometimes it's nice to have the printed page—especially when I'm reading in bed!

- **The New York Times:** Some of the best health and lifestyle columnists around—read it online **www.nytimes.com**

- **Nutrition Action Newsletter**, published by The Center for Science in the Public Interest (CSPI) (**www.cspinet.org**): A non-profit consumer advocacy organization whose twin missions are to conduct innovative research and advocacy programs in health and nutrition, and to provide consumers with current, useful information about their health and well-being.

- **Tufts Health and Nutrition Letter** (**www.healthletter.tufts.edu**): An independent, expertly-written health and nutrition newsletter from the faculty of Tufts University.

- **Environmental Nutrition** (**www.environmentalnutrition.com**): Founded in 1977, this independent monthly newsletter (no advertisements) is edited by registered dietitians and other nutrition experts—I look to it for reliable and timely information on food and nutrition.

Online News and Information Resources:

I just typed "nutrition" into my Web browser and instantly see 182 million websites. So where to start? Here are just a few of the websites I reference often:

- **ADA Knowledge Center:** American Dietetic Association Daily News (**www. eatright.org/dailynews**):   ADA members can register and have the latest information on food, nutrition, and health sent directly to their inbox. Non-members can visit the site daily for the daily issue. If you are currently working in the dietetics field or plan to become a nutrition professional, the ADA invites you to join—there are lots of benefits to membership, such as seminars, certifications, and professional networking.

- **Food and Nutrition Information Center** (**www.nal.usda.gov/fnic**): From this United States Department of Agriculture website, you can browse by subject, ranging from Dietary Guidance to Dietary Supplements, and be connected to a free reference library. I can't say enough about this website—it is chock full of information on food, fitness, and general health information. Find articles, books, magazines, and research studies—it's just a click away, and I use it often when I'm writing articles and need credible references.

- **National Restaurant Association:** Link to their free industry newsletter, SmartBrief, at **www.restaurant.org**. I keep up with the trends and new products and services in the U.S. and abroad. Of course, I take their opinions with a grain of salt—the restaurant industry has an agenda that is sometimes in conflict with my personal philosophy of staying thin naturally. But it's important to stay current, because it's what you don't know that can hurt you—and knowledge is power.

- **Nutrition.gov** is a service of the National Agricultural Library and provides links to tons of info about nutrition, healthy eating, physical activity, and food safety for consumers.

- **Oldways Preservation Trust** (**www.oldwayspt.org**):   A nonprofit food issues advocacy group—these are the guys who invented the Mediterranean Food Guide Pyramid and many more ethnic food pyramids, which are fun to reference. Log on for easy-to-understand info about health and just plain enjoying good food.

- **Shape Up America** (**www.shapeup.org**):   A nonprofit organization committed to raising awareness of obesity as a health issue and to providing responsible information on healthy weight management.

- **WIN—the Weight-control Information Network** from the U.S. Department of Health and Human Resources (**www.win.niddk.nih.gov**): Provides science-based information on weight control, obesity, physical activity, and related nutritional issues.

Cooking & Recipes

I have a repertoire of favorites and often create meals from what's fresh at the farmer's market or on sale at the grocery store. Practice, practice—and keep it simple; grilled vegetables and fish; beans and legumes; salads and my pizza are my favorites.

Print:

- **Joy of Cooking**, by Irma S. Rombauer and Marion Rombauer Becker. Scribner, 1985.

- **1,001 Low-Fat Recipes:** Quick, Easy, Great-Tasting Recipes for the Whole Family (1,001), 2nd edition, by Sue Spitler and Linda R. Yoakam. Surrey Books, 1998.

- **Cook's Illustrated:** www.cooksillustrated.com The print version contains no advertising, lots of great pictures and illustrations—a lot of great information about food and wine, and not necessarily "low fat" cooking, but I modify the recipes!

- **American Diabetes Association's Diabetes Forecast**: http://www.diabetes.org/diabetes-forecast.jsp

Online:

- **Online recipes:** Simply type "healthy recipes" into your Web browser. The best ones allow you to search by low calorie, ingredient, nutrient, or even calories per serving.

  o Startcooking.com with Kathy Maister: How to Measure Food www.startcooking.com

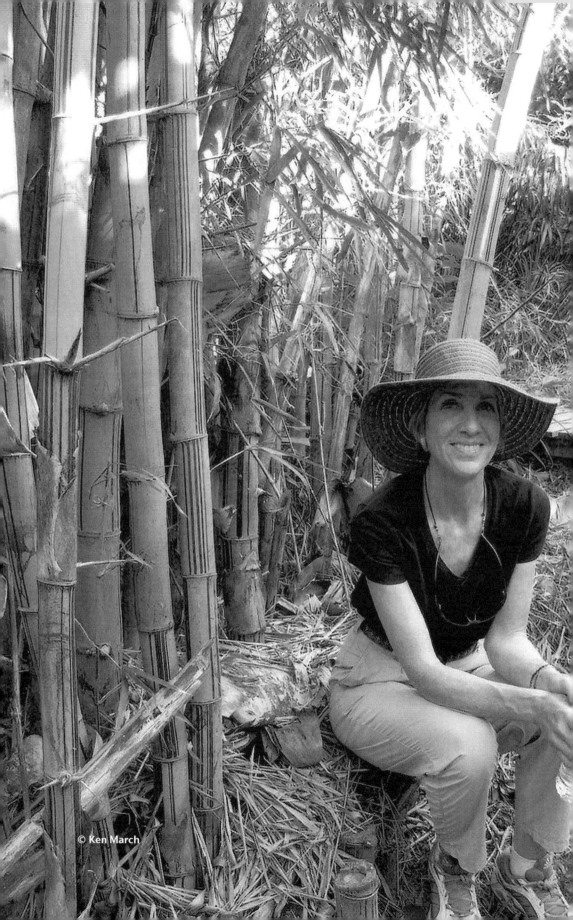

Chapter 11

Now You!
Your Second Nature You

You have to have confidence in your ability,
and then be tough enough to follow through.
—Rosalynn Smith Carter

M y rebellious nature has proven successful for me. I challenge the new *normal* and I reject the eat-all-you-can mentality. I have overcome equating food with comfort or love.

I love food—I love to eat and I like to cook, but I have rebelled against the foods that made me fat—especially fatty, fried foods, refined white flour products, and huge portions. I don't customarily overeat, and I try to do deliberate activity every day. These second nature behaviors reinforce my ability to maintain my weight.

It didn't happen overnight—at the beginning, it was tough to break my habit of using food to deal with stress, because I didn't realize that I had to *replace* that old behavior with *naturally thin* new ones. It took me about six months to not feel anxious about food, and probably a good year to make the habits normal. It was not a straight line to today—I regained almost ten pounds in my late 30s but I rebounded, and went back to eating simply, increased my exercise, and maintained my fitness. The regain reinforced what I knew—and what I had conveniently ignored—until I tried on those pair of favorite jeans, which suddenly didn't fit. I had been overeating and under-exercising, but since I wasn't monitoring my weight, it was easier to ignore the weight gain.

DEFINITION

Rebel

-noun

   1. Someone who exhibits great independence in thought and action
      (synonym: maverick)

-verb

   1. Take part in a rebellion; renounce a former allegiance

   2. Break with established customs

Monitoring your weight and facing your body changes helps you focus on good behaviors. Once I put those jeans in the front of my closet and saw them on a daily basis, they helped me remember to eat well and stay active.

See, I don't obsess about my weight, which is just a number on the scale and does not indicate fitness. A scale can be motivational, especially at the beginning of a weight loss program, because it is easy to "see" and graph progress toward a weight goal. But weight is just part of the picture---to be *naturally thin* is reflected in the way you feel, how much energy you maintain, how you feel about what you're eating, how your clothes fit, and the way your muscles feel.

Yes, certain medical conditions and medications may make it hard to lose weight— some may cause you to easily *gain* weight. Many women will attest to the frustration that is menopause, when you may feel like you're doing everything right, but still feel bloated and unfairly getting nowhere. But eating well, staying active, and reducing stress helps you feel better; and building lean muscle makes you feel great.

There's plenty of evidence that weight isn't the only indicator of health, and you can definitely be healthy even if your weight isn't within the normal BMI. You may be "underweight" and be small-boned and very lean, with a low 18.0 range. You may be heavy-boned and muscular with a BMI over 25, and still be healthy. Underweight has problems all its own. If you're eating fewer calories than you need to maintain your fitness, you'll undo all the work you did to achieve "thin." Insufficient nutrition means low energy, possible vitamin and mineral deficiency, lowered immunity, and possible muscle loss.

When I was overweight and out of control about overeating, there was no critical health issue that motivated me to change. My blood pressure was normal, my cholesterol was normal, and my blood glucose was normal. There is no type 2 diabetes in my immediate family, and I realized I resembled my father, who lived with obesity for years without any symptoms.

But he was miserable. He constantly complained about being overweight, he went on diets, he even used to question, "Why can't I lose weight?" And just like him, I didn't like what I saw, but I rebelled against the norm that was my family history, and decided to take control. I did enough research to realize that I was using food to hide from the challenge of eating differently. I used food to distract myself from the problem at hand—that managing my weight would take work and deliberate, conscious decisions every day.

I finally learned why I was blessed with such a rebellious nature—and made it work for me. I rejected my natural tendencies to overeat and under-exercise. And I continue to reinforce this revolutionary way of living by practicing every day. What long ago was a structured plan turned into daily choices that have now become second nature.

It is natural—when exposed to huge portions of tasty food—to eat more of it. It is natural that if we have labor-saving devices, we use them. But what is human nature winds up conspiring against our best interests, and eating more means weight gain— and moving less means more weight gain.

Thus, being naturally thin is a myth for most—it's certainly more natural to be overweight in our current environment. Rebel against the status quo, and don't let others make decisions for you. Invite your family, your friends, and your peers to join you. Read package labels back to front—ingredients first, and don't be fooled by advertising. Reject the message that unhealthy foods are sexy or fun. Rebel against products that purport to give you energy—wait until you experience the energy that comes from staying fit!

There is a big difference between thin and fit. You can be too thin, but you can never be too fit. This is how I think about my weight. Thin is a reflection of the work I put into being fit. I feel best when I eat enough calories to maintain energy, strength, and muscle.

Take the challenge and break with the established customs that make overweight so easy and fitness hard to achieve. Make deliberate food choices, and treat your body as your life machine—you need to take care of it so it will get you where you want to go, and that means moving every day. Start by examining what your *usual* diet is—and pinpoint the changes that will make it better. Monitor your weight or waist, and track your progress. Adopt your second nature behaviors, and stay thin naturally.

When I get up, I think about the end of the day and how good I'll feel by staying in control and making healthy choices. Weight control happens: One meal, one snack, one day at a time.

I Practice What I Preach

I gain weight as easily as anyone else. So the reason I weigh roughly what I did when I graduated from high school is not good luck—it's because I practice what I preach!

I work out every day for at least 40 minutes. I often hear from people that they don't have the time to exercise. My feeling is I don't have the time NOT to. Exercise keeps me energetic, motivated, and, therefore, more productive. I invest an hour a day in exercise, and get back hours, days, weeks, and years of energetic productivity in return. I consider the return on investment highly favorable.

Eating well is equally important, but a bit more complicated. I can eat well because I know how, in spite of the challenges of the modern food supply. I do all I can to share my knowledge so that others have comparable "skill power" for practicing good nutrition. Skill power is essential, because it provides the way.

But it does not provide the will, and that, too, is important. Wanting to eat well and not knowing how is frustrating. Knowing how and not bothering is a wasted opportunity! Food is the fuel that powers up the human body; a high performance body—thin or otherwise—requires high performance fuel. I think everyone should care passionately about the quality of fuel they put into themselves, not to mention their kids.

Being thin or healthy is mostly about what you know, and how you put that knowledge to work. There is some luck involved, of course, but we can greatly influence the probability of health outcomes, good or bad, by the choices we make. The choices I make every day are designed to tip the odds in my favor.

David L. Katz MD, MPH, FACPM, FACP,
director of the Yale Prevention Research Center, and author of
The Way to Eat: A Six-Step Path to Lifelong Weight Control
(2002, Sourcebooks, Inc)

Top Habits of Permanent Weight Maintainers

The National Weight Control Registry (www.nwcr.ws/Research) studies successful weight maintainers (on average, participants have lost 60 pounds and kept it off for five years).

- Although some have lost the weight on their own, more use a structured program, and having a support system is valuable.

- Most modified their diet and added daily physical activity to lose weight.

- Successful maintainers average about an hour of activity daily, and walking is one of the most popular forms of exercise.

- Most maintain their weight by making smart choices and monitoring their portions. Most cut calories by limiting fried foods and sweets.

- Almost all successful weight maintainers eat breakfast.

- Most monitor their weight, and if they regain, they go back to what worked to lose the weight immediately.

- They turned off the tube! Most watch less than 10 hours a week.

- They like their lifestyle and don't think of it as a diet.

- And best of all, the longer you do it, the better it gets; the more you enjoy your new food choices and your strong body, the more it becomes second nature.

Chapter 12

84 Tips
for Living Thin Naturally:
Living, Eating, Moving

Happiness is not a station you arrive at, but a manner of traveling.
—Margaret B. Runbeck

Living Tips

1. Get Ready: If you are ready for action, then go for it! If you aren't ready for a lifestyle makeover, then get your calendar and mark down one action item each week for the next four weeks. For instance, eat a salad with dinner, drink fewer sodas (or wine, coffee, etc.) daily, walk for 20 minutes (or more) three times a week, or do leg lifts while watching television.

2. Get Help: Support is what allowed me to adopt naturally thin habits. Connect with either an individual or group—keep it consistent, especially for the first six months to one year. It works.

3. All Diets Work: But the only diet that works permanently is **your** diet. You can go on any diet to lose weight, but keeping it off takes permanent change.

4. Get Smart: Use the American Dietetic Association's MyPyramid.gov or other calorie-counting tool or book, and get smart about how much you're usually eating by simply logging your usual diet for a week. The more you know, the easier it is to make good choices.

5. Neutral: Food is not bad or good. Food doesn't have human qualities. Food is either healthy, fatty, high in fiber, or high in calories. You choose—you have the power to say yes or no, based on your goals.

6. Make Your Body Your Hobby: Consider *you* your hobby, and invest resources in improving it.

7. De-Stress: Stress can be fattening! Studies show that chronic stress wreaks havoc on your health, including promoting weight gain. Take time to relax and get enough sleep.

8. Don't Weight! Aim for fat loss, not weight loss. And replace fat with lean muscle—so you can keep the weight off more easily.

9. Get Measured: Measure your progress in two ways—a scale is a real simple way of clicking off the numbers, especially at the start. But stay focused on physique—measure inches, waist size, or dress or pants size.

10. Lifetime Guide: Adopt a new anti-diet attitude. Let the new diet and exercise plan that you used to lose weight be your guide to permanent weight maintenance.

11. Get Real: Instead of setting an intimidating, unrealistic goal, such as "I will lose 20 pounds by Christmas," set small, achievable goals, such as, "Within four weeks by sticking to my diet and exercise plan, I expect to lose between two and five pounds."

12. One-Step Substitutions: New *steps* mean smart substitutions—not eliminations. *Switch* from whole milk to reduced fat for one week, then to nonfat the next. *Stop* adding fat, and instead, add more flavor with new herbs and spices.

13. Just the Facts, Please: Read the package from back to front, and ignore the manufacturer's claims. Just because there's a picture of fruit on the package doesn't mean there is fruit in the product. Some examples of this misleading packaging are fruit roll-ups, fruit juice drinks, and fruit-flavored cereals.

14. Keep it Simple: The shorter the ingredient list, the more natural the product. Compare breakfast cereal labels—you'll be surprised at the number of unnatural additives, preservatives, flavors, and colors in cereals that picture whole grains on the front of the box.

15. Prepare to Succeed—Part 1: Write down your menu for the week, which takes all the guesswork out of weight management. Include any meals you plan to eat out—write down what you plan to eat at the restaurant, too.

16. Prepare to Succeed—Part 2: Go shopping! Create a shopping list with your meal plan, having all your foods for the week when you shop takes the guesswork out of healthy eating.

17. Your Story: The change happens when you write it down. Each evening, work on tomorrow's story by writing in your journal. Then, make a record and log what you did today—your food, activities, and feelings. Create scenarios to overcome any obstacles.

18. I *Can*, I *Will*, I *Must*: Create your own affirmations—sayings that you repeat often, that are positive and strengthen your resolve, and that keep you reminded of your progress. I put mine on my bathroom mirror, my car dashboard, and my refrigerator!

19. Exercise Your Will: Physical exercise is critical, but so is mental strength—to say "no" to all the temptations around you. As with any exercise, you become more proficient as you practice.

20. Eat to Live: Instead of living to eat. Do you have a favorite food that doesn't fit into your weight loss plan? Modify, improve, and lose. For instance, if you find it difficult to say "no" to pizza, make it fit by eating one slice and a big salad, instead of three slices.

21. My Request Rule: I politely tell my server how I'd like it prepared. "On the side, please," for sauces, gravies, and salad dressing is essential when dining out.

22. Learn the Code for Calories: "Crunchy" restaurant food usually means deep-fried; "crispy" cereals usually mean added sugar.

23. Read Labels: Read *Serving Size* first, since the first line on the Nutrition Facts label sets the stage for calories. The calories listed represent only one serving. Soda is a great example: A 20-ounce bottle has 2.5 servings—if you finish the bottle, you take in almost 500 calories.

24. My Weight Loss Mantra: When tempted by something I know I like—but that I don't need, especially after a satisfying meal, I think, "so it tastes great—been there, done that".

25. Explore: I've gotten into a habit of exploring every new neighborhood I visit. I get up early, walk around during lunch, try to see my surroundings, and expand my horizons while getting some exercise.

26. Portion distortion: Most people underestimate their daily caloric intake. Break out the food diary, and don't be afraid to write everything down. Make adjustments, if necessary, based on your meal plan.

27. Slow it down: Eating too fast usually means eating more than you need. Give your brain time to catch up with your stomach. It takes about 20 minutes to feel the food, so savor your food—when you enjoy it more, you'll be satisfied with less.

28. Energy: Health experts warn that overweight and obesity increase your risk for heart disease, type 2 diabetes, and stroke, but there's also the toll excess weight has on your energy. Overweight not only makes you feel sluggish, but it's hard on your joints, muscles and tendons.

29. Practice saying "No, thank you": You have the choice to eat it—or not. You're not obligated just because you're offered.

30. Full Stop: Resign from the "Clean Plate Club," because you don't have to finish if you're full. Take the rest for a snack or meal the next day.

31. R & R: The average person requires 7.2 hours of sleep to feel rested. There are exceptions—Bill Clinton needs only four to five hours, but Albert Einstein needed about 10 hours. There is something to be said for dreaming! Too little sleep may increase stress and overweight. Whatever you need...be sure to get it.

32. Hydrate Often: Fluids are necessary to process foods, absorb nutrients, regulate your body temperature, and eliminate waste. Water is a good habit to learn. Instead of a can of soda, reach for a glass of water.

33. Save and Spend: Instead of spending your hard earned cash on overpriced (and potentially high calorie) coffee drinks, take the money you save and buy a new pair of high quality athletic shoes.

34. Leave a Little: Some have success by always leaving something behind—a psychological strategy to lower calories while still indulging.

35. Thank YOU: Reward yourself for a job well done. When you reach each goal, enjoy your just reward—make it support your lifestyle, like a new workout outfit or athletic shoes or a massage—because you deserve it!

Activity Tips

36. Move: If you're lethargic, it could be because you're not active. Feeling sluggish? Breathe. Your body needs oxygen; you'll be amazed at how energetic you'll feel by doing some deep breathing exercises. Stretch: Roll your shoulders, tense your muscles, and then relax; this will increase blood flow and energize you immediately. Increase your heart rate by fast walking, dancing, or even stepping in place—instant energy.

37. Your Buddy: Walking is more fun with someone—or something, like a dog! A buddy motivates you to go longer. If no friend is available, use your personal stereo to listen to your favorite tunes or talk show.

38. Anatomy is <u>not</u> destiny: Even if your mother, father, and siblings are overweight, you can outsmart your genes with a healthy diet and exercise. Light weight training will slim your body—a toned torso displays clothes better.

39. Build muscle: Replace fat stores with lean muscle and improve your fat-burning naturally. Start gradually and work up to at least three days a week of training with resistance bands and light weights. Consult with your doctor if you've not worked out before.

40. Salsa: Dance the salsa, feel sexy, and be beautiful! Oh, don't you just love those shows where celebrities dance with professional dancers? They work it!

41. Sit On a Ball: I alternate sitting on a balance ball with sitting in an ergonomic chair in front of my computer. Wear sneakers and change positions about every 20 minutes.

42. Your Lifestyle: Instead of paying someone else to wash your car or clean your house, make household chores aerobic. Put the money saved doing it yourself toward a new bathing suit (and burn calories too!)

43. Breathe: Go for a walk—a brisk walk, for just 15 minutes, twice a day, and deliberately breathe deeply. It's not hard—it takes commitment, but in a month, there goes a pound!

44. Television: Instead of sitting for hours in front of the television, get on your exercise bike and pedal. Each time a commercial comes on, pedal! Put the treadmill—or your balance ball and bands—in front of the TV. Burn about 200 calories per hour of viewing and do it at least five evenings per week during your favorite program. You can burn enough calories to see the scale drop five or more pounds in a month.

Eating Tips

45. Calories versus Portions: Although calories count, focus on counting portions instead. Know the approximate number of portions you need daily, and mentally tally how you eat.

46. Eat: Don't eat too little! Poor nutrition decreases energy and can depress immunity. Too few calories can play havoc with your metabolism. Lose weight in a healthy way, with a balanced meal plan and sufficient calories to fuel your engine.

47. Break the fast: Start your day with breakfast. Studies show that those who eat breakfast have more energy for the rest of the day. People who skip breakfast are not as alert, not as productive, and tend to be more overweight compared to people who do eat breakfast.

48. Start Smart: Studies point to healthy-type cereal eaters as the most successful weight-maintainers. Eat a non-sweet or just slightly sweetened cereal (maximum four to six grams of sugar per serving) every morning for breakfast. My boxed favorites include Kashi GoLean and the wheat 'n bran version of spoon-sized shredded wheat. Just switch from your usual sweetened raisin bran cereal to bran flakes and add your own naturally sweet raisins (two tablespoons). Switch from 2% to 1% milk, or nonfat, and reduce the calories in your usual breakfast enough to lose a pound per month.

49. New Breakfast: Don't like breakfast foods? Try a sandwich—make it a lean one, such as turkey on whole wheat bread. A fruit smoothie made with yogurt and fruit is delicious and balanced. Choose 1% or fat-free; low or no-sugar yogurts.

50. A Hot Start: Instead of instant oatmeal or even quick oats, hot whole oatmeal packs more energy with a lower glycemic impact. Simply microwave a half-cup of oats with one cup of water for approximately two minutes.

51. Lighten' Up: What you add to coffee and tea can easily tip over your diet. Two tablespoons of half-and-half have about 50 calories—I drink my coffee black and save my calories for frozen yogurt.

52. Bring Lunch: Buying lunch everyday is a budget buster, and it's more difficult to control your calories. Save money by bringing healthy lunch and snacks to work or school, and put the money toward a reward that enhances your health, such as a new bike or a gym membership.

53. Light Dinner: Have a satisfying salad for dinner. Add a drained 3.5 oz. can of wild salmon to a bowl of mixed greens. Add a cup each of chopped tomato, onion, cucumber, broccoli, shredded carrots, and any other crunchy vegetable you like.

54. Portion Control: Today's "mega" plates make average-sized portions look smaller. I serve everything on salad plates, which helps avoid portion distortion.

55. Better Brew: Although a cup or two of coffee can perk you up in the morning, lower your caffeine dose by switching to decaf in the afternoon. Or have tea, which has less caffeine. Both green and black teas contain antioxidants, but to avoid caffeine, choose decaffeinated.

56. Plate-portion: Practice portion control by using measuring cups to learn what a cup of cereal or rice or fruit looks like; use measuring spoons to visually define a tablespoon of hummus or nuts or mayonnaise; use a scale to define what a cooked serving of meat or fish looks like; then you can take your *natural diet* with you everywhere.

57. Drink to Your Health: A glass of wine with dinner may have health benefits but alcohol has calories, so if you drink, men—limit to two; women—stay with one. Exceptions to wine include pregnant women or if your doctor advises you to abstain.

58. Whole Grains: Have more nutrition, taste, fiber, and make you fuller. Read the nutrition panel on the package—the first ingredient should be "whole wheat" or other whole grain. "Wheat" or enriched flour doesn't make it whole wheat.

59. Veggie Power: Snack on quick and easy (and nutritious) vegetables. Eat crunchy veggies—they're full of fiber and have only 25 calories per whole cup.

60. Green snacks: If I'm hungry and don't want to add too many calories to my day, I microwave three cups of frozen, crunchy veggies (broccoli, squash, or okra are my favorites). Sprinkle with some herbal seasonings or dehydrated butter flakes.

61. Don't Whiten Foods: Avoid "white," prepared salads, dips, and casseroles full of mayonnaise, cream cheese, and sour cream.

62. Switch to Whole: Whole grains, unpeeled fruit, and lots of salads and vegetables contain fiber that helps you maintain your weight, and unprocessed foods taste better, too.

63. Make it Easy: Eat fresh but conveniently by stocking bags of pre-washed and cut vegetables and salad greens. Toss with grilled chicken strips or a can of salmon for a quick, filling, tasty, and nutritious dinner.

64. Sweet Promise: Swear off all sweetened bottled beverages forever. Soda, sweetened teas, and bottled juice drinks add hundreds of empty calories, and consumption is linked to increased rates of obesity. Even sports drinks are mainly quick calories—best for long-distance and extreme exercise. If you usually drink regular soda...Stop! Lose more than two pounds in just one month without trying (estimating about 10 cans per week). One 12-ounce can of soda has 150-170 calories...and no nutrition. Have ice cold water or a can of diet soda, if you like...but limit the diet stuff to one can per day.

65. Chips: Change the potato chips to pretzels—then to baby carrots. One serving of chips has 60 more calories than pretzels and 10 times more fat grams. Just changing this snack will help you lose approximately a half pound this month. Next month, make it baby carrots—and lose another half-pound.

66. Fat: Stop adding fat to your food. I used to do it, and now this is my number-one naturally thin tip—don't do it. Do you add butter to your bread? Do you add mayo to your tuna? Do you drink full-fat milk? How about full-fat ice cream? Just switch products. Newly formulated low fat mayonnaise is tasty, and you'll never miss the extra calories. Lower fat ice cream or nonfat frozen treats have only about 100 calories per serving.

67. Set Aside the Sugar: Your morning coffee can undo all the good efforts of the day before! A mocha latte with syrup and whipped cream has all the hallmarks of a decadent dessert and can add 420 calories before you've even eaten breakfast. Instead, have a cappuccino with nonfat milk and a sprinkle of cinnamon...and lose up to three pounds in a month—and save a lot of money besides.

68. Ditch Deep-Fried: Effortlessly change your waistline by choosing smart cooking techniques. Eat broiled chicken instead of fried chicken; baked fish instead of fried fish; grilled meat instead of fried burgers. All savings add up to calorie deficits. Bake, broil, grill, or sauté with broth, wine, or water in a non-stick pan.

69. Fast Food: Wean from fast food by ordering differently. Order a "Whopper Junior" with extra tomato and "hold the mayo". The Junior-sized sandwich (400 calories) is plenty for most folks—the original has 700 calories—enough for two. Just eliminate the mayonnaise and save 390 calories. Assuming you eat out at least twice a week, you'll drop nearly one pound in a month just by switching to a smart-sized sandwich.

70. Red Power: Switch from ketchup to salsa for excellent antioxidants. Make your own: Add to a cup of chopped, seeded tomatoes to two tablespoons *each* of chopped red onion, seeded cucumber, red pepper, and cilantro (optional). Whisk and add to vegetables: Two tablespoons of balsamic vinegar, one teaspoon of olive oil, one teaspoon of lime juice, one garlic clove, minced, and a quarter teaspoon of black pepper.

71. Make it Crunchy: Nix the store-bought croutons (usually high in fat and often trans fat) and add fiber and antioxidants from chopped walnuts, almonds, or sunflower seeds. Use your measuring spoon—one tablespoon of dry roasted seeds or nuts has about 50 calories.

72. Reduce white sugar: Eating sugar when you're feeling low creates a rebound effect that makes you crave more sugar. Eating small, balanced meals every few hours helps you maintain energy so you won't need that sugar stimulation.

73. Sweet snack: Plan for a sweet snack that's good for you, approximately 100 calories. A perfect treat is a six-ounce cup of calcium-rich lite yogurt.

74. Pop Some Corn: My hot air popcorn popper is faster than microwave popcorn, and hot air means no nasty chemicals for the best fiber-rich, guilt-free snack without trans fat or cholesterol.

75. Real Tea: Avoid bottled sweetened teas, even if they're labeled "natural." Most have water and high fructose corn syrup as the first two ingredients—and about 200 calories per serving.

76. Cravings: Head off chocolate cravings and keep it nutritious with a calcium-fortified sugar-free hot chocolate, only about 50-60 calories, or a cup of nonfat chocolate pudding made with nonfat milk.

77. Sweet and Tart: My best before-bed snack is a warm cup of chamomile tea sweetened with a little honey plus a sliced-thin crisp Granny Smith apple. The combination of tart and sweet is infinitely satisfying.

78. Roast Vegetables: Scrub and chunk eggplant, squash, onions, and peppers: Toss in one tablespoon olive oil with mixed herbs and bake at 400 F for 40 minutes, stirring frequently.

79. Grill a Baked Potato: Jazz up your potato by splitting and either grilling or broiling—serve with salsa.

80. Make Pizza: Use your mixer to knead quick dough, or buy whole wheat crust; top with veggies, salmon, sardines, and some low fat cheese.

81. Stock shrimp: Thaw frozen, cooked shrimp. Chop coarsely, then toss lightly with a half-and-half blend of nonfat yogurt and nonfat mayo plus a dash of celery salt and lemon juice. Serve with a tossed salad and whole-grain crackers.

82. Take a Multivitamin: Daily—and choose one with extra calcium and magnesium—minerals that are often deficient in diets, even when you're not restricting calories. Your body can best take advantage of all the foods you eat when you have all the vitamins and minerals necessary to complete the chemical reactions needed for energy.

83. Unwanted Habits: Do you drink too much (choose as many as apply to you) Coffee? Alcohol? Soda? The effects of caffeine are cumulative and some sodas—even clear ones have as much caffeine as a cup of coffee. Excess alcohol provides excess calories, may interrupt sleep, and has possible negative health consequences.

84. Change Patterns: Challenge yourself and break out of your weight loss meal plan routine. For one week, eat dinner for breakfast on Tuesday and Saturday; the next week, eat breakfast for dinner on Wednesday and Sunday.

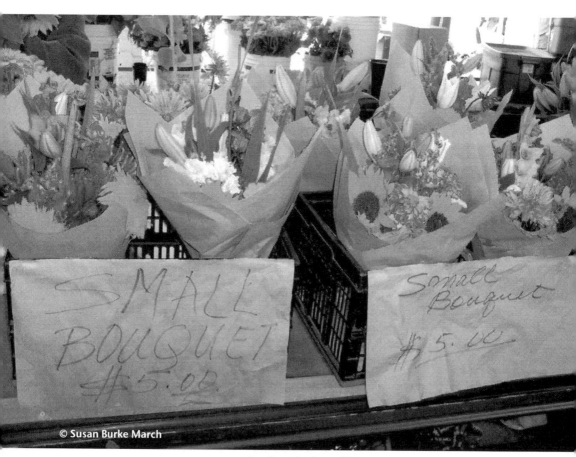

© Susan Burke March

Small can be beautiful

References

Introduction

1. Adam, T.C., and E.S. Epel. July 24, 2007. Stress, eating and the reward system. *Physiology & Behavior* 91: 449-458.

Chapter 1

1. Wang, Y., and M.A. Bevdoun. January 1, 2007. The obesity epidemic in the United States—gender, age, socioeconomic, racial/ethnic, and geographic characteristics: A systematic review and meta-regression analysis. *Epidemiologic Reviews* 29: 6-28.

2. Centers for Disease Control and Prevention. n.d. *About BMI for Children and Teens.* http://www.cdc.gov/nccdphp/dnpa/bmi/childrens_BMI/about_ childrens_BMI.htm

Chapter 2

1. c1-1 Trust for America's Health. 2007. *F as in Fat: How Obesity Policies are Failing in America.* Support from the Robert Wood Johnson Foundation. http://www.rwjf.org/newsroom/newsreleasesdetail.jsp?id=10512

2. Wang, Y., and M.A. Bevdoun. January 1, 2007. The obesity epidemic in the United States—gender, age, socioeconomic, racial/ethnic, and geographic characteristics: A systematic review and meta-regression analysis. *Epidemiologic Reviews* 29: 6-28.

3. United States Department of Health & Human Services. 2007. *Overweight and Obesity: At a Glance.* http://www.surgeongeneral.gov/topics/ obesity/calltoaction/fact_glance.htm

4. Waters, E.B., and L.A. Baur. 2003. Childhood obesity: Modernity's scourge. *The Medical Journal of Australia* 178: 422-423.

5. Nader, P., et al. 2006. Identifying risk for obesity in early childhood. *Pediatrics* 118: e594-e601.

6. Freedman, D.S., L.K. Khan, M.K. Serdula, W.H. Dietz, S.R. Srinivasan, and G.S. Berenson. 2005. The relation of childhood BMI to adult adiposity: the Bogalusa heart study. *Pediatrics* 115: 22-27.

7. Nielsen Media Research. n.d. *Nielsen Media Research Reports Television's Popularity is Still Growing.* http://www.nielsenmedia.com/nc/portal/site/ Public/ menuitem.55dc65b4a7d5adff3f65936147a062a0/ ?vgnextoid=4156527aacccd010VgnVCM100000ac0a260aRCRD

8. Kaiser Family Foundation. March 28, 2007. *New Study Finds that Food is the Top Product Seen Advertised by Children—Among All Children, Tweens See the Most Food Ads at More than 20 a Day.* http://www.kff.org/entmedia/entmedia032807nr.cfm

9. Tomkinson, G.R., and T.S. Olds. 2007. Secular changes in pediatric aerobic fitness test performance: The global picture. *Medicine and Sport Science* 50: 46-66.

10. International Diabetes Federation. June 25, 2004. *Diabetes and Obesity Epidemic in Children: International Call to Action.*

11. Christakis, N.A., and J.H. Fowler. 2007. The spread of obesity in a large social network over 32 years. *New England Journal of Medicine* 357: 370-379.

12. Parker-Pope, Tara. March 4, 2008. A one-eyed invader in the bedroom. *New York Times.* http://www.nytimes.com

13. Robinson, T.N. October 27, 1999. Reducing children's television viewing to prevent obesity: A randomized controlled trial. *Journal of the American Medical Association* 282: 1561-1567.

14. Striegel-Moore, R.H., D. Thompson, S.G. Affenito, D.L. Franko, E. Obarzanek, and B.A. Barton, et al. 2006. Correlates of beverage intake in adolescent girls (the National Heart Lung and Blood Institute Growth and Health Study). *Journal of Pediatrics* 148: 183-187.

15. Wansink, B., and P. Chandon. 2006. Meal size, not body size, explains errors in estimating the calorie content of meals. *Annals of Internal Medicine*: 326-332.

16. *High Rate of Overweight and Obesity Found in Children Having Surgery.* January 17, 2007. University of Michigan Health System.

17. Davis, M.M., D.C. Singer, and S.J. Clark. December 2007. Parental concerns about childhood obesity: time for a reality check? *C.S. Mott Children's Hospital National Poll on Children's Health, University of Michigan* 2. http://www.med.umich.edu/mott/research/chearbmi.html

18. Campaign for a Commercial-Free Childhood. n.d. http://www.commercialfreechildhood.org

Chapter 3

1. *What is MI?* 1998-2008. Motivational Interviewing: Resources for clinicians, researchers and trainers. http://www.motivationalinterviewing.org

2. Miller, W.R., and S. Rollnick. 1991. *Motivational Interviewing: Preparing People to Change Addictive Behavior.* New York: Guilford.

3. Prochaska, J.O., C.C. DiClemente, and J.C. Norcross. 1992. In search of how people change. *American Psychology* 47: 1102-1104.

4. Miller, W.R., and S. Rollnick. 1991. *Motivational Interviewing: Preparing People to Change Addictive Behavior.* New York: Guilford.

5. American Society for Reproductive Medicine. n.d. *Weight and Fertility: Patient's Fact Sheet.* http://www.asrm.org

6. National Heart, Lung and Blood Institute: National Institutes of Health. n.d.b. *What is Metabolic Syndrome?* http://www.nhlbi.nih.gov/health/dci/Diseases/ms/ms_whatis.html

7. Schwartz, M.B., L.R. Vartanian, B.A. Nosek, and K.D. Brownell. 2006. The influence of one's own body weight on implicit and explicit anti-fat bias. *Obesity* 14: 440-447.

Chapter 4

1. Bolles, Richard Nelson. 2008. *What Color is Your Parachute? A Practical Manual for Job-hunters and Career-changers.* 2nd ed. Ten Speed Press.

2. Center for Science in the Public Interest. n.d. http://www.cspi.org

3. Rooney, B.L., C.W. Schauberger, and M.A. Mathiason. December 2005. Impact of perinatal weight change on long-term obesity and obesity-related illnesses. *Obstetric Gynecology* 106: 1349-1356.

4. Boney, C.M., A. Verma, R. Tucker, and B.R. Vohr. March 2005. Metabolic syndrome in childhood: Association with birth weight, maternal obesity, and gestational diabetes mellitus. *Pediatrics* 115: e290-296.

Chapter 5

1. Weight Control and Diabetes Research Center, The. n.d. *LITE Study: Living Lean in a Toxic Environment.* http://www.lifespan.org/services/ clintrials/general/lite.htm

2. United States National Library of Medicine and National Institutes of Health. n.d. *Body Mass Index: Medical Encyclopedia: Medline Plus.* http://www.nlm. nih.gov/medlineplus/ency/article/007196.htm

3. BMI Table: Weight-control Information Network (WIN); the U.S. Department of Health and Human Services: National Institutes of Health: http://win.niddk. nih.gov/statistics/index.htm#table

Chapter 6

1. Gardner, C.D., A. Kiazand, and S. Alhassan, et al. 2007. Comparison of the Atkins, Zone, Ornish, and LEARN diets for change in weight and related risk factors among overweight premenopausal women. The A to Z weight loss study: A randomized trial. *Journal of the American Medical Association* 297: 969-977.

2. Oldways Preservation Trust. n.d. *The Mediterranean Diet Pyramid.* http:// www.oldwayspt.org/ med_diet.html

3. United States Environmental Protection Agency. n.d. *Fish Advisories: Consumption Advice.* http://www.epa.gov/waterscience/ fishadvice/factsheet.html

Chapter 7

1. Mann, T., A.J. Tomiyama, E. Westling, A.M. Lew, B. Samuels, and J. Chatman. 2007. Medicare's search for effective obesity treatments: Diets are not the answer. *American Psychologist* 62: 220-233.

2. Smith, C.F., and R.R. Wing. 2000. New directions in behavioral weight-loss programs. *Diabetes Spectrum* 13: 142-148.

3. Gold, B.C., S. Burke, S. Pintauro, P. Buzzell, and J. Harvey-Berino. 2007. Weight loss on the web: A pilot study comparing a structured behavioral intervention to a commercial program. *Obesity* 15: 155-164.

4. Tate, D.F., R.R. Wing, and R.A. Winett. 2001. Using internet technology to deliver a behavioral weight loss program. *Journal of the American Medical Association* 285: 1172-1177.

5. Harvey-Berino, J., S. Pintauro, P. Buzzell, and E.C. Gold. 2004. Effect of internet support on the long-term maintenance of weight loss. *Obesity Research* 12: 320-329.

6. USDA Center for Nutrition Policy and Promotion. n.d.b. *Steps to a Healthier You.* http://www.mypyramid.gov

7. American Heart Association. n.d. *Alcohol, Wine and Cardiovascular Disease.* http://www.americanheart.org/presenter.jhtml?identifier=4422;

8. USDA Center for Nutrition Policy and Promotion. n.d.a. *Does Alcohol Have a Place in a Healthy Diet?* http://www.cnpp.usda.gov/Publications/ NutritionInsights/insight4.pdf

9. *Caloric Values of Alcoholic Beverages.* n.d. Rochester: The University of Rochester Health Service. http://www.rochester.edu

10. Center for Food Safety and Applied Nutrition. September 2003. *Office of Nutritional Products, Labeling, and Dietary Supplements.* http://www.cfsan. fda.gov/~dms/lab-hlth.html

11. Maister, Kathy. n.d. *How to Measure Food.* http://www.startcooking.com

Chapter 8

1. Miller-Kovach, Karen, MS, RD. 2007. *She Loses, He Loses: The Truth About Men, Women, and Weight Loss.* New Jersey: John Wiley & Sons.

2. Schmitz, K.H., M.D. Jensen, K.C. Kugler, R.W. Jeffery, and A.S. Leon. 2003. Strength training for obesity prevention in midlife women. *International Journal of Obesity* 27: 326-333.

3. Jurca, R., M.J. LaMonte, T.S. Church, C.P. Earnest, S.J. Fitzgerald, C.E. Barlow, A.N. Jordan, J.B. Kampert, and S.N. Blair. 2004. Associations of muscle strength and aerobic fitness with metabolic syndrome in men. *Medical Science Sports Exercises* 36: 1301-1307.

4. American College of Sports Medicine. n.d.b. *Selecting and Effectively Using a Pedometer.* http://www.acsm.org/AM/ Template.cfm?Section=Brochures2&CONTENTID=7530&TEMPLATE=/CM/ ContentDisplay.cfm

5. Tudor-Locke, C., and Bassett, D.R., Jr. 2004. How many steps/day are enough? Preliminary pedometer indices for public health. *Sports Medicine* 34: 1-8.

Chapter 9

1. Huckabee, Mike. 2005. *Quit Digging Your Grave With a Knife and Fork: A 12-Step Program to End Bad Habits and Begin a Healthy Lifestyle.* Time Warner Book Group.

2. National Restaurant Association. 2008. *Industry Facts: 2008 Restaurant Industry Overview.* http://www.restaurant.org/research/ind_glance.cfm

3. National Heart, Lung and Blood Institute. n.d.a. *Portion Distortion! Do You Know How Food Portions Have Changed in 20 Years?* http://hp2010.nhlbihin.net/portion

4. Wansink, B., and J. Kim. 2005. Bad popcorn in big buckets: Portion size can influence intake as much as taste. *Journal of Nutrition Education & Behavior* 37: 242-245.

5. Warshaw, Hope S. 2006. *What to Eat When You're Eating Out.* 1st ed. American Diabetes Association.

6. Center for Science in the Public Interest. January/February 1997. What's at steak? *Nutrition Action Newsletter.* http://www.cspinet.org/nah/steak-jf.html

7. Powell, L., F. Chaloupka, and Y. Bao. October 2007. The availability of fast-food and full-service restaurants in the United States associations with neighborhood characteristics. *American Journal of Preventive Medicine* 33: S240-S245.

8. Lopez, R.P. 2007. Neighborhood risk factors for obesity. *Obesity* 15: 2111-2119.

9. Pereira, M.A., A.I. Kartashov, C.B. Ebbeling, L. Van Horn, M.L. Slattery, D.R. Jacobs, Jr., and D.S. Ludwig. 2005. Fast-food habits, weight gain, and insulin resistance (the CARDIA study): 15-year prospective analysis. *Lancet* 365: 36-42.

10. National Alliance for Nutrition and Activity, The. n.d. *From Wallet to Waistline: the Hidden Costs of 'Supersizing.'* http://www.preventioninstitute.org/portionsizerept.html

11. Young, L.R. and M. Nestle. 2002. The contribution of expanding portion sizes to the U.S. obesity epidemic. *American Journal of Public Health* 92: 246-249.

12. Centers for Disease Control and Prevention. 2006. *Research to Practice Series No. 2: Portion Size.* Division of Nutrition and Physical Activity.

13. Roast and Post Coffee Company, The. n.d. *Consumption Facts.* http://www.realcoffee.co.uk

More Information

American College of Sports Medicine. n.d.a. *Guidelines for Healthy Adults Under Age 65.* http://www.acsm.org

Binge Eating Disorder. 2008. Weight Control Information Network. http://win.niddk.nih.gov/publications/binge.htm

Centers for Disease Control and Prevention. 2003-2004. *Data on the Prevalence of Overweight and Obesity Among Adults: United States National Health and Nutrition Examination Survey.* http://www.cdc.gov/nccdphp/dnpa/obesity/trend/index.htm

Centers for Disease Control and Prevention. 2007. *Overweight and Obesity; Childhood Overweight; Overweight Prevalence.* http://www.cdc.gov/nccdphp/dnpa/obesity/childhood/prevalence.htm

Lappé, Frances Moore. 1971. *Diet for a Small Planet.* Ballantine Books.

National Center for Overcoming Overeating. 2008. http://www.overcomingovereating.com

National Eating Disorders Association. 2008. http://www.nationaleatingdisorders.org

Sothern, Melinda S., T. Kristian Von Almen, and Heidi Schumacher. 2001. *Trim Kids™: The Proven 12-Week Plan that has Helped Thousands of Children Achieve a Healthier Weight.* New York: HarperCollins.

Tate, D.F., E.H. Jackvony, and R.R. Wing. 2003. Effects of internet behavioral counseling on weight loss in adults at risk for type 2 diabetes: A randomized trial. *Journal of the American Medical Association* 289: 1833-1836.

USDA Center for Nutrition Policy and Promotion. n.d.c. *Vegetarian Diets.* http://www.mypramid.gov/tips_resources/vegetarian_diets.html

USDA Economic Research Service. 2008. *Briefing Rooms: Food Consumption.* http://www.ers.usda.gov/Briefing/Consumption

Vegetarian Resource Group. n.d. *Vegetarianism in a Nutshell.* http://www.vrg.org/nutshell/nutshell.htm

Weiner, S. 1998. The addiction of overeating: Self-help groups as treatment models. *Journal of Clinical Psychology* 54: 163-167.

Index

Acknowledgments

I've always been good at sales, and enjoyed the challenge. For years, most of my jobs involved selling something—either goods or services—sometimes both. I clerked at a beer and wine store while in college, the first time around; was licensed to sell real estate in Florida, and had a small insurance brokerage back in New York. But, in 1990, I began what I think now as the second—and better half of my life as I know it. At age 36, I went back to school, and started my career anew.

I'm lucky to have had the opportunity to begin again. And I was smart and persistent too—I challenged myself to change and to learn. After graduating, my first job was in the senior healthcare center of what is now Mount Sinai Hospital of Queens. For the first time, I felt like I made a difference. It wasn't all about me making the sale—it was about my being an important part of a professional team effort.

Thank you, Richard Bengis, who as Food & Nutrition Director promoted me to chief nutritionist—I think Richard's example of smart and compassionate leadership set me on the path toward success.

Dr. David Rabinowitz, director of pathology, became my mentor and friend, and generously provided his expertise, support and guidance. In collaboration with his staff, we improved patient assessment and diagnoses.

Nine years after graduating and firmly on track as a clinical nutrition manager, my first marriage was winding down. I decided to move to Florida from New York, and had lined up interviews for clinical or management positions. The day before I was to leave I got a phone call from a recruiter—would I be interested in working for an online company? "What's that?" I asked. Online weight loss?

In 1999 the world was such a very different place—I knew only one or two people with their own cell phones; no one had a GPS, and the world was just beginning to log on to the Internet daily. Dialup was the only service available, and since nobody I knew used email, "online" wasn't on my radar.

I must admit I didn't fully appreciate what working online entailed and could have played it safe, and accepted a position as a hospital clinical manager—my first interviews had produced two job offers, but...Dave Humble, eDiets.com's founder and CEO, interviewed me, and asked why I wanted to work for eDiets. Well—that was an interesting question—why indeed? I said, almost instinctively, "Because I think that this job involves selling good nutrition...and I'd like to combine my sales background with my clinical experience—it just jives perfectly". Dave, thanks for the opportunity— you are a pioneer. The next seven years were challenging, but fascinating.

I quickly expanded my responsibilities and soon created a new nutrition support, then services department, and worked with the development, marketing and business teams to create and launch new programs and products. I met some very special people— especially in development of digitized "partner programs"—with special thanks to Dr. Melinda Sothern of Louisiana State University, co-author of Trim Kids; Colette Heimowitz of Atkins Nutritionals, and dietitian Pat Groziak of Slim-Fast, and contributors Dr. David Katz from Yale University Obesity Research Center, and dietitians and diabetes educators Hope Warshaw and Janis Roszler. Special thanks for their friendship and expertise go to my dietetic colleagues Beth Casey Gold of the University of Vermont's VTrim program and Christine Miller, certified diabetes educator, and to Dr. Barbara Wilson of Tesco Diets. I'd like to acknowledge marketing experts Merilee Kern, Georgianne Brown and Harriet Gallu; writer and editor Glenn Mueller and professional experts Kandee Biren, Ellen Delalla, Dr. Matthew Anderson and Dr. John Sklare. Thanks to my former nutrition support staff at eDiets—online and on the phone, they offered calm compassion and expertise.

Finally, former editor in chief John McGran could always make me (and his readers!) laugh. As "mein editor" for my favorite gig as "chief nutritionist" John edited many of my weekly, then daily e-columns.

To my friends and colleagues who generously contributed your personal expertise for this book—you made this book better. This book's guiding message comes from you, from dietetic professionals and health experts, and from people with everyday challenges who take the steps necessary to stay healthy and "naturally thin" without dieting.

To my friends and peers who helped by reviewing the manuscript and offering constructive criticism, thank you. Thanks to my colleagues at the American Dietetic Association's Weight Management Dietetic Practice Group and Florida Dietetic Association—for the opportunity to serve. Volunteers enjoy unanticipated benefits and opportunities as interact with many of the most accomplished experts in the field of nutrition and weight management.

Thanks to Mansion Grove House publisher Uday Kumar for your enthusiasm, expertise, patience and persistence, and thanks to Ken Dawes for his creative design.

Thanks to my dear friend Barbara Read and my niece Stephany March. The photos of their active kids having fun are just perfect!

And finally, all my love to my best friend Charlotte Tomic, who always believed and stayed close.

Be Empowered!

More Breakthrough Books from Mansion Grove House

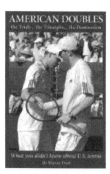

AMERICAN DOUBLES

A close-up view that is intriguing, exciting and impossible to put down. Many fans and journalists lament the state of American tennis, wondering when the next great players will hit the scene. What the critics may not realize is that Americans have dominated the doubles scene for decades and the future looks bright.

ISBN-13 9781932421163

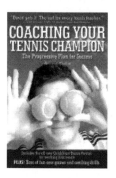

COACHING YOUR TENNIS CHAMPION

Want new games to get your 8-year old excited about tennis? No problem. David's Coaching Your Tennis Champion uses the new QuickStart Tennis format and lays out progressive game plans organized day-by-day and for each age group. Simply turn to the appropriate page..voila! you have your bright new idea for Game of the Day! You will love it! Your juniors will adore it! Big time-saver for coaches. Fun know-how for parents!

ISBN-13 9781932421156

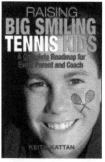

RAISING BIG SMILING TENNIS KIDS

Whether you are a tennis playing parent or a parent curious about tennis, this book will empower you to raise kids who swing the tennis racket with as much aplomb as their happy smiles. The best age to get your kid started in tennis. How to motivate kids to go back, practice after practice. When to focus exclusively on tennis. Save on lessons, find scholarships and sponsors. How to pursue a career in professional tennis. Gain insight into tennis organizations and agents. Have fun along the way at the best tennis camps and resort.

ISBN-13 9781932421118

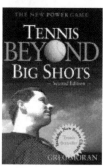

TENNIS: BEYOND BIG SHOTS

Greg Moran brings to this book his wealth of experience, spanning decades as a competitive player and much sought-after tennis teaching professional. Award winning Pro and Director of Tennis at The Four Seasons Racquet Club, Wilton, CT, Greg enthusiastically teaches top ranked players, working warriors as well as eager beginners. A prolific contributing writer for leading tennis magazines, he has also appeared on television to share his strategies for winning, playing longer and enjoying more. Greg is a member of the Wilson Advisory Staff and a national speaker for the Cardio Tennis program launched by the US Tennis Association and the Tennis Industry Association.

ISBN-13 9781932421170

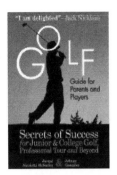

GOLF GUIDE FOR PARENTS AND PLAYERS

Jack Nicklaus acclaimed guide unveils the secrets of success for junior and college golf, the professional tour and beyond. Golf pros Jacqui and Johnny, offer exclusive guidance and new ideas on: How to motivate kids to go back, practice after practice. When to focus exclusively on golf. Save on lessons, find scholarships and sponsors. How to pursue college golf and a career in professional golf. Gain insight into golf organizations and agents. Have fun along the way at the best golf camps and resorts.
ISBN-13 9781932421149

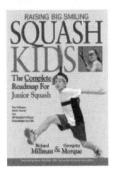

RAISING BIG SMILING SQUASH KIDS

Stanford University recently added Squash to its athletics, joining Yale and Cornell. Forbes magazine rates Squash as the number one sport for fitness. With courts and college programs springing up across the country. Richard Millman, world-class coach and Georgetta Morque, a prolific sportswriter, offer a complete roadmap for parents, professionals and kids. The best age to get started in squash; how to motivate kids; the road to top colleges; and attractive career options. Plus: cultivating friendships, character building and achieving a lifetime of fitness.
ISBN 1932421432

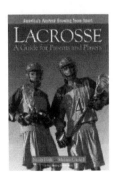

LACROSSE: A GUIDE FOR PARENTS AND PLAYERS

Lacrosse is America's fastest growing team sport. Action-packed and fun, lacrosse is a game anyone can play — the big and small, boys and girls. Lacrosse offers a positive outlet, a place to fit in at school, motivation to excel, and opportunities for team travel. Whether your kid is 8 or 18, experienced or just starting, this book is the complete guide to all that lacrosse has to offer. Empower yourself with practical answers and unique ideas, whether you are new to lacrosse or once were a player. Make lacrosse an exhilarating part of your family life.
ISBN 1932421076

Available Worldwide

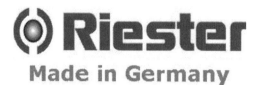
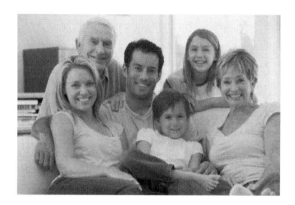
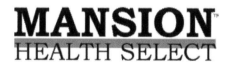

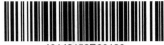

Made in the USA
Charleston, SC
29 March 2015